White Lesions

Brown Lesions

Yellow lesions

Red Papules and Nodules

PED

COLOR TEXTBOOK OF
PEDIATRIC DERMATOLOGY

SECOND EDITION

WILLIAM L. WESTON, M.D.
Professor and Chairman
Department of Dermatology
Professor of Pediatrics
University of Colorado
Health Sciences Center
Denver, Colorado

ALFRED T. LANE, M.D.
Associate Professor of Dermatology and Pediatrics
Stanford University School of Medicine
Stanford, California

JOSEPH G. MORELLI, M.D.
Associate Professor
Department of Dermatology
Professor of Pediatrics
University of Colorado
Health Sciences Center
Denver, Colorado

with 531 illustrations

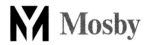

St. Louis Baltimore Boston Carlsbad Chicago Naples New York Philadelphia Portland
London Madrid Mexico City Singapore Sydney Tokyo Toronto Wiesbaden

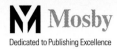

Mosby
Dedicated to Publishing Excellence

A Times Mirror
Company

Publisher: Anne S. Patterson
Editor: Susie Baxter
Developmental Editor: Ellen Baker Geisel
Project Manager: Linda Clarke
Production Editor: Veda King
Manufacturing Manager: J.A. McAllister
Cover Designer: Carolyn O'Brien
Designer: Lisa Diercks
Electronic Composition Artist: Christine H. Poullain

SECOND EDITION
Copyright © 1996 by Mosby–Year Book, Inc.
Previous edition copyrighted 1991

Printed in the United States of America

Composition by Mosby Electronic Publishing, Philadelphia
Color photographs by Color Associates
Printing/binding by Von Hoffman

Mosby–Year Book, Inc.
11830 Westline Industrial Drive
St. Louis, MO 63146

Library of Congress Cataloging-in-Publication Data

Weston, William, L.
  Color textbook of pediatric dermatology / William L. Weston, Alfred T. Lane, Joseph G. Morelli. — 2nd ed.
    p.   cm.
  Includes bibliographical references and index.
  ISBN 0-8151-9201-0
  1. Pediatric dermatology.   I. Lane, Alfred T.   II. Morelli, Joseph G.   III. Title.
  [DNLM: 1. Skin Diseases—in infancy & childhood.   WS 260 W536c 1996]
  RJ511.W46   1996
  618.92'5—dc20
  DNLM/DLC
  for Library of Congress   95-20703
                                                CIP

      98   99   00   /   9   8   7   6   5   4   3   2

Dedication

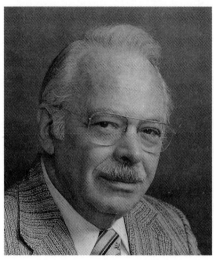

Alvin H. Jacobs, M.D.

Alvin Jacobs, M.D., is the "very best friend ever" to pediatric dermatology. Like a child in the formative years, pediatric dermatology struggled to find its way as a field of medicine. Al Jacobs was always there to help, to guide, to listen. Any pediatrician worth their salt knows the name of Alvin Hirsch Jacobs, M.D. He has presented hundreds of lectures on pediatric dermatology to national, regional, and local meetings, with never a negative comment. We can think of no others in the field who can match that accomplishment. His seminars on neonatal dermatology are classic, and often the most popular at national pediatric or dermatology meetings. Anyone who hears Al Jacobs talk knows they have heard the master. There are thousands of pediatricians whose first—and often *only*—formal teaching in pediatric dermatology came from Al Jacobs.

We decided to dedicate this book to Al Jacobs for another aspect of his professional career: his work behind the scenes in pediatric dermatology. For a complete appreciation of his contributions we must first examine the man. He was born in Reno, Nevada, and spent his boyhood among the ponderosa pines and broad valleys below the Comstock lode. This was still the Wild West, an invigorating life for an ambitious young man. After receiving the gold medal at graduation from the University of Nevada in 1933, he ventured east to the famous Johns Hopkins University School of Medicine, where he received his medical degree in 1937. After internship in Pittsburgh, he spent a year in child neurology at the Neurological Institute of New York. He returned west for training in pediatrics and infectious disease at San Francisco County Hospital, then served as chief resident in pediatrics at Stanford University. It was then June 1942, his country was at war, and Dr. Jacobs joined the Navy and was assigned to Navy Medical Research Unit Number 1. By 1946 he was a Lieutenant Commander and ready to return to the practice of pediatrics. In his private practice of pediatrics in San Francisco, Al quickly recognized that 20% of his patients had primary skin complaints and that he was poorly prepared to deal with them. He found his colleagues in pediatrics similarly unprepared, and decided to remedy the situation. After a year's fellowship in dermatology at Stanford he joined the Stanford faculty, and established a career in pediatric dermatology that has spanned three decades. He is now Professor of Dermatology and Pediatrics, Emeritus (active) at Stanford University. He still pursues his love of pediatric dermatology with his usual vigor.

Al Jacobs was a founder of the Society for Pediatric Dermatology and served as its first president. In many ways Al Jacobs was to pediatric dermatology what George Washington was to the establishment of the United States. It is so crucial that the leaders at the founding have the wisdom and vision to create an organization that will grow and be flexible enough to accommodate the changes needed in future generations. The advice and counsel of Al Jacobs was critical for the field of pediatric dermatology.

It is Al Jacobs the man who has endeared himself to so many in pediatrics and pediatric dermatology. He avoided the arrogance that often accompanies positions of importance in academic medicine, and remained the kind, considerate, warm man who always had time to listen to your needs or your problems. It has been his accessibility that has made the field of pediatric dermatology accessible for all who are interested. Who could resist that big smile beneath the cookie-duster moustache or those kind, twinkling eyes? Any personal encounter with Al Jacobs makes one feel they are with their best friend.

It is said that the fulfillment of life is to love, be loved, and have useful work. Al Jacobs loves his charming wife, Opal; his children; his chosen field of pediatric dermatology. In turn, he is loved by his wife and children and the hundreds of physicians whose lives he has touched.

This book is also dedicated to our families: Dr. Janet Atkinson Weston, Betsy and Kemp Weston; Maureen, Amy, Andy, Jeremy, Jordan, and Matthew Lane. We appreciate their support and willingness to provide photographs for this text from their family albums.

William L. Weston, M.D.
Alfred T. Lane, M.D.

Preface

How is the second edition of *Textbook of Pediatric Dermatology* different from the first edition? We have not changed the goals. We are still determined to meet the specific needs of the clinician responsible for the primary care of children. We incorporated the advice of clinicians, house staff, and students to improve this textbook from the first edition. We have greatly increased the number of color photographs and improved their quality. We added a third author, Joseph G. Morelli, M.D., Associate Professor of Dermatology and Pediatrics, to assist us with this edition. Dr. Morelli brings his special expertise in hemangiomas, vascular malformations, pigmentary disturbances, and photobiology to this edition. All three authors are board certified in pediatrics and dermatology.

All three authors wrote specific sections, but each section was reviewed by all three. Each author strongly believes that a textbook should not be written from other textbooks, but rather from original articles. Thus, this edition was written as a unique resource, as was the last. We all believe that the book should be written in the simplest, most understandable manner for the clinician. We have tried to hold to these beliefs, even as we incorporated the latest information, including the latest genetic discoveries, by explaining their importance in the pathogenesis of disease.

We retained a number of unique features that were included in the previous edition. The Problem-Oriented Differential Diagnosis Index was retained on the inside of the front and back covers to allow the busy clinician rapid access when the diagnosis is not clear. A concise formulary specific for pediatric patients is still available in the appendix. All the useful tables throughout the text were retained and several new ones added. The same organization for each disease was retained except for the change that references appear at the end of each condition and are now cited within the text. New to this edition are Patient Education Information sheets provided in the appendix. (These may be copied and used in your practice.) There are two new chapters. In Chapter 13, hemangiomas and vascular malformations are now considered separately. In Chapter 19, genodermatoses are also considered separately in view of the incredible advances in the genetics of skin disease over the past few years. We have tried to provide the busy clinician with concise, decisive information.

Without the encouragement of our own mentors, this book would not be possible. We have rededicated this second edition to Alvin Jacobs, M.D. who, at a time when the world had less than a handful of pediatric dermatologists, had the vision of the creation of a new discipline. He provided the impetus to so many young people hesitant to enter the uncertain world of a discipline yet undefined. A special tribute to Dr. Jacobs appears on the dedication pages. We thank Drs. Robert Goltz, W. Mitchell Sams, and Lowell Goldsmith for their guidance, protected time, and generous support of our careers. We also thank the officers and members of the Society of Pediatric Dermatology, who provided us with collegiality, clinical expertise, scientific interest, and nurture. We trust that with this book we are in some way again repaying the great debt we owe our colleagues.

William L. Weston, M.D.
Alfred T. Lane, M.D.
Joseph G. Morelli, M.D.

Contents

COLOR TEXTBOOK OF
PEDIATRIC DERMATOLOGY

SECOND EDITION

1

Structure and Function of the Skin

A firm understanding of normal skin structure and function is necessary for recognition and treatment of skin disease. Those providing medical care for children should apply the principles of skin biology to the pediatric patient and master essentials of the embryology and development.

THE EPIDERMIS

Keratinization

The epidermis functions as a barrier, preventing penetration from outside and retaining substances inside. Over 95% of epidermal cells are keratinocytes. The process of keratinocyte replication and maturation is called *keratinization*. The major keratinocyte proteins are keratins, which provide scaffolding to determine keratinocyte shape. The process of keratinization begins with proliferation of new keratinocytes in the region of the basal cell layer, near the dermal-epidermal junction (Fig. 1-1). As keratinocytes differentiate, they accumulate granules called *keratohyaline granules* in their cytoplasm and the type of keratin bundles within the cells becomes thicker.[1] The exact function

of the keratohyaline granules is unknown, but they are believed to be important in the organization and formation of a thickened cornified cell membrane. Keratohyaline granules appear within epidermal cells as they emigrate outward from the basal layer and reach the granular layer. Within the granular layer the cells lose their cylindrical and cuboidal shapes and begin to flatten as they go through the process of terminal differentiation or programmed cell death (*apoptosis*). Cell nuclei are lost and the keratinocytes flatten like stacks of plates. This final layer is called the *horny layer*, or *stratum corneum*. The stratum corneum cells accumulate like bricks on a wall, separated by intercellular lipids, which function like mortar. The intercellular lipids are an integral part of the epidermal barrier function.

Individual keratinocytes are bound together by desmosomes and adherens junctions. The desmosomes contain membrane glycoproteins desmocollins and desmogleins, and cytoplasmic proteins desmoplakins and plakoglobin.

The process of keratinization is continuous within the skin. The newly formed keratinocytes of the basal layer mature and are shed from the skin over an interval of approximately 28 days. Skin diseases may be associated with variation in the speed and process of keratinization.

Epidermal barrier

It is said that the skin is the interface between humans and their environment. Indeed, the most important function of the epidermis is to provide a skin barrier against microorganisms and irritating chemicals, as well as to impede the exchange of fluids and electrolytes between the body and the environment. This barrier function resides in the stratum corneum, where the terminally differentiated keratinocyte develops a tough cell envelope beneath the plasma membrane. The process of envelope formation involves biochemical processing of *involucrin*, the major cytoplasmic protein precursor of the cell envelope. The epidermal barrier is completed by extracellular lipid layers surrounding the terminally differentiated keratinocytes.

Although the skin, including the epidermis and dermis, is 1.5 to 4.0 mm thick, the epidermal barrier is only 0.05 to 0.1 mm thick. By the daily shedding of one to two cell layers of stratum corneum, or scale, the epidermal barrier prevents excessive colonization of the skin surface. In addition to continuous shedding, the flattened stratum corneum cells are tightly adherent to each other, so that to obtain entrance into the lower epidermis and dermis, chemicals or microorganisms must pass between tightly compacted epidermal cells.

The water content of the environment greatly influences the epidermal barrier (see Chapter 22). Both an excessive and an inadequate water content in the epidermal barrier will cause microscopic and macroscopic breaks in the barrier.

In response to friction or other forms of repeated trauma such as ultraviolet light (UVL) or chemical injury, stratum corneum is formed in amounts greater than usual, as can be noted on the palms and soles. The stratum corneum is thinnest over the eyelids and scrotum.

Pigmentation and ultraviolet light

Four biochromes in the skin are responsible for clinical pigmentation: melanin, beta carotene, oxyhemoglobin, and reduced hemoglobin. The brown-black pigment melanin is the dominant pigment of the skin. It is the pigment closest to the observer's vision and darkest in color. In dark-skinned individuals, it is difficult to recognize yellow pigment (beta carotene), red pigment (oxyhemoglobin), and blue pigment (reduced hemoglobin). Melanin is produced by the pigment-forming cell, the melanocyte, which is located in the epidermis. Different skin regions contain different numbers of melanocytes. For example, three

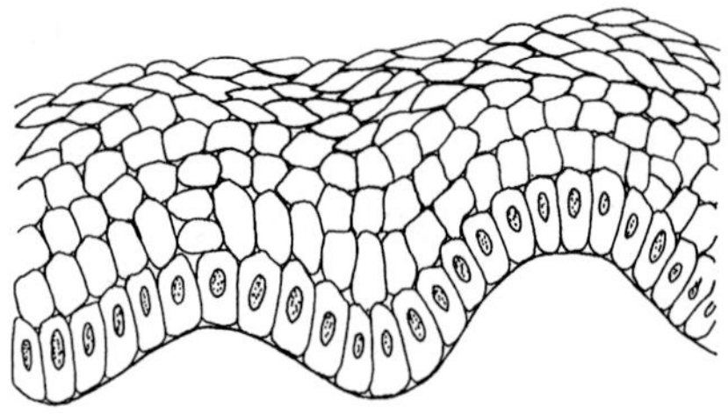

Fig. 1-1
Normal epidermis. The germinative layer with prominent nuclei is at the base of the epidermis and within the same compartment as the fully differentiated cells. As these basal cells differentiate, they migrate up toward the skin surface, shed their nuclei, become flattened, and are shed from the skin surface.

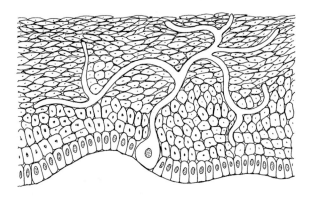

Fig. 1-2
Melanocyte-keratinocyte unit. The dendritic melanocyte, shown here as a clear cell with many branches, provides melanin pigment to many keratinocytes.

times as many melanocytes are found in the epidermis of the forehead as in the abdominal skin. Numbers of melanocytes per unit area of skin are the same despite racial differences in pigmentation.

Each epidermal melanocyte has dendritic cytoplasmic extensions that make contact with 35 to 45 epidermal cells. This melanocyte-keratinocyte unit (Fig. 1-2) is responsible for clinical pigmentation. The brownish-black polymer melanin is produced within the melanocytes in special membrane-bound organelles called melanosomes. The enzymes, including tyrosinase, that are crucial for melanin production are contained within the melanosome membrane. Melanosomes develop in stages. Tyrosinase and other enzymes convert the colorless chemical tyrosine to an oxidized quinone compound, which in turn becomes polymerized into the brownish-black compound melanin. Clinical pigmentation depends on the stage of the melanosome produced and dispersion of melanosomes from melanocytes to keratinocytes. Keratinocytes actively phagocytize the melanosomes. In black skin, melanosomes are single units of advanced-stage melanosomes, whereas in lighter-skinned persons, the melanosomes are aggregated and of earlier developmental stages. Thus the major difference in black and white skin is the stage of the melanosome development and the ability to transfer and disperse melanin pigment, not the number of melanocytes per unit area of skin.

The function of melanin is to protect the deoxyribonucleic acid (DNA) structure of epidermal cell nuclei from damage by UVL irradiation. Melanin dispersed within the cytoplasm of keratinocytes forms a protective cap over the keratinocyte nucleus when the keratinocytes are exposed to UVL (Fig. 1-3). Melanin pigment is lost by the daily shedding of stratum

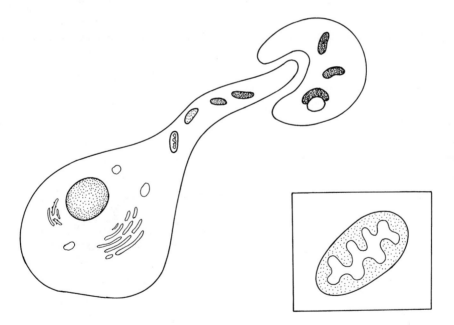

Fig. 1-3
Melanin production and transfer. Melanosomes (inset) are organelles formed in the rough endoplasmic reticulum and Golgi area of melanocytes. Their membranes contain the enzyme tyrosinase, responsible for the formation of the brown-black polymer, melanin. At the end of the dendrite, the melanocytes are shown transferring pigment to the keratinocyte, where the melanin moves to form a cap of the keratinocyte nucleus as protection against ultraviolet injury.

corneum cells. Melanin within the dermis, such as that found in dermal melanocytic birthmarks, has no such mechanism available for its elimination.

UVL from the sun increases melanin pigmentation by first oxidizing preformed melanin, increasing cross-linking of the melanin polymer and darkening the color. This effect occurs within minutes after exposure and is called *immediate pigment darkening*. During the 4 to 6 days following UVL exposure, both increased melanin production and melanin transfer to keratinocytes produce tanning.

Sunlight

The sun produces UVL of numerous wavelengths, which, based on their biologic effects, are arbitrarily divided into three groups: ultraviolet A (UVA), ultraviolet B (UVB), and ultraviolet C (UVC) (Table 1-1). Incoming UVL from the sun is scattered by small molecules in the atmosphere and absorbed by the ozone layer; all UVL below 290 nm is absorbed, so that virtually no UVC reaches the earth's surface.

Sunburn is caused by wavelengths of light from 290 to 320 nm. Photons of UVL are absorbed by electrons of chemicals with double bonds and ring structures, such as nucleic acids, DNA, and proteins, producing excited electron states within these molecules or free-radical formation. Beta carotene and melanin act by stabilizing the free radicals and are natural photoprotective chemicals found in skin. About 10% of UVB passes through the epidermis and reaches the dermis. The erythema and pain of sunburn are mediated via prostaglandins and other mediators. The sunburn wavelengths of UVL are blocked by window glass. The tanning and thickening of the epidermal barrier that result from exposure to sunlight impair the penetration of UVL into the lower epidermis and dermis. Wavelengths of light from 320 to 400 nm (UVA) are responsible for the photosensitivity seen in the many drug photoallergies and psoralen phototoxicity. Light of these wavelengths passes through window glass and is emitted from fluorescent lamps such as those used as overhead lighting in schools.

Epidermal basement membrane

The junction between the epidermis and dermis is the epidermal basement membrane. This structure is composed of the basal keratinocyte, the lamina lucida, the lamina densa, and the sublamina densa. Keratins in the basal keratinocyte attach into the electron-dense plaques associated with the hemidesmosomes. Anchoring filaments extend from the hemidesmosome through the lamina lucida into the lamina densa. The lamina densa consists of a lattice of structural proteins that are anchored to the dermis by the anchoring fibrils of the sublamina densa.

Two bullous pemphigoid antigens are recognized by sera from patients with bullous pemphigoid. Bullous pemphigoid antigen 1 is associated with the cytoplasmic portion of the basal cell hemidesmosome, and bullous pemphigoid antigen 2 is a transmembrane portion of the hemidesmosome. Laminins 5 and 6 are associated with the anchoring filaments. Laminin 1, nidogen, and type IV collagen are associated with the lamina lucida and lamina densa. The anchoring fibrils of the sublamina densa are composed of type VII collagen.[2]

Autoantibodies against basement membrane structures or genetic defects of these structures cause a variety of diseases. Correlation of the function of specific structures of the basement membrane and disease-associated defects has helped to increase understanding of the epidermal-dermal junction.

Table 1-1.
Biologic Effects of Ultraviolet Light

Group	Wavelength (nm)	Biologic effects
UVC	200-290	Cytotoxic (bactericidal, retinal injury)
UVB	290-320	Sunburn, sun tanning, systemic lupus erythematosus, skin cancers
UVA	320-400	Drug photoallergies, porphyria, phytophotodermatitis, psoralens photoaging, PUVA therapy

PUVA, psoralen ultraviolet A-range.

THE DERMIS

The dermis is composed predominantly of collagen fibers and elastic fibers enclosed in a gel continuum of mucopolysaccharides. This fibrous complex gives the dermis its great mechanical strength and elasticity, allowing the skin to withstand severe frictional stress yet still be extensible over joints. Elastin, collagen, and mucopolysaccharide gel are all produced and secreted by fibroblasts. Types I, III, IV, and VII are the predominant collagens in the skin.

Although the principal mass of the dermis consists of collagen fibers and is acellular, numerous other elements are present, including mast cells, inflammatory cells, blood and lymph vessels, and cutaneous nerves. These elements are responsible for regulation of heat loss, the host defenses of the skin, nutrition, and other regulatory functions.

Collagen, elastin, and mechanical properties

Most of the mechanical strength of the skin is derived from the fibrous protein collagen, a macromolecule with a large hydroxyproline content. Mature collagen structure becomes rigid with cross-linking of adjacent protein chains, and young collagen that is without significant cross-linking fails to limit skin distention. Defective collagen results in extensive and excessive distensibility of the skin, as seen in Ehlers-Danlos syndrome, or severe blisters, as seen in recessive dystrophic epidermolysis bullosa. Elastin fibers, which are composed of both an amorphous and a fibrillar portion, are responsible for the reversible distensibility that allows the skin to be restored to normal size after stretching. Defective elastin production results in extreme wrinkling and redundant skin as seen in cutis laxa.

Cutaneous vasculature

Cutaneous arteries course through the subcutaneous fat and give rise to two vascular plexuses that run parallel to the epidermis. These vascular plexuses contain arteriovenous shunts to divert blood from the skin and provide nutrition to it, to regulate heat loss, and to participate in the defense against foreign substances. The epidermis contains no blood vessels and receives its nutrition via the diffusion of plasma into the intercellular epidermal spaces. The stratum corneum has no such nutritive process.

Heat regulation and sweating

Skin is important in the control of body temperature. Heat generated in organs and muscles is rapidly transported to the skin vasculature. The cutaneous circulation acts as a "radiator." Varying the rate and volume of blood flow through the skin controls heat loss from this radiator. The blood flow is controlled by the autonomic nervous system. Heat from the skin surface is lost by evaporation of water in the form of eccrine sweat. Heat loss or gain by convection or radiation depends on environmental temperature. At comfortable temperatures, body heat can be regulated by the cutaneous vasculature alone, without sweating. In hot, dry environments the core body temperature may rise slightly but is stabilized by heat loss via sweating. In hot, humid environments evaporation of water from the skin surface is restricted, and heat gain occurs in the child's body. If this condition is allowed to continue over a period of time, high fever, dehydration, and sodium depletion may occur. In children born with deficient numbers of eccrine sweat glands (hypohidrotic ectodermal dysplasia), heat gain occurs during hot weather or overheating and recurrent high fever is often a presenting feature of the condition.

Cutaneous nerves

Sensory nerve endings in the skin can elicit all of the principal sensations: touch, pain, itch, warmth, and cold. The skin is supplied by myelinated branches of spinal nerves. Nerve branches enter the dermis from the subcutaneous fat and form both a superficial and a deep nerve plexus. Unmyelinated branches from either plexus terminate in nerve endings that may be simple or specialized. Terminals from a single axon may serve an area as broad as 1 cm^2 and overlap with nerve endings from other axons. Inflow of cutaneous sensory information is strongly controlled and modulated by the cerebral cortex. The skin has a high sensitivity to rapid mechanical stimulation, with positional movements of less than 1 μm detectable. Sensations of cold persist continuously when skin temperature is below 30° C, and sensations of warmth persist continuously when it is above 37° C. Changes in temperature of 0.03° C can be detected, especially if the skin temperature changes faster than 0.007° C/sec. Thermal sensitivity is highest on the face.

At temperatures below 18° C and above 45° C, pain is produced. Pain may also be induced by pressure greater than 50 g/mm² and by disruption of skin. A number of chemicals injected into the skin may also elicit pain. Itch is a sensation related to pain and is greatest close to transitions of mucous membranes. Histamine is considered to be the most important mediator of itch, but many other mediators are capable of producing this sensation.

HOST DEFENSES OF THE SKIN

When breaks in the epidermal barrier occur, microorganisms invade the upper epidermis. Plasma proteins—such as complement proteins and immunoglobulins that normally bathe the intercellular epidermal space—initiate an inflammatory response. Cutaneous vasodilatation (erythema) occurs early after this initial process, with diffusion of more plasma proteins, followed by the migration of neutrophils, T lymphocytes, B lymphocytes, and monocyte-macrophages into the dermis and later the epidermis. Such cells initially accumulate around dermal blood vessels, but may migrate to the epidermis through the dermal-epidermal junction and between epidermal cells. For example, in impetigo large numbers of neutrophils accumulate just beneath the stratum corneum. Mast cells containing histamine, heparin, and platelet-activating factors are located around cutaneous blood vessels and play a regulatory role in the immune response of the skin by their influence on cutaneous vascular responses.

The initial response of the skin to invasion by microorganisms consists primarily of migration of neutrophilic leukocytes, but by 18 to 24 hours it is characterized by the appearance of lymphocytes and monocyte-macrophages in the dermis. Microorganisms or

foreign substances not initially destroyed by neutrophils are presumably further digested by macrophages or destroyed by direct lymphocytotoxicity. A rich lymphatic system is also found in the dermis, and foreign substances are carried to regional lymph nodes, where specific immune responses are generated by T lymphocytes and B lymphocytes. Some antigen recognition probably occurs in the skin, since antigen-processing cells (Langerhans cells) are found in the epidermis and direct Langerhans-T lymphocyte contact occurs that may be important in the recognition of foreign antigens.

The epidermal barrier remains the primary defense of the skin, but microorganisms that pass through the barrier are destroyed within the midepidermis as the skin defenses attempt to keep them out of deeper tissue.

EPIDERMAL APPENDAGES

Epidermal appendages, which are modifications of epithelium, include hair follicle structures, sebaceous glands, nails, and the apocrine and eccrine sweat glands.

Hair growth

The hair growth cycle has three phases: the growing phase, anagen; the regressing phase, catagen; and the resting phase, telogen. The cells of anagen hairs have a high mitotic rate and are among the most rapidly replicating cells in humans. The hair growth originates from the hair bulb, which is located in the lower dermis. Human scalp hair grows about 1 cm a month. When growth of the hair ceases, the catagen phase occurs, resulting in cessation of mitosis and upward migration of the hair bulb into the middermis. The hair shaft becomes clubbed at the bottom, causing the catagen hair to become a telogen hair (also called club hair). The telogen hair remains in the follicle for 2 to 3 months and is pushed out when the new hair grows.

There are great differences in the hair growth cycle among the different hair types found in the various body regions. Ambisexual hair follicles are common to both sexes and are androgen dependent. At puberty, androgen converts vellus hairs to terminal hairs in the axilla and the lower pubic triangle. Conversely, conversion of terminal scalp hairs to vellus hairs occurs in the temporal area of the scalp at puberty. Male sexual hair is responsive to high androgen levels, which convert vellus hairs to terminal hairs in the beard area, ears, sternum, and upper pubic triangle. In the occipital and bifrontal areas of the scalp, androgen levels result in a conversion of terminal to vellus hairs, resulting in androgenetic alopecia.

Hair cycles are asynchronous and vary within body sites. In the scalp at any point in time, about 85% of the hairs are growing (anagen), 14% are resting (telogen), and 1% are regressing (catagen). Newborns convert most of their hairs to telogen hairs within the first 6 months of life. Some newborns take several months to develop new anagen hairs, resulting in a "bald baby." Other infants develop new anagen hairs so rapidly that they appear not to lose their hair. After acute febrile diseases children or adults can have many hairs convert from anagen to telogen hairs with a subsequent period of months with markedly thinned hair (telogen effluvium).

Sebaceous glands

Sebaceous glands are present everywhere on the human skin except for the palms, soles, and dorsa of the feet. Generally they are associated with hair follicles and empty through a short duct into the canal of the hair follicle. The sebaceous sweat glands are holocrine glands that produce sebum, a semiliquid mixture of glandular cell debris containing glycerides, free fatty acids, wax esters, squalene, cholesterol, and cholesterol esters. The largest and most numerous sebaceous glands are found on the face, scalp, chest, and back.

Sebum production is androgen dependent and begins at puberty in skin regions with abundant sebaceous follicles. Sebaceous gland volume, sebaceous cell size, and secretory capacity are all directly androgen dependent. Obstruction of the sebaceous gland is associated with acne in humans.

Eccrine glands

Humans each have 2 to 5 million eccrine glands. These glands function to cool the body through evaporative heat loss of eccrine sweat. In addition, these glands may help to moisten the frictional surfaces of the skin.

Apocrine glands

Apocrine sweat glands are in the axilla, mons pubis, areola of the breast, circumanal area, and the scalp. They are located deep in the subcutaneous tissue and usually open into a hair follicle. Apocrine glands secrete a yellowish, sticky fluid after puberty. The secretion is produced in response to stress or sexual stimulation. In lower animals, these glands function as sex attractors and territorial markers.

Nails

Nails are formed by the fifth fetal month. The nail matrix contains epithelial cells responsible for the production of the nail plate. The nail matrix occupies an area beneath the proximal nail fold, a portion of which may be seen as the lunula. Fingernails grow approximately 1 cm in 3 months and toenails grow slower. Newborn nails are spoon-shaped and thin and may remain so until 2 or 3 years of age.

SUBCUTANEOUS FAT

The subcutaneous fat lies just beneath the dermis and is composed principally of lipocytes. It serves as a cushion to trauma, a heat insulator, and a highly important source of energy and hormone metabolism. Premature infants have poorly developed subcutaneous tissues, contributing to thermal instability and metabolic difficulties.

DEVELOPMENT OF SKIN

Periderm

Knowledge of the structure and function of developing fetal skin is invaluable in understanding abnormalities observed in newborn and infant skin. The single layer of ectodermal cells overlaying the developing fetus interacts with the mesoderm below to form the epidermis and dermis, respectively. Through this interaction the appendages develop, and the unique properties of skin at different body sites result.

Between 4 and 5 weeks gestation, the single layer of ectodermal cells of the fetal epidermis is covered by a layer of flattened cells called the *periderm*. The periderm cells expand across the developing epidermis by active mitosis, becoming rounded bulging cells uniformly covered by microvilli. The stratum corneum forms beneath the periderm cells during the fifth to sixth month. At this time periderm cells regress and become shrunken remnants that slough into the amniotic fluid and become one component of the vernix caseosa.

The morphologic characteristics of these cells suggest a transport function for periderm cells. The periderm may transport fluids, electrolytes, and sugars into the developing embryo.

Epidermal development

After 8 weeks gestation an intermediate cell layer develops between the basal cells and the periderm. In time this layer stratifies and adds additional cell layers. By 24 weeks gestation granular and cornified cells are present on almost all regions of the body. From this time until birth, the stratum corneum matures and thickens so that at birth, the term infant's skin barrier function is comparable to that of an adult. Depending on the gestational age at birth, the premature infant's barrier function is more deficient the earlier the premature birth.

The sequence of development of the keratins, the development of the basement membrane zone, the development of the desmosomes, hemidesmosomes, and the antigens of the epidermis have been catalogued.[1,2] The epidermis follows a sequence of development that is being intensively studied to understand the cellular interactions of normal development and the errors that occur in skin diseases.

Cells that migrate into the epidermis

Although the epidermis is ectodermal in origin, cells from other sources migrate into the epidermis.

Langerhans cells are present within the epidermis by 6 weeks gestation, but they may not be functionally mature until after 12 weeks gestation. The melanocyte is derived from the neural crest and migrates to the epidermis before the twelfth gestational week. By 16 weeks gestation melanocytes with melanosomes capable of synthesizing melanin are noted, and by 20 weeks gestation the epidermis has its full complement of melanocytes. Merkel's cells appear in the epidermis of the fingertips, glabrous skin, and nail beds by 12 weeks gestation and serve as special sensory organs. These cells may develop within the epidermis rather than being an immigrant cell as previously thought.

Epidermal appendages

Hair follicle or sweat gland development begins earlier in the scalp, palm, and sole than in other body areas. The hair germ begins in the scalp by 12 weeks gestation as a proliferation of keratinocytes above a collection of fibroblasts. These cells proliferate and invaginate into the dermis, forming the hair peg and the subsequent hair follicle. Granular cells are present within the hair follicle after 14 weeks gestation, a full 6 to 10 weeks before they are seen in the interfollicular skin. Hair grows at an oblique angle to the skin surface such that hair will erupt caudally, causing the hair to point downward.

Anlagen of eccrine glands may be present on the sole as early as 10 weeks gestation. The eccrine gland secretory coil forms on the sole at about 16 weeks gestation, and the secretory and myoepithelial cells differentiate at 22 weeks gestation. The sebaceous gland primordia develop off the hair follicle after 16 weeks gestation. Steroid hormone stimulation of sebaceous glands is so great that these glands are considerably larger in the third trimester fetus than those of a child. Apocrine glands, the last of the appendages to develop, first appear during the sixth month of fetal development.

Nails and volar pads

Development of the fetal nail, the volar pads, skin ridges, and sweat glands are tied together in the developing digit. These structures form simultaneously at 8 weeks gestation, just after the digits separate from one another. By 12 weeks gestation the proximal and distal nail folds have formed, and the volar pads are formed from mounds of mesenchyme and an increased intermediate layer of the epidermis. The distal nail fold is the first epithelial structure to keratinize, beginning at 12 weeks gestation. A nail plate covers the nail bed by 17 weeks gestation. Primary dermal ridges appear at 12 weeks gestation, and secondary dermal ridges at 16 weeks gestation. Sweat gland buds appear in the fingertips at 12 weeks gestation, but sweating does not occur until after 32 weeks gestation.

Influences of the dermis on epidermal growth and differentiation

The fetal dermis plays an overwhelmingly predominant role in transformation of the ectoderm into epidermis and maintenance of controlled epidermal appendage development. The continued interaction between the epidermis and dermis maintains the continued presence of the thickened skin of the palms and soles or the thinner skin of the face. The epidermal appendages are maintained by epidermal-dermal interaction, and once full-thickness injury occurs, the re-formed scar tissue appears unable to regenerate new appendages. Skin diseases associated with thickening or thinning of the epidermis may be associated with abnormal epidermal-dermal communications.

The dermis

The primordial dermis begins as a cellular mesenchyme that is watery and without fibrous structure. By 6 weeks of age a fine meshwork of collagen fibrils underlies the dermal-epidermal junction and adheres to the dermal mesenchymal cell surfaces. Extracellular collagen increases with age, and fibrils associate into collagen fiber bundles. Cells of the dermis become spaced farther apart, and their elongated axes become oriented parallel to the skin surface. The fine collagen network persists at the dermal-epidermal junction and ensheathes epidermal appendages as they project downward. The dermis increases in thickness from 0.1 mm at 7 weeks to 0.7 mm by 20 weeks of gestation. As the epidermal appendages project deeply into the der-

mis at 16 weeks of age, the dermis organizes two distinct regions: the papillary dermis with fine fibrillar collagen and the reticular dermis with large collagen bundles. By 20 weeks of age the fetal dermis is similar to that of the adult in structure, although still smaller in total thickness. Preliminary studies have demonstrated the 8-week-old fetus to contain fibronectin and types I, III, and V collagen within the dermis. By 14 weeks recognizable fibroblasts, mast cells, endothelial cells, Schwann cells, and histiocytes are found in the fetal dermis. By 60 days of gestation anchoring filaments are associated with the basal lamina at the dermal-epidermal junction. At 22 weeks of age the elastic fibers form, but well-developed elastic fiber networks are not observed until after 32 weeks, and the adult form of mature elastic fibers does not occur until after 2 years of age.

Few rigorous studies have been performed on the other components of the dermis, including vasculature, lymphatics, and nerves. Fat initially forms with discrete areas within the dermis at 16 to 18 weeks, then demarcation of a distinct fat layer that coincides with the development of hair follicles and their projection into the lower dermis.

Overall, newborn epidermal, hair, sweat, and sebaceous structures are nearly identical to adult structures. The dermis is less mature than adult dermis, being thinner with less organization of collagen and elastic fibers, with a less organized vascular network and cutaneous nerves. The newborn dermis appears as a transition between fetal and adult structures.

References

1. Fuchs E: Genetic skin disorders of keratin, *J Invest Dermatol* 99:671, 1992.
2. Marinkovich P: The molecular genetics of basement membrane diseases, *Arch Dermatol* 129:1557, 1993.

General Reference

Goldsmith LA, editor: *Biochemistry and physiology of the skin*, ed 2, New York, 1991, Oxford University Press.

2

Evaluation of Children with Skin Disease

T
he language of dermatology frequently inhibits students, house officers, and practitioners dealing with children from using the correct terminology for skin disease.[1] It is neither proper nor helpful to simply use the term *rash*. This chapter describes the correct approach to the presenting features, signs, and initial laboratory findings when evaluating children with cutaneous disease. One should memorize the primary lesions. Particular attention should be paid to the presence of vesicles, pustules, scaling, and color changes. These four morphologic features will allow the identification of the major morphologic groups, which is essential for proper diagnosis and differential diagnosis.[2] A problem-oriented algorithm is included in this chapter to allow determination of the morphologic groups of skin disease by their cutaneous appearance. Mastering this information will aid in communication with others delivering medical care to children.

MEDICAL HISTORY

The history obtained regarding a child's skin condition should be considered in the same fashion as a general medical history. The onset and duration of each symptom should be recorded. Associated systemic symptoms should be sought, along with a thorough review of systems. A medical history, complete family history, and information on recent medications should also be obtained.

Health care advice is sought for children for three major concerns regarding their skin: itching (pruritus), scaling, and cosmetic appearance.

Pruritus

Persistent itching in the skin often provides the impetus to seek medical attention. The examiner should note whether the itching is localized or generalized and whether it is associated with skin lesions. Itching without skin lesions suggests biliary obstruction, diabetes mellitus, uremia, lymphoma, or hyperthyroidism. If the pruritus is associated with skin lesions, dermatophytosis, scabies, and the many types of dermatitis should be considered.

Scaling

Normally one cell layer of stratum corneum, composed of flattened nonviable remnants of keratinocytes packed with protein (keratin), is shed daily.

This is not usually visible. Acute injury and resultant separation of 10 to 20 cell layers of stratum corneum result in clinically visible white sheets of scale, such as that seen in desquamation after a sunburn or thermal burn. Overproduction of stratum corneum by proliferating epidermis, as in psoriasis, results in visible accumulation of excess scale. The scale in psoriasis is thick in contrast to thin (pityriasis) scale.

Cosmetic appearance

Parents may be concerned about color change in the child's skin. A history of the time of appearance of skin lesions, sequence of color changes, and course of skin changes should be obtained.

EXAMINATION OF THE SKIN

The evaluation of skin lesions requires careful inspection of the entire cutaneous surface, and many skin diseases are diagnosed only by their morphologic appearance. Examination of the skin should consist of identification of the primary lesion (the earliest lesion to appear) and secondary changes, and a description of the color, arrangement, and distribution of lesions. Often, however, one sees children with secondary skin changes without primary lesions. For correct diagnosis, a rigorous search should be made for a primary lesion.

Primary skin lesions

1. A *macule* (Fig. 2-1) is a color change in the skin that is flat to the surface of the skin and not palpable (e.g., a tan macule, café-au-lait spot, white macule, vitiligo).

2. A *papule* (Fig. 2-2) is a solid, raised lesion with distinct borders 1 cm or less in diameter (e.g., lichen planus, molluscum contagiosum).

3. A *plaque* is a solid, raised, flat-topped lesion with distinct borders and an epidermal change larger than 1 cm in diameter (e.g., psoriasis).

4. A *nodule* (Fig. 2-3) is a raised, solid lesion with indistinct borders and a deep palpable portion. A large nodule is termed a tumor (e.g., rheumatoid nodule, neurofibroma). If the skin moves over the nodule, it is subcutaneous in location; if the skin moves with the nodule, the nodule is intradermal.

5. A *wheal* (Fig. 2-4), an area of tense edema in the upper dermis, produces a flat-topped, slightly raised lesion (e.g., urticaria).

6. A *vesicle* (Fig. 2-5) is a raised lesion filled with clear fluid (e.g. varicella, herpes simplex) that is less than 1 cm in diameter. A *bulla* is a raised lesion larger than 1 cm and filled with clear fluid.

7. A *cyst* (Fig. 2-6) is a raised lesion that contains a palpable sac filled with solid material.

8. A *pustule* (Fig. 2-7) is a raised lesion filled with a fluid exudate, giving it a yellow appearance (e.g., acne, folliculitis).

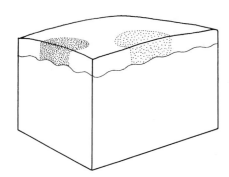

Fig. 2-1
A *macule* is a color change in the skin that is flat to the surface of the skin and not palpable (e.g., a tan macule, café-au-lait spot, white macule, vitiligo).

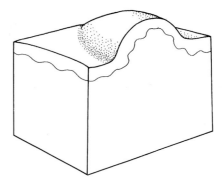

Fig. 2-2
A *papule* is a solid, raised lesion with distinct borders 1 cm or less in diameter (e.g., lichen planus, molluscum contagiosum).

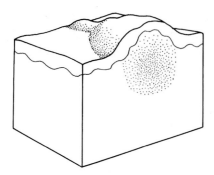

Fig. 2-3

A *nodule* is a raised, solid lesion with indistinct borders and a deep palpable portion. A large nodule is termed a *tumor* (e.g., rheumatoid nodule, neurofibroma).

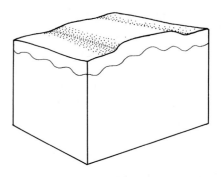

Fig. 2-4

A *wheal,* an area of tense edema in the upper dermis, produces a flat-topped, slightly raised lesion (e.g., urticaria).

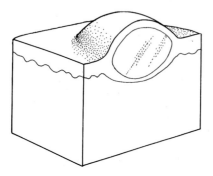

Fig. 2-5

A *vesicle* is a raised lesion filled with clear fluid (e.g. varicella, herpes simplex) that is less than 1 cm in diameter. A *bulla* is a raised lesion larger than 1 cm and filled with clear fluid.

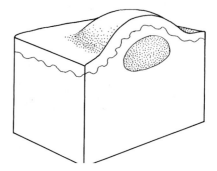

Fig. 2-6

A *cyst* is a raised lesion that contains a palpable sac filled with liquid or semisolid material (e.g., epithelial cyst).

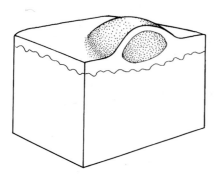

Fig. 2-7

A *pustule* is a raised lesion filled with a fluid exudate, giving it a yellow appearance (e.g., acne, folliculitis).

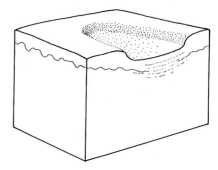

Fig. 2-8

In *atrophy* the skin surface is depressed because of thinning or absence of the dermis or subcutaneous fat (e.g., atrophic scar, fat necrosis).

Secondary changes

1. *Erosions and oozing.* A moist, circumscribed, slightly depressed area represents a blister base (*erosion*) with the roof of the blister removed (e. g., burns, dermatitis). Because the action of chewing or sucking easily removes the thin blister roof (oral mucosa lacks a stratum corneum), most oral blisters present as erosions (e.g., aphthae, herpes simplex stomatitis).

2. *Crusting* represents dried exudate of plasma combined with the blister roof, which sits on the surface of skin following acute dermatitis (e.g., impetigo, contact dermatitis).

3. In *scaling*, whitish plates are present on the skin surface (e.g., psoriasis, ichthyosis). *Desquamation* refers to peeling of sheets of scale following an acute injury to skin (e.g., burn, toxic drug reaction, scarlet fever).

4. In *atrophy* (Fig. 2-8) the skin surface is depressed because of thinning or absence of the dermis or subcutaneous fat (e.g., atrophic scar, fat necrosis). If the epidermis is thinned, it appears as fine wrinkling.

5. *Excoriations* are oval to linear depressions in the skin with a complete removal of the epidermis, exposing a broad section of red dermis. Excoriations are the result of fingernail removal of the epidermis and upper dermis.

6. *Fissures* are characterized by linear wedge-shaped cracks in the epidermis extending down to the dermis, and narrowing at the base.

Disruption of the skin surface

The presence of weeping, crusting, cracking (fissures), or excoriations is characteristic of disruption of the skin surface.[2] Disruption is seen in eczematous lesions but is absent in papulosquamous lesions, and is an important feature in distinguishing the two.

Mobility of skin

By grasping the skin between thumb and forefinger, the skin should be mobile. Excessive stretching indicates a type of Ehlers-Danlos syndrome, immobility suggests scleroderma (see Chapter 19).

Color

The color of a skin lesion should be described as skin-colored, brown, red, yellow, tan, or blue. Particular attention should be paid to whether the red or red-brown lesion completely blanches (e.g., petechiae do not blanch). Red or red-brown color in skin is dependent on the pigment oxyhemoglobin, which is found in red blood cells within superficial cutaneous blood vessels. Compressing the superficial vascular plexus by direct pressure forces red blood cells into deeper vascular channels, and blanching of the skin is observed. If the skin does not blanch with pressure, red blood cells are outside the vascular channels and located in the adjacent dermis.

Melanin is the dominant pigment in the skin. Since it is located in the outer layer of skin closest to the observer's eye, melanin may obscure other pigments located in deeper layers. In dark-skinned infants and children, one must use a disciplined approach to detect erythema, cyanosis, or jaundice. First, determine the normal skin color, then compare the involved skin area with the normal skin. Erythema will appear dusky red or violet. Cyanosis will appear black. Jaundice will appear diffusely darker, and one must examine the sclera to detect the presence of this disease. Carotenemia will appear golden-brown. The examiner may observe melanin as brown, blue-black, or black shades.

Arrangement of lesions

1. *Discrete.* Lesions are distinct and discretely separated from one another.

2. *Linear.* Lesions found in a straight line are called linear (e.g., lichen striatus).

3. *Annular.* Lesions found in a circular arrangement are called annular (e. g., granuloma annulare).

4. *Grouped.* Vesicles, papules, or nodules found closely adjacent to each other in a localized skin area are considered to be grouped (e.g., herpes simplex, herpes zoster).

Distribution of lesions

It is useful to note whether an eruption is generalized, acral (hands, feet, buttocks, and face), or localized to a specific skin region, such as a dermatome.

RECORDING OF SKIN LESIONS IN THE HEALTH RECORD

Skin lesions should be described in an orderly fashion: distribution, arrangement, color, secondary changes, and primary lesion. For example, guttate psoriasis could be written as generalized, discrete, red, scaly papules. If altered, mobility of skin, hair changes, or nail changes should also be recorded.

THE PROBLEM-ORIENTED ALGORITHM

After mastering the description of skin lesions the clinician can prepare a logical series of steps toward a correct diagnosis, even if the disease is initially unrecognized. Lynch has developed a problem-oriented algorithm for the nondermatologist (as modified in Table 2-1).[2] It can be applied to infants and children with skin disease, where it has been found to be most useful. Lynch's algorithm defines morphologic groups of dermatologic disease, which will allow the differential diagnosis and eventual correct diagnosis of a skin condition. These groups and the chapters in which they are found are listed in Table 2-2. (See the Problem-Oriented Differential Diagnosis Index, located at the front of this book.)

The problem-oriented algorithm requires that three initial objective findings be determined: Are blisters present? Are the lesions red? Are the lesions scaling? A series of 11 additional determinations completes the algorithm.

The detection of blisters is the crucial initial step in this diagnostic exercise.[2] If even a single blister is detected, no matter what form of other skin lesions may be observed, one should consider first the possibility of a blistering disease and proceed to determine whether the blister fluid is clear or pustular. If no blisters are observed, one should next determine if the skin lesions observed are red. If they are not red, it should be determined whether they are skin-colored or another color such as brown (which includes blue-black or black shades), yellow, or white.

The algorithm is particularly helpful if lesions are red.[2] If the skin lesions observed are red, it should be determined whether the individual lesions themselves are scaling or nonscaling. If they are red and nonscaling, it should be determined whether the surfaces of individual lesions are dome-shaped papules or flat. If lesions are red, nonscaling, and flat, vascular reactions should be considered. If lesions are red or raised, it should be determined whether they are firm or compressible. If compressible, vascular lesions should be considered. If firm, the morphologic group called inflammatory papules and nodules should be considered. If lesions are red and scaling, it should be decided whether there is surface disruption. If lesions have surface disruption, eczematous lesions should be considered. If they are red, scaly dome-shaped papules, papulosquamous lesions should be considered.

Changes in skin mobility should be determined. This includes skin that can be stretched excessively or is fixed to the underlying fascia or deeper structures and cannot be moved. Finally, any changes to hair or nails should be described.

Starting with 3 initial determinations, and then adding up to 11 more, one can place the skin disease observed into 1 of 13 morphologic groups. Grouping the skin disease observed in this fashion increases the likelihood of finding a precise diagnosis. One can determine the proper diagnosis with use of the Problem-Oriented Differential Diagnosis Index.

LABORATORY FINDINGS

Exfoliative cytology

Exfoliative cytology is indicated in any blister-forming disease to detect acantholytic cells (pemphigus) or epidermal giant cells (herpes simplex or herpes zoster). Scrape the blister base with a No. 15 blade and place on a glass microscope slide. Allow to dry, and stain with Wright's stain or Giemsa stain and examine under the 40× objective of a microscope.[3,4]

Table 2-1.
The Problem-Oriented Algorithm

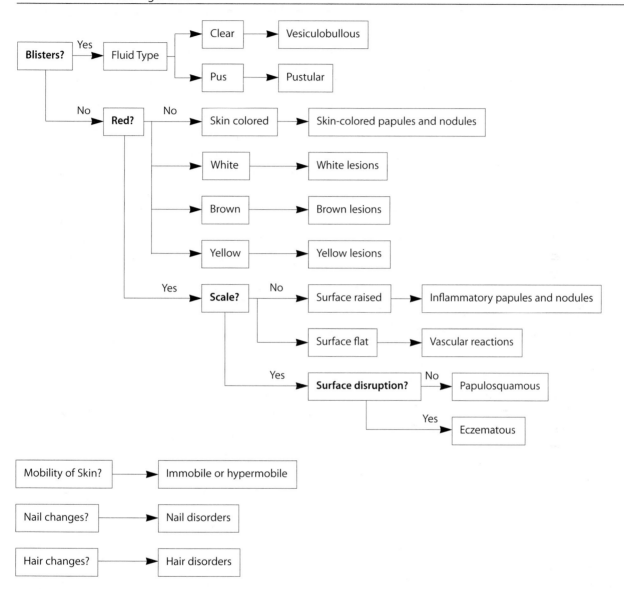

Modified from Lynch PJ: Dermatology for the house officer, ed 3, Baltimore, 1994, Williams & Wilkins, p 99.

Table 2-2.

Groups of Dermatologic Disease

Morphologic group	Chapter
1. Vesiculobullous diseases	4, 5, 7, 8, 9, 11, 18
2. Pustular diseases	3, 5, 6
3. Skin-colored papules and nodules	7
4. White lesions	16
5. Brown lesions	16
6. Yellow lesions	7, 16
7. Inflammatory papules and nodules	3, 5, 6, 7, 9, 18
8. Vascular reactions	13
9. Papulosquamous diseases	9
10. Eczematous diseases	4, 18
11. Hair changes	14
12. Nail changes	15
13. Immobile and hypermobile skin	19

Skin biopsy

Any skin tumor, palpable purpura, persistent dermatitis, or blister that is not diagnosed by morphologic appearance should be examined by biopsy for a histopathologic diagnosis.[4]

Punch biopsy

Cleanse the skin to be biopsied with alcohol. Inject 0.1 to 0.2 ml of lidocaine 1% intradermally using a tuberculin syringe and 30-gauge needle.[4,5] A 4-mm Keys' punch is pressed firmly downward into the skin, which is stretched perpendicular to wrinkle lines. The punch is rotated until the soft subcutaneous fat is penetrated. The specimen is removed with forceps and scissors and placed in buffered formalin 10% for histologic examination.[4,5] For immunofluorescence testing, the specimen should be frozen at −70° C or in liquid nitrogen, or placed in special skin immunofluorescence transport media.

Shave biopsy

After local anesthesia is achieved as previously described, a small elevated lesion may be shaved off with a sterile No. 15 blade or razor blade.[4]

Fungal scraping

Any red, scaly skin or scaly scalp should be scraped to evaluate the possibility of dermatophyte infection, which can mimic a wide variety of skin disorders (see Chapter 6). Fine scales are scraped from the edge of a lesion onto a glass slide.[4] A drop of potassium hydroxide (KOH) 20% added to the scale will dissolve the stratum corneum cells but not the hyphae. A coverslip is placed on the slide, and the scrapings are examined under the 10× objective of the microscope for long, thin, branching hyphae or spores.

References

1. Burton JL: The logic of dermatological diagnoses, *Clin Exp Dermatol* 6:1, 1981.
2. Lynch PJ: *Dermatology for the house officer,* ed 3, Baltimore, 1994, Williams & Wilkins, p 99.
3. Oranje AP, Folkers E: The Tzanck smear: old, but still of inestimable value, *Pediatr Dermatol* 5:127, 1988.
4. Arndt KA: *Manual of dermatologic therapeutics. II. Procedures and operations,* Boston, 1989, Little, Brown, p 171.
5. Lynch PJ: *Dermatology for the house officer,* ed 3, Baltimore, 1994, Williams & Wilkins, p 62.

3

Acne

ACNE VULGARIS

Clinical features

The common variety of acne, acne vulgaris, is the most prevalent skin condition observed in the pediatric age group. The common forms of acne occur during two major ages: the newborn and the adolescent. Neonatal acne is a response to maternal androgen and first appears at 2 to 4 weeks of age, and lasts until age 4 to 6 months. The lesions are primarily on the face, upper chest, and back, in a distribution similar to that in adolescent acne. The individual lesions seen are the same as described for adolescent acne. An oily scalp or face is often seen. It is believed that severe adolescent acne will develop in infants with severe forms of neonatal acne.[1] Persistence of neonatal acne beyond 12 months of age may be associated with endocrine abnormalities.

Early lesions of acne in the form of microcomedones develop in 40% of children ages 8 to 10 years, primarily on the face. Acne vulgaris peaks in late adolescence and may continue until the late twenties or early thirties. Many authorities believe acne is one of the earliest signs of puberty.[2,3] Eventually 85% of adolescents will develop acne. Acne occurs in sebaceous follicles (Fig. 3-1). There are several types of follicular channels present in skin. The sebaceous follicles have large, abundant sebaceous glands and a small vellus hair. They are located primarily on the face, upper chest, back, and penis (Fig. 3-2).

Obstruction of the sebaceous follicle opening produces the clinical lesions of acne.[4] If the obstruction occurs at the follicular mouth, a wide, patulous opening develops that is filled with a plug of stratum corneum cells. This is the *open comedone,* or *blackhead* (Fig. 3-3). Open comedones are the predominant clinical lesion in early adolescent acne. The black color results from oxidized melanin within the stratum corneum cellular plug, not from dirt. Open comedones do not often progress to inflammatory lesions.

Obstruction of the sebaceous follicle just beneath the follicular opening in the neck of the sebaceous follicle produces a cystic swelling of the follicular duct just beneath the epidermis. The stratum corneum produced accumulates continuously within the cystic cavity. This is seen clinically as the *microcomedone* (*closed comedone,* or *whitehead*) (Fig. 3-4). These

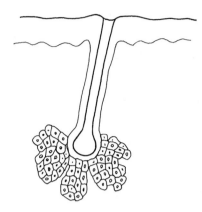

Fig. 3-1
Normal sebaceous follicles. Large sebaceous glands excrete sebum into cylindrical sebaceous channel.

microcomedones may be the precursors to inflammatory acne. Children 8 to 10 years of age often have microcomedones for many months before red papules or pustules are observed. If open and closed comedones are the predominant lesions seen in adolescent acne, it is designated as comedonal acne.

Inflammatory lesions in acne prompt the adolescent to seek medical attention. These lesions include firm red papules, pustules, nodules, cysts (Fig. 3-5), and, rarely, interconnecting draining sinus tracts. Most adolescents will have a mixture of microcomedones, red papules, pustules, and blackheads at the time of examination. Inflammatory acne can be classified as mild, moderate, or severe. Mild inflammatory acne consists of a few to several inflammatory papules, pustules. and no nodules. Patients with moderate inflammatory acne will have several to many inflammatory papules, pustules, and a few to several nodules, whereas those with severe inflammatory acne will have numerous and/or extensive inflammatory papules, pustules, and many nodules.[5] Excoriation of acne papules and microcomedones is common and scarring may result. Usually, multiple shallow erosions or crusts are found.

Adolescents with cystic acne require prompt medical attention, since ruptured cysts or sinus tracts result in scar formation. New acne scars are highly vascular and have a red or purplish hue. Such

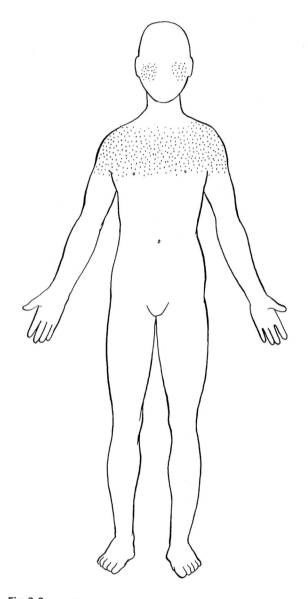

Fig. 3-2
Distribution of sebaceous follicles.

scars eventually regain normal skin color after several years. Acne scars may be depressed beneath the skin level, raised, or flat to the skin. In adolescents with a tendency toward keloid formation, keloidal scars can occur following acne lesions, particularly over the sternum. Hypertrophic scars may also occur, even in those without keloids. In typical adolescent acne several different types of lesions are

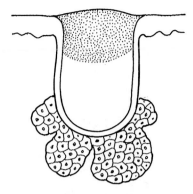

Fig. 3-3
Open comedone. Wide, patulous opening of sebaceous channel with plug of stratum corneum cells in follicular mouth.

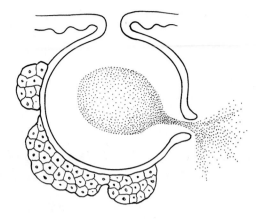

Fig. 3-5
Inflammatory papule. Overgrowth of bacteria and rupture of the wall, producing a foreign body reaction surrounding the follicle.

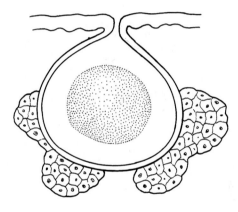

Fig. 3-4
Microcomedone (closed comedone). Obstruction of the follicular channel just beneath the opening.

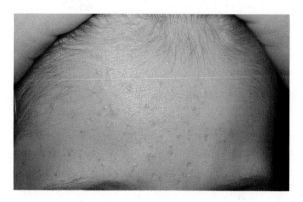

Fig. 3-6
Comedonal acne. Multiple microcomedones on the forehead of an 8-year-old female.

present at one time, such as open and closed comedones (Fig. 3-6), inflammatory papules (Fig. 3-7) and pustules (Fig. 3-8), excoriated lesions (Figs. 3-9 and 3-10), and nodulocystic acne (Fig. 3-11). Neonatal acne (Fig. 3-12) is characterized by inflammatory papules on the face and chest, with all the lesions in a similar stage.

Drug-induced acne should be suspected if all the lesions are in the same stage at the same time, with involvement of the abdomen, lower back, arms, and legs (Fig. 3-13), as well as the usual acne areas (see Box 3-1). The presence of unusual acne, hirsutism,

premature pubarche or androgenic alopecia, especially when associated with obesity and/or menstrual irregularities, should prompt an endocrine evaluation.[6] The most common causes of hyperandrogenism in females are functional ovarian and functional adrenal hyperandrogenism. Laboratory screening for hyperandrogenism is evaluated by obtaining blood levels of free testosterone, dehydroepiandrosterone, and androstenedione. If any of these are elevated, the source of the excess androgens can then be determined by measuring the response of free testosterone, dehydroepiandrosterone, and cortisol to dex-

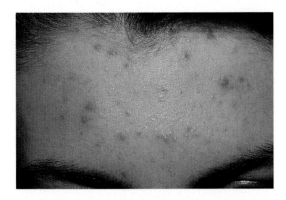

Fig. 3-7
Mild inflammatory acne. Several inflammatory papules.

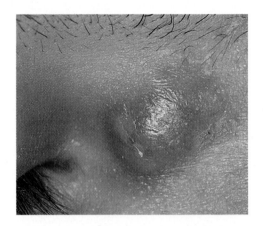

Fig. 3-9
Excoriated acne. Oozing from red papule that has been squeezed.

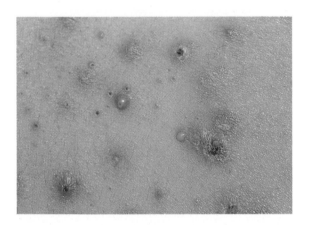

Fig. 3-8
Severe inflammatory acne. Extensive papules/pustules on the back.

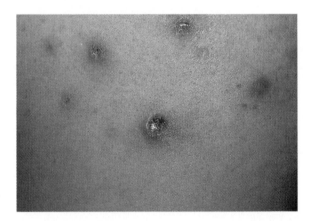

Fig. 3-10
Excoriated acne. Atrophic scar from attempted fingernail removal of acne lesion.

amethasone suppression testing. Treatment options for hyperandrogenism include oral contraceptives, low-dose glucocorticoids, and antiandrogens.

Several variants of acne occur in adolescence. Frictional acne from headbands, football helmets, tight bras, or other tight-fitting garments occurs predominantly under the skin area where the garment is worn. Oil-based cosmetics may also be responsible for a predominantly comedonal acne, and hair sprays and oil-based mousse produce acne along the scalp hair margin.

Differential diagnosis

Conditions to be considered in the differential diagnosis of acne are listed in Box 3-2. Rosacea in children can be confused with acne vulgaris. In addition to acne papules and pustules, prominent telangiectasia and a persistent flush to cheeks, nose, or chin are observed. In many instances rosacea in children results from the use of potent topical glucocorticosteroids on the face (Fig. 3-14).

Nevus comedonicus, which may be confused with neonatal acne, is a birthmark consisting of a linear

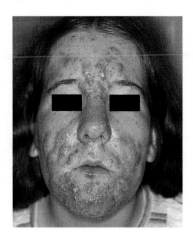

Fig. 3-11
Nodulocystic acne. Deep nodules and cysts on the face of an adolescent.

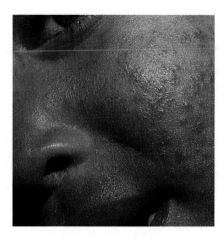

Fig. 3-13
Steroid acne. Red papules all in the same stage in a adolescent treated with systemic steroids.

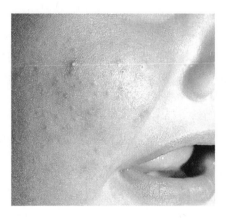

Fig. 3-12
Neonatal acne. Predominantly comedones on the face of a 3-month-old infant.

Box 3-1 Drugs responsible for acne
Androgens
Adrenocorticotropic hormone (ACTH)
Glucocorticoids
Hydantoins
Isoniazid

arrangement of open comedones. It is present from birth and is usually unilateral. The anatomic abnormality of nevus comedonicus may also result in obstruction of the sebaceous follicle, with resultant red papules, pustules, or cysts, with inflammatory lesions restricted to the birthmark. Miliaria may also mimic neonatal acne, although the lesions are transient, lasting less than 48 hours, in contrast to neonatal acne lesions, which persist for weeks.

Flat warts occurring on the face are sometimes confused with acne. They are papular, flat-topped, and skin-colored to slightly darker. The angiofibromas seen in tuberous sclerosis may be confused with acne. They are erythematous, soft papules seen in the nasolabial folds and on the cheeks and chin. The onset of these lesions is typically at 5 or 6 years of age. The absence of comedones is an important clue to the diagnosis of angiofibroma, as is the presence of leaf-shaped white macules, seizure disorders, and connective tissue nevi.

Molluscum contagiosum may occasionally be mistaken for acne lesions, but careful inspection will reveal the central umbilication at the top of the papule characteristic of this disease.

Pathogenesis

It is accepted that the primary event in acne is obstruction of the sebaceous follicle. Ordinarily the

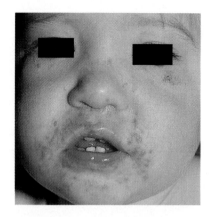

Fig. 3-14
Perioral dermatitis aggravated by topical steroid use. Toddler with perioral red papules and pustules from prolonged daily therapy with topical steroid.

lining of such follicles contains one to two layers of stratum corneum cells, but in acne the stratum corneum is overproduced. This phenomenon is androgen dependent in adolescent acne. The sebaceous follicles contain an enzyme, testosterone 5α-reductase, which converts plasma testosterone to dihydrotestosterone (DHT). DHT is a potent stimulus for sebaceous follicle cell nuclear division and, subsequently, of excessive cell production. Thus obstruction requires the presence of both circulating androgens and the converting enzyme. The interplay of circulating and skin factors is felt to be crucial to the genesis of clinical acne. After the production or the administration of androgens, one would expect a delay of 2 to 4 weeks until cellular proliferation occurs and follicular obstruction appears. This, indeed, is what is seen in androgen-induced acne as well as acne vulgaris. The majority of patients that have only acne vulgaris do not have endocrinologic abnormalities.

The pathogenesis of inflammatory acne is not well understood. Undoubtedly, manipulation of a closed comedone could lead to rupture of the cavity contents into the dermis, with a subsequent inflammatory response (Fig. 3-5). Spontaneous inflammation also occurs in obstructed follicles, but the reasons are unclear. A currently attractive hypothesis is that overgrowth of gram-positive bacteria in the obstructed follicle, either *Propionibacterium acnes* or *Staphylococcus epidermidis,* might produce bacterial chemotactic peptides, enzymes, or other factors that initiate inflammation. Although overproduction of sebum frequently accompanies acne, sebum or metabolites of sebum are unlikely as a cause of inflammation in acne as presently understood. Rupture of the comedonal contents into the dermis induces a foreign body reaction, which may heal with fibrosis.

Treatment
Topical keratolytic agents
The mainstay of antiacne therapy is the use of potent topical keratolytic agents applied to the skin to relieve follicular obstruction. Two classes of potent keratolytic agents—retinoic acid and benzoyl peroxide—have been found to be the most efficacious agents for the treatment of acne. Either agent may be used alone once daily, or the combination of retinoic acid applied to acne-bearing areas of skin once daily, in the evening, and benzoyl peroxide applied in the morning may be used. Since the two classes of keratolytics work by different mechanisms, they are synergistic. Topical keratolytic regimens will control 80% to 85% of adolescent acne. Retinoic acid and benzoyl peroxide are most effective in the gel forms; lotions and solutions, particularly the over-the-counter (OTC) preparations, have less efficacy. Dryness to the skin from using an alcohol- acetone-containing gel may be

Table 3-1.

Quick guide to initial acne therapy

Clinical appearance	Treatment
Comedones only (Fig. 3-6)	Retinoic acid 0.025% cream or benzoyl peroxide 5% gel once daily
Red papules, few pustules (Fig. 3-7)	Retinoic acid 0.025% cream in the evening plus benzoyl peroxide 5% or 10% gel in the morning
Red papules, many pustules (Fig. 3-8)	Retinoic acid 0.025% cream in the evening, benzoyl peroxide 5% or 10% gel in the morning, plus oral antibiotics: either tetracycline or erythromycin 500 mg twice daily
Red papules, pustules, cysts, and nodules (Fig. 3-11)	Retinoic acid 0.05% cream once daily plus benzoyl peroxide 10% gel twice daily plus oral tetracycline or erythromycin 1 to 1.5 g daily

severe. The adolescent will often not use the prescribed gel medication because of the dryness experienced. Alternative strategies designed to reduce dryness are use of a noncomedogenic moisturizer such as Moisturel, Purpose lotion, or Neutrogena Moisture after application of the gel; use of the gel every other day; or use of the cream preparations. Topical keratolytic therapy is recommended as the primary therapy for comedonal and mild papular forms of acne. Continuous use for several months is often required. There is debate as to whether tretinoin should be avoided in pregnancy because of the potential of photoisomerization to isotretinoin, but a recent retrospective study did not demonstrate an increase in birth defects in children whose mothers used tretinoin in the first trimester of pregnancy.[7] For papular acne use benzoyl peroxide gel once or twice daily; for comedonal acne use retinoic acid once daily as initial therapy. If no improvement occurs over 4 to 6 weeks, the other form of keratolytic can be added. In inflammatory acne topical keratolytics plus oral antibiotics are recommended as initial therapy. Topical keratolytics are not used when oral retinoids, such as isotretinoin, are required.

Antibiotics

Topical antibiotics are used to avoid systemic side effects caused by systemic antibiotics. Antibiotics are less effective given topically than systemically and at best are equipotent to 250 mg of oral tetracycline taken once a day. Clindamycin phosphate 1% is the most efficacious of all topical antibiotics. Some percutaneous absorption may rarely occur with this drug, resulting in diarrhea and colitis. Topical erythromycin 1%, 1.5%, and 2% solutions, 2% ointment, and 3% gel are quite effective, as is 1% meclocycline cream; topical tetracycline 1% or 2.2% is minimally efficacious (Tables 3-1 and 3-2). Topical antibiotics are most useful for maintenance therapy after improvement from 1 to 2 months of oral antibiotics is observed. Oral antibiotics can be discontinued and improvement maintained with topical antibiotics plus topical keratolytics.

Oral antibiotics that are concentrated in sebum, such as tetracycline and erythromycin, are very effective in inflammatory acne. The usual dose is 500 mg to 1 g of tetracycline or erythromycin taken daily divided in two doses. Tetracycline should be taken on an empty stomach for reliable absorption. Oral antibiotics should be continued for 1 to 3 months until the acne lesions are suppressed. Topical keratolytics should be used in combination with oral antibiotics. Therapy for a period of at least 4 to 6 weeks is required for clinical improvement. Routine laboratory monitoring is unnecessary during antibiotic therapy.[8]

Table 3-2.

Selected Acne Treatment Products

Product			Size
Topical keratolytics (apply once or twice daily)			
Retinoic acid (tretinoin)			
Retin-A	0.025% cream		20 g; 45 g
	0.05% cream		20 g; 45 g
	0.01% gel		15 g; 45 g
	0.025% gel		15 g; 45 g
Benzoyl peroxide			
Desquam-X 5% and 10% gel			42.5 g; 85 g
Desquam-E 5% and 10% emollient gel			42.5 g; 84 g
Persa-gel 5% and 10% gel			45 g; 90 g
Persa-gel W 5% and 10% gel			45 g; 90 g
Benzac 5% and 10% gel			60 g
Benzac W 5% and 10% gel			60 g; 90 g
Benzac AC 5% and 10% gel			60 g; 90 g
Topical antibiotics (apply twice daily)			
Clindamycin phosphate 1% solution (Cleocin T)			60 ml
Meclocycline sulfosalicylate 1% cream (Meclan)			20 g; 45 g
Erythromycin 2% solution (T-Stat, Erycette, ATS)			60 ml
Systemic antibiotics (one or two capsules twice daily)			
Tetracycline hydrochloride			250-mg capsule; 100/bottle
Erythromycin			250-mg capsule; 100/bottle
Oral retinoids (40-mg capsule twice daily for 16-20 weeks)			
Isotretinoin (Accutane)			10- and 40-mg capsule

Oral retinoids

The oral retinoid isotretinoin (13-*cis*-retinoic acid) has been very efficacious in nodulocystic acne resistant to standard therapeutic regimens (Fig. 3-11). It is not recommended that isotretinoin be used as the drug of first choice for acne.[9,10] The precise mechanism of action is unknown, but decreased sebum production, follicular obstruction, and skin bacteria as well as general antiinflammatory activities have been described. The initial dosage is 40 mg once or twice daily (0.5 to 1.0 mg/kg/day) for 4 months, then the drug is stopped. Isotretinoin is neither designed for nor efficacious in comedonal acne or in other mild forms of acne. Side effects include dryness and scaliness of the skin, dry lips, and occasionally dry eyes and nose. Up to 10% of patients experience mild hair loss, but it is reversible. Elevated levels of liver enzymes and blood lipids have rarely been described. Oral retinoids are the most efficacious treatment of severe cystic acne. Teratogenicity restricts the use of isotretinoin in females of childbearing potential.[11] The isotretinoin teratogen syndrome is characterized by malformations of the central nervous system, and has been reported in 25% of women who became pregnant while taking isotretinoin. Usage in young women of childbearing age is not recommended, and a negative pregnancy test should be obtained before the drug is considered, with careful adherence to the guidelines provided by the manufacturer, including monthly contraceptive counseling and pregnancy tests. Patients should be

Box 3-3   Nonacnegenic cosmetics and moisturizers

Cosmetics

Allercreme
  Matte-Finish Makeup
  Waterbase, Oil-Free
Almay
  Fresh-Look Oil-Free Makeup for Oily Skin
  Smooth Coverup Makeup for Blemish-Prone Skin
  Oil Control Makeup
  Teen Oil-Free Makeup
Charles of the Ritz
  T-Zone Controller
Chanel
  Teint Pur Oil-Free Makeup
  Teint Pur Matte
Clarion
  Oil-Free Liquid Makeup
Clinique
  Pore Minimizer Makeup, Fragrance- and Oil-Free
  Stay True Makeup, Fragrance- and Oil-Free
  Stay True Oil-Free—designed for sensitive skin—
    SPF 15
Coty
  Glowing Finish
Covergirl
  Fresh Complexion, 100% Oil-Free
Dermage
  Sheer Foundation Base
  Opaque Foundation Base
  Sunscreen Foundation Base
Elizabeth Arden
  Extra Control Makeup

Estee Lauder
  Tender Matte Makeup, Fragrance- and Oil-Free
  Lucidity Makeup
  Simply Sheer
  Fresh Air Makeup Base, Oil-Free
  Demi-Matte Makeup, Fragrance- and Oil-Free
Lancome
  Maquicontrol, Oil-Free Liquid Makeup
L'Oreal
  Mattique Illuminating Makeup
Mary Kay Cosmetics
  Oil-Free Foundation, Fragrance- and Oil-Free
Maybelline
  Shine-Free Oil-Control Liquid Makeup
  Shade of You Oil-Free Makeup
Max Factor
  Shine-Free Makeup
Monteil
  Habitat Natural Light Makeup
Nuskin
  No Colour Oil-Free Moisturizing Finish
Physician's Formula
  Oil-Control Matte Makeup
Revlon
  Spring Water Matte Makeup
  Color Style Natural Color Oil-Free Makeup
Shisheido
  Pureness Oil-Control Makeup.
Ultima II
The Nakeds: The Foundation Oil-Free Formula

Moisturizers

Moisturel
Cetaphil lotion

encouraged to enroll in the pregnancy prevention program of the manufacturer. Treatment for longer than 4 months is not recommended. At least a 4-month rest period off the drug is recommended before a second treatment course is considered.

Other acne treatments

There is no convincing evidence that dietary management, mild drying agents, abrasive scrubs, oral vitamin A, ultraviolet light, cryotherapy, or incision and drainage have any beneficial effects in the management of acne. Oral hormonal therapy should be reserved for patients with documented endocrine abnormalities or hirsutism. Topical antiandrogens are now under investigation, but so far have been demonstrated to be only modestly effective.[12]

Factors that aggravate acne vulgaris

Acne can be aggravated by a variety of external factors, resulting in further obstruction of partially occluded sebaceous follicles. Avoidance of oil-based cosmetics, hair-styling mousse, face creams, and hair sprays may alleviate the comedonal component of acne 4 to 6 weeks after use of the cosmetics is discontinued. A list of nonacnegenic cosmetics and moisturizers is found in Box 3-3. Change of habits such as changing tight-fitting garments may be helpful. Stopping drugs that induce acne should be attempted, if possible.

Patient education

Acne therapy requires that adequate time and explanation accompany any treatment program. It is important to explain the mechanism of acne and the treatment plan to the adolescent patient. Specifically explain that not much improvement can be expected for 4 to 8 weeks. Time should be set aside at the first visit to answer the patient's questions about acne. One should be certain to inquire what the patient's peers, relatives, and others have advised. Written

Table 3-3.

Grading System for Acne

		Follow-up		
	Baseline (Date)	1 (Date)	2 (Date)	3 (Date)
Location and Grade				
(0–3)				
Face				
Comedones				
Papules				
Pustules				
Cysts				
Chest				
Comedones				
Papules				
Pustules				
Cysts				
Back				
Comedones				
Papules				
Pustules				
Cysts				

0 = no lesions; 1 = 1–19 lesions; 2 = 20–39 lesions; 3 = 40 or more lesions.
Grade each category (comedones, papules, pustules, cysts) for each location (face, chest, back).

patient education handouts and lists of useful moisturizers and cosmetics are extremely valuable. The presence of excoriations should prompt an explanation regarding how attempted fingernail removal of acne usually results in scars that are permanent (Figs. 3-9 and 3-10). Suggestions as to relieving the nervous habit are useful.

Follow-up visits

Follow-up visits should initially be every 4 to 6 weeks. The criterion for ideal control is a few new lesions every 2 weeks. Do not expect to completely prevent any new acne lesions from appearing. Reexplain what the medications you are using are intended to achieve, and question the patient to determine whether the medications are being used properly. At the first visit a baseline evaluation grading comedones, papules, pustules, and cysts in each affected skin region should be entered on the patient's record to assist with objective measure-

ment (Tables 3-3 and 3-4). At each subsequent visit the same scoring system should be used for comparison. Objective and subjective evaluations are more likely to differ than correlate in acne patients, and one must rely on objective findings to properly evaluate response to therapy. Most authorities recommend treatment with oral antibiotics for at least 1 to 3 months. At the follow-up visit a decision to stop oral antibiotics is made when 90% improvement in red papules and pustules is observed and documented by the scoring system listed in Tables 3-3 and 3-4. When oral antibiotics are stopped, improvement can be maintained by twice-daily application of topical antibiotics. At each follow-up emphasize that therapeutic response is slow in acne and is evaluated over weeks to months, not days. Be certain that the red-purple scars, which require 6 to 12 months to fade, are not the lesions that determine alterations in treatment strategy. Scars are not influenced by antibiotics or keratolytics.

Table 3-4.
Evaluation of Acne Patients (Example)

		Follow-up		
	Baseline (10/1/97)	1 (11/3/96)	2 (12/8/96)	3 (1/28/96)
Location and Grade				
(0–3)				
Face				
Comedones	2	1	1	0
Papules	1	1	0	0
Pustules	0	0	0	0
Cysts	0	0	0	0
Chest				
Comedones	0	0	0	0
Papules	0	0	0	0
Pustules	0	0	0	0
Cysts	0	0	0	0
Back				
Comedones	1	1	1	1
Papules	2	2	2	1
Pustules	1	0	0	0
Cysts	0	0	0	0

0 = no lesions; 1 = 1–19 lesions; 2 = 20–39 lesions; 3 = 40 or more lesions.
Grade each category (comedones, papules, pustules, cysts) for each location (face, chest, back).

PERIORAL DERMATITIS AND STEROID ROSACEA

Clinical features

Erythema, slight scaling, telangiectasia, and red papules characterize these closely related conditions.[13] In perioral dermatitis and steroid rosacea, lesions are found in the nasolabial folds, just beneath the nose and on the chin (Fig. 3-14). Often lesions begin as red macules with a slight scale and are misdiagnosed as dermatitis. A topical steroid is used, and the lesions get progressively worse, with redder, telangiectatic skin and red papules or pustules seen. Frequently the child received the steroid from a relative in the health care field or used an OTC steroid. Superpotent topical steroids are most often associated with steroid rosacea after a few weeks of use, but low-potency steroids, if used daily over many weeks, will also induce the condition. Infants and adolescents are most often involved, although the exact prevalence is not known.

Occasionally pustules and red papules will be found on the lower eyelids in addition to the perioral skin (Fig. 3-15). Rarely the perioral lesions will have a granulomatous histology and reveal closely spaced, skin-colored micronodules in a perioral distribution.[14,15]

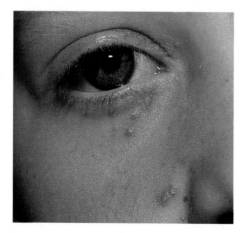

Fig. 3-15
Lower eyelid lesions in a child with perioral dermatitis.

Differential diagnosis

At the onset of disease a dermatitis such as seborrheic or contact dermatitis is suspected, although careful examination will not detect disruption of the skin surface. This misdiagnosis leads to therapy that worsens the condition. Acne vulgaris may also be restricted to the perioral skin, but the presence of comedones, which are usually absent in rosacea, will help differentiate. Rarely tinea faciei (see Chapter 6) will involve perioral skin. Scrapings for microscopic identification of fungus and fungal culture will differentiate.

Pathogenesis

Although many authorities feel that perioral dermatitis and steroid rosacea are related to acne, the pathogenesis is unclear. Sebaceous gland hyperplasia, obstructed sebaceous follicles, and prominent telangiectasias are pathologic features. In steroid rosacea the role of topically applied steroids is well established, although the exact mechanism is unknown. Although there is speculation that yeast species have a role, it is as yet unproven.

Treatment

The treatment protocols used for common acne are effective in perioral dermatitis and steroid rosacea. Topical steroid preparations must be discontinued, recognizing that the condition will worsen for about 1 week. In mild cases topical keratolytics or topical antibiotics alone will suffice. With many red papules and pustules present, oral erythromycin for 4 to 6 weeks may be required. Topical metronidazole 0.75% gel has also been shown to be effective.[13]

Patient education

Many patients are reluctant to stop topical steroids, because their skin is improved for 2 or 3 hours after each application. Insist that topical steroids be stopped, and advise that the child's skin will worsen for 1 week before it begins to improve. Caution not to use steroids to treat the predicted worsening. It is important to emphasize that this is a form of acne, and treatment is similar to acne treatment. Providing advice that only certain children are susceptible is useful.

Follow-up visits

A visit in 4 weeks to evaluate the response to therapy is recommended.

References

1. Chew EW, Bingham A, Burrows D: Incidence of acne vulgaris in patients with infantile acne, *Clin Exp Dermatol* 15:376, 1990.
2. Lucky AW, Biro FM, Huster GA, et al: Acne vulgaris in premenarchal girls: an early sign of puberty associated with rising levels of dehydroepiandrosterone, *Arch Dermatol* 130:308, 1994.
3. Lucky AW, Biro FM, Huster GA, et al: Acne vulgaris in early adolescent boys, *Arch Dermatol* 127:210, 1991.
4. Winston MH, Shalita AR: Acne vulgaris: pathogenesis and treatment, *Pediatr Clin North Am* 38:889, 1991.
5. Pochi PE, Shalita AR, Strauss JS, et al: Consensus statement. Classification of acne, *J Am Acad Dermatol* 24:495, 1991.
6. Rosenfield RJ, Lucky AW: Acne, hirsutism, and alopecia in adolescent girls. Clinical expressions of androgen excess, *Endocrinol Metab Clin North Am* 8:347, 1993.
7. Jick SS, Terris BZ, Jick H: First trimester topical tretinoin and congenital disorders, *Lancet* 341:1181, 1993.
8. Driscoll MS, Rothe MJ, Abrahamian L, Grant-Kels JM: Long-term oral antibiotics for acne: is laboratory monitoring necessary?, *J Am Acad Dermatol* 28:595, 1993.
9. American Academy of Pediatrics Committee on Drugs: Retinoid therapy for severe dermatological disorders, *Pediatrics* 20:119, 1992.
10. Layton AM, Cunliffe WJ: Guidelines for optimal use of isotretinoin in acne, *J Am Acad Dermatol* 27:S2, 1992.
11. Dai WS, LaBraico JM, Stern RS: Epidemiology of isotretinoin exposure during pregnancy, *J Am Acad Dermatol* 26:599, 1992.
12. Lookingbill DP, Abrams BB, Ellis CN, et al: Inocoterone and acne, *Arch Dermatol* 128:1197, 1992.
13. Manders SM, Lucky AW: Perioral dermatitis in childhood, *J Am Acad Dermatol* 27:688, 1992.
14. Frieden IJ, Prose NS, Fletcher V, Turner ML: Granulomatous perioral dermatitis in children, *Arch Dermatol* 125:369, 1989.
15. Smitt JH, Das PK, Van Ginkel JW: Granulomatis perioral dermatitis (facial Afro-Caribbean childhood eruption [FACE]), *Br J Dermatol* 125:399, 1991.

4

Dermatitis

Dermatitis is inflammation of the superficial dermis and epidermis, leading to disruption of the skin surface. The characteristic disruption of the skin surface is recognized as crusting, weeping, excoriation, and cracking (fissures). Dermatitis is a common disorder among children and adolescents. The prevalence of dermatitis between 1 and 5 years of age is 34.5 per 1000; between 6 and 11 years, 26.7 per 1000; and between 12 and 17 years, 35.5 per 1000.[1] About 80% of infants may have dermatitis in the first month of life.[2] The terms *dermatitis* and *eczema* are used interchangeably, although eczema was initially used to refer to blistering dermatitis, being derived from a Greek term meaning "to boil over." Dermatitis may vary in intensity from an acute condition, with vesicle formation, oozing, and crusting, to a chronic form, with epidermal thickening, a shiny flattened epidermal surface, and exaggerated skin creases. In an intermediate form, called *subacute dermatitis*, both vesiculation and epidermal thickening are present. *Acute dermatitis* implies an intense stimulus, whereas *chronic dermatitis* suggests a stimulus of low potency repeatedly occurring over a period of time. All forms of dermatitis characteristically involve the epidermis, with inflammation and disruption of epidermal integrity.

The categories of dermatitis are traditional and imprecise. Except for the various forms of contact dermatitis, the pathogenesis is unknown. Therefore it may be best simply to describe the lesions as dermatitis rather than to apply modifying adjectives such as atopic when the etiology is unclear. Some traditional terms are used in this section to avoid confusion with the previous medical literature.

ATOPIC DERMATITIS

Clinical features

Atopic dermatitis is a hereditary disorder associated with either a family or a personal history of asthma, allergic rhinitis, or atopic dermatitis. *Atopy* is from the Greek, meaning "without place, unusual," and was first employed in 1923 by Coca and Cooke to denote inherited human hypersensitivity as exemplified by asthma and hay fever.

A variety of terms have been used in literature to designate the condition. Atopic eczema, allergic eczema, Besnier's prurigo, eczema, and circumscribed neurodermatitis are terms less acceptable and less widely used than atopic dermatitis. Up to 50% of patients with dermatitis compatible with the diagnosis of atopic dermatitis also have respiratory manifestations of atopy, such as extrinsic asthma or allergic rhinitis. Very rarely does a patient have all three manifestations of the atopic triad.

The diagnosis of atopic dermatitis is a clinical one. The clinical appearance of atopic dermatitis may represent a phenotype resulting from different mechanisms. There is no single diagnostic criterion for the phenotype we appreciate as atopic dermatitis; rather, a combination of features must be considered. The major features listed in Box 4-1 are useful in the diagnosis.[3-5] Although many other features may be noted, such as facial pallor, Denny's lines under the eyes, intolerance to wool or occlusive clothing, associated ichthyosis, cataracts, and eosinophilia, they are not considered diagnostic of the disease or necessary for the diagnosis.

Atopic dermatitis commonly begins before the age of 6 months.[6] At the onset the distribution is primarily on the cheeks, face, trunk, and extensor surfaces of the arms and legs (Fig. 4-1). Frequently the dermatitis seen in the first months of life is a subacute dermatitis characterized by thickened shiny skin and oozing. Although atopic dermatitis develops in infancy in most affected persons, it develops during early childhood in some. By adolescence over 90% of atopic dermatitis patients will already have the disorder. Of all infants in whom atopic dermatitis develops, only a third will continue to have the disease during childhood. Similarly, of those who still have dermatitis during childhood, only a third will have difficulties at adolescence. Thus one ninth of those who had infantile dermatitis will still have the features and problems of dermatitis in adolescence.[7]

Itching has long been recognized as a significant feature of atopic dermatitis. It commonly occurs in paroxysms and can be severe. In most patients itching is most severe in the evening, and scratching continues while the child is sleeping.[8] The threshold for itching in atopic dermatitis patients is lowered, and their itching is more prolonged than that in normal persons. Scratching frenzies may be reported. The propensity for itching and the resultant trauma from scratching are central to the genesis of atopic dermatitis (Fig. 4-2).

The distribution of dermatitis is largely age dependent (Fig. 4-1). Infantile atopic dermatitis, distributed largely on the cheeks (Figs. 4-3 and 4-4), face, trunk, and extensor surfaces of extremities, evolves into the childhood phase, with dermatitis on the feet and in the flexural areas, such as the antecubital fossa, popliteal fossa (Figs. 4-5 and 4-6), and neck. By adolescence the distribution has become that seen in older adults, with bilateral involvement of the flexural areas and hand eczema. Involvement of the eyelids is common in all phases of atopic dermatitis and may help to make the diagnosis. Foot involvement is common in school-age children and adolescents and may be associated with atopic dermatitis or juvenile plantar dermatosis (JPD).

The primary clinical lesion of atopic dermatitis has not been described. In fact, many observers believe that all visible skin lesions in atopic dermatitis are secondary to scratching. Intense erythema and oozing are absent except in patients with secondary bacterial infection. During exacerbation, dark-skinned patients may demonstrate follicular papules (Fig. 4-7), especially on the trunk. In black skin, hyperpigmented, lichenified nodules are commonly found on the lower arms and legs in addition to flexural involvement (Fig. 4-6).

Dry skin is strongly associated with atopic dermatitis. Patients with atopic dermatitis have reduced water content of the stratum corneum despite greater water

---

Box 4-1   Cardinal features of atopic dermatitis in children

Presence of an itchy rash
Visible flexural dermatitis
Onset under age 2
History of flexural dermatitis

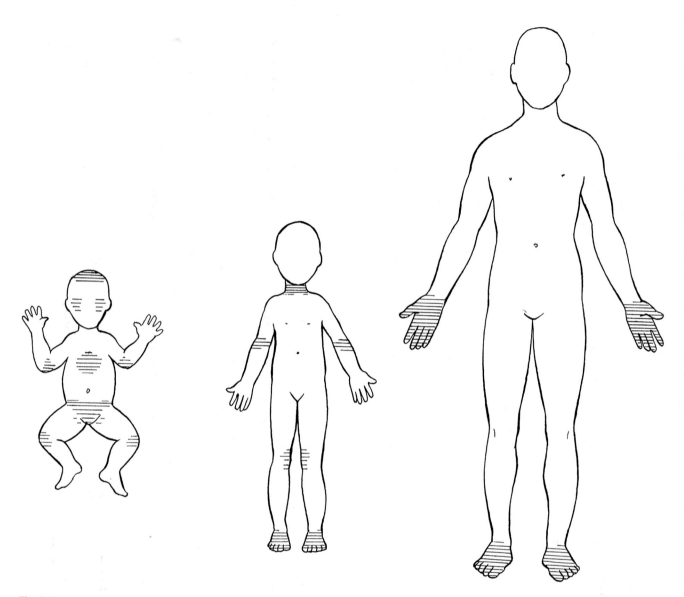

Fig. 4-1

Age-dependent distribution of atopic dermatitis. Involvement of the face, scalp, trunk, and extensor surfaces of extremities as seen in infants, flexural skin in toddlers, and hands and feet in preteens and adolescents.

loss through the skin.[9] Secretion of sebum and sweat may be suppressed in some patients with atopic dermatitis. Dry skin and horny follicular papules (keratosis pilaris) are common findings, particularly on extensor surfaces. Microscopic fractures of the stratum corneum during drying result in loss of the epidermal barrier and increased susceptibility to irritants and infection. There is little doubt that dryness of the skin during the winter months in cool climates is a significant factor in exacerbation of atopic dermatitis. Dry, slightly scaly, hypopigmented patches seen in mild atopic dermatitis are called *pityriasis alba* (Fig. 4-8)

Abnormal vasomotor responses are found in a minority of children with atopic dermatitis. The vari-

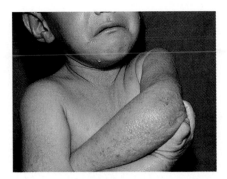

Fig. 4-2
Itching frenzies may be severe, as seen in this unhappy child.

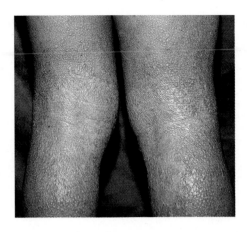

Fig. 4-5
Flexural involvement of popliteal fossa in atopic dermatitis.

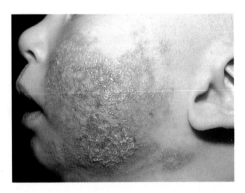

Fig. 4-3
Acute dermatitis of the cheeks with oozing and crusting in an infant with atopic dermatitis.

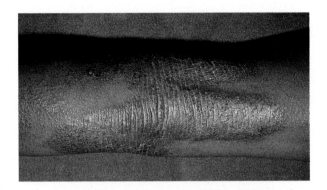

Fig. 4-6
Lichenification of the popliteal fossa from chronic rubbing of the skin in atopic dermatitis.

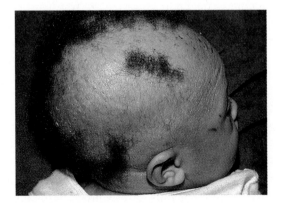

Fig. 4-4
Alopecia associated with atopic dermatitis; note the lichenification of the face and scalp.

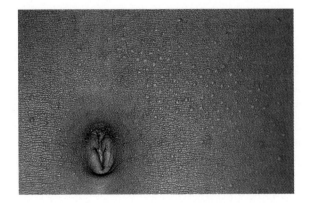

Fig. 4-7
Follicular hyperkeratosis seen on the abdomen of an adolescent with atopic dermatitis.

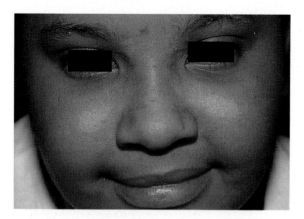

Fig. 4-8
Hypopigmented, slightly scaly patch of mild dermatitis is referred to as pityriasis alba.

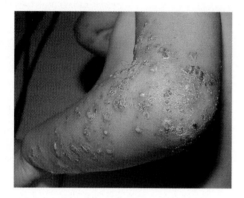

Fig. 4-9
Secondarily infected atopic dermatitis with multiple pustules and areas of crusting.

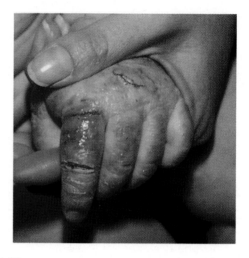

Fig. 4-10
Fissures and many breaks of the skin in atopic dermatitis, with secondary bacterial infection.

ety of vasomotor reactions in atopic dermatitis patients suggests a tendency toward vasoconstriction of the skin. The facial skin, particularly that about the nose, appears pale, and the peripheral extremities may have a lower skin temperature than that of normal persons. The skin reacts to cold stimuli with marked vasoconstriction. White dermatographism, the production of a white line with surrounding blanching after stroking erythematous skin with a blunt instrument, is seen in some children with atopic dermatitis. This blanching is thought to represent edema. There is also a diminished response of atopic skin to intradermal injections of histamine.

Children with atopic dermatitis may be extremely sensitive to certain contact irritants. They may experience bouts of itching and subsequent exacerbation of dermatitis when wool or an irritant chemical contacts the skin. Detergents and frequent soaping of the skin often result in prolonged itching. Sensitivity to contactants may partially explain localization of dermatitis in certain areas, particularly on the hands and feet.

Emotional stress indisputably leads to increased scratching. This occurs frequently in children, from either heightened awareness of itching or a habit of scratching. The child experiences transient relief after a scratching frenzy. Atopic dermatitis worsens during such episodes. It is important for patients or their parents to recognize that scratching the skin is a means of expressing anxiety. Secondary skin infection with bacteria such as *Staphylococcus aureus* may worsen the dermatitis (Figs. 4-9 and 4-10) and worsen itching.

Differential diagnosis

Differential diagnosis should include any disorder manifested by dermatitis. Thus contact dermatitis of the primary irritant and allergic type, seborrheic dermatitis, nummular eczema, scabies, molluscum contagiosum, JPD, polymorphous light eruptions, the dermatitis of human immunodeficiency virus (HIV) infection or immunodeficiency and tinea constitute the major considerations in the differential diagnosis of atopic dermatitis in childhood. In infants, seborrheic dermatitis may be impossible to distinguish from atopic dermatitis. Serum immunoglobulin E (IgE) levels may be elevated in infantile atopic dermatitis, but they are of no diagnostic or prognostic value.

Pathogenesis

Although there are a number of hypotheses as to the mechanism of the generation of atopic dermatitis in children, the exact pathogenesis is unknown. Various forms of both antibody and cellular immunodeficiency, abnormal β-adrenergic receptors and responses, food allergies, and aeroallergens such as house dust mites have been evoked, but there is no convincing evidence to substantiate any of these hypotheses. The dermatitis can be exacerbated by xerosis, irritation of the skin, or epicutaneous application of a contact irritant or allergen.

Treatment

Atopic dermatitis is a chronic disease, frustrating for both child and parents. Weeks of effective control can be followed by a sudden, severe relapse. It is tempting for the physician to focus on one or several factors as causes and to regard their elimination as curative. The patient or the family should be told that there is no immediate cure for atopic dermatitis but that spontaneous remissions do occur, and that this disorder can be controlled by therapy. Patients and family should pay careful attention to factors aggravating atopic dermatitis, which are listed in Box 4-2. The mainstays of therapy are topical steroids, lubricants, wet dressings, oral antibiotics, and avoidance of factors that aggravate the dermatitis. General care instructions are listed in Box 4-3.

Sweating and heat intolerance can be managed by avoiding occlusive clothing, airtight occlusive dressings such as Saran Wrap, and overheating. Dry skin can be managed by rehydration of the skin with water and covering the skin generously with a lubricant. Irritant contact sensitivity can be managed by washing infants without soap when possible and, when using soap, by limiting the time the soap is in contact with the skin by rinsing the child quickly after the soap has been applied. Direct contact with wool clothing, home cleaning agents, or irritating chemicals should be avoided. Secondary bacterial infection by *S. aureus* or *Streptococcus pyogenes* resulting from the frequent breaks in the skin and the excoriations caused by scratching is treated with systemic antibiotics (Figs. 4-9 and 4-10). If lymphadenopathy is present, or if the lesions are crusted and weeping, antibiotics are recommended.

Stress and anxiety can be difficult to manage. Stress increases the sense of pruritus. Parents usually do not intentionally intend to accelerate stress for their children, and all stresses cannot be removed. The stress and anxiety of the atopic dermatitis condition may require therapeutic intervention and discussion with parents who already blames themselves for the child's condition. Emphasize to the parents that the

---

Box 4-2   Factors that aggravate atopic dermatitis
Dry skin
Sweating
Contact sensitivity
Stress and anxiety
Secondary bacterial infection

Box 4-3   General instructions for long-term management of atopic dermatitis
Keep the skin lubricated.
Wear loose-fitting cotton clothing.
Keep fingernails trimmed short.
Avoid overheating of skin.
Always use a soap substitute.
Limit time of soap substitute exposure to the skin.

primary problem is the skin condition. Removal of stress may be beneficial, but treatment of the skin is most important.

Relief of itching is the cornerstone of therapy for atopic dermatitis. Itching may be relieved by removal of the factors aggravating atopic dermatitis, by the use of topical glucocorticosteroids of low or moderate potency, or by antihistamines. Significant antihistamine sedation often must be achieved before relief of pruritus occurs. The mainstay of therapy for atopic dermatitis remains topical steroid preparations and lubrication. They are central to most treatment strategies for atopic dermatitis. For initial care (see Boxes 4-4 and 4-5), select a low- or moderate-potency topical steroid.[10,11] Steroid creams are not as lubricating as the ointments and are more easily covered with a lubricant. Ointments may sting less when applied to inflamed skin. For infants and nonlichenified skin, a low-potency topical steroid may be adequate. The face and genital areas should be treated only with a low-potency steroid.

Management of acute severe dermatitis
Steroids and wet dressings

Acute weeping dermatitis is best treated by the application of wet dressings, the methodology for which is outlined in Box 4-6. Often such patients have multiple excoriations, crusting, and secondary bacterial infection; thus the use of wet dressings in combination with systemic antibiotics is necessary. It may be difficult to treat such patients successfully without the use of antibiotics. Apply a moderate-potency steroid ointment or cream (see Box 4-8) to affected areas; cover with a damp cotton dressing followed by a dry cotton dressing. In 6 hours remove all dressings and reapply steroids. Follow by applying a redampened dressing, then a dry dressing. Continue this procedure for 24 to 72 hours, then switch to a long-term management strategy. An alternate strategy is to use wet dressings and steroids overnight for 7 to 10 consecutive nights, then use maintenance therapy. Since the evaporation of water results in cooling, be certain to keep the child's room warm when using wet dressings. Use systemic antistaphylococcal antibiotics to treat secondary infection, and oral antihistamines to relieve pruritus.

Box 4-4   Instructions for topical care of atopic dermatitis

1. Wet the skin for 5 to 10 minutes twice a day.
2. Towel off the beads of water and quickly apply the steroid preparation to wet skin twice daily. Apply the steroid only on the area of dermatitis.
3. Apply a lubricant to the entire body immediately after the topical steroid. The lubricant may be applied over the steroid if the steroid is a cream. The lubricant should be applied while the skin is still wet twice a day.
4. Reapply the lubricant through out the day if the skin appears dry.
5. As the skin improves, continue the lubricant twice a day or more frequently. Decrease the topical steroid to once a day or less frequently as needed. You may also be able to decrease the potency of the topical steroid.
6. With further improvement, the frequency of wetting the skin and lubrication can be decreased.

Box 4-5 Systemic therapy for atopic dermatitis

1. Use of diphenhydramine (3 to 5 mg/kg/day) or hydroxyzine (1 to 2 mg/kg/day) may decrease the sensation of pruritus. One dose given 1 hour before bedtime may be most effective.
2. For crusted, oozing, infected-appearing lesions, antistaphylococcal oral antibiotics are beneficial (e.g., dicloxacillin, 12 to 25 mg/kg/day, or cephalexin, 25 to 50 mg/kg/day) three to four times a day for 14 days or more.

Box 4-6 Instructions for wet dressings

Materials needed
1. Prescription for moderately potent steroid ointment or cream
2. Two pairs or more of cotton or mostly cotton sleepers or long johns
3. Warm water in a sink or basin

Technique
1. Apply steroid ointment to rash.
2. Wet one pair of cotton sleepers in warm water; wring out until damp.
3. Place damp sleepers on child, the dry sleepers over the damp ones.
4. Be certain room is warm enough and child does not chill.

Duration of treatment (Use 1 or 2)
1. Use overnight for 5 to 10 nights.
2. Change every 6 hours for 24 to 72 hours (e.g., reapply steroid; redampen damp sleepers).

Box 4-7 Instructions for maintenance care of atopic dermatitis

1. Wet skin once or twice a day and lubricate immediately
2. Lubrication can be applied several additional times a day to dry skin.
3. Use antihistamines at bedtime for itching as necessary.
4. If flare up occurs, re-treat as described in Boxes 4-4 and 4-5.

Box 4-8 Topical steroids for use in childhood atopic dermatitis

Low potency
    Hydrocortisone 1% and 2.5%
    Desonide 0.05%
Moderate potency
    Fluocinolone acetonide 0.025% (Fluonid, Synalar)
    Hydrocortisone valerate 0.2% (Westcort)
    Mometasone furoate 0.1% (Elocon)
    Triamcinolone 0.1% (Kenalog, Aristocort)

Long-term management of atopic dermatitis
In addition to the methods of skin care listed in the Boxes 4-4 and 4-7, cetyl alcohol lotion cleanser can be used as a soap substitute or in place of the bath. Bathe the child only once a week, and apply a lubricant cetyl alcohol lotion liberally to the body three or or four times a day. Additional lubricants can be applied throughout the day as needed.

Topical steroids and lubricants are discussed in detail in Chapter 22. Boxes 4-8 and 4-9 give a short list of commonly used products. In more humid climates lotions and creams may be effective. In a drier climate greasy lubricants and ointments may be more effective. The choice of the vehicle will depend on the clinical condition, the environment, and the preference of the patient.

Referral for special therapy

Children who are not responding to treatment may be referred to a dermatologist for further treatment.

Often therapeutic failures result from not following the treatment plan or in the child who has unrecognized and untreated secondary bacterial infection or scabies. Phototherapy with ultraviolet B (UVB) sunlamps or photochemotherapy with psoralen and ultraviolet light (PUVA) may be efficacious in children with atopic dermatitis who have failed standard therapy. Phototherapy should be supervised by trained, experienced dermatologists.

Alternative therapies

Although many parents or physicians are convinced that foods induce exacerbation of atopic dermatitis, scientific evidence to reproduce dermatitis by foods is unconvincing for most children.[12-18] This should not

---

Box 4-9 Lubricants useful for atopic dermatitis

Hydrophilic petrolatum (Vaseline)
Aquaphor
Eucerin
Moisturel
Cetyl alcohol lotion (Cetaphil)

---

become an emotional issue between parents and treating physician. Restrictive diets have no long-term benefits in atopic dermatitis and may eventuate in nutritional deficiency if too restrictive. Evening primrose oil, desensitization shots, PUVA, interferon, Chinese herbs, and a number of other remedies have been advocated.[19-22] The risks and benefits of these therapies require further study. Oral steroids may produce temporary benefits, but high doses are required, and they have no role in management of a chronic disease because of side effects with long-term use.

Patient education

It is helpful to instruct the child and parents in the method of application of the topical medications. One may choose to explain that the child has "sensitive" skin, that heredity plays a role in determining this tendency, but the cause is not known. Emphasize to the parents the extreme pruritus associated with this condition. The severity of the itching sensation is so great that the child will produce painful, deep excoriations in an effort to relieve the pruritus. It should be stressed that a cure is not possible, but that good control can be achieved, so that the child can live a comfortable and normal life. Preventing further skin irritation is also helpful (see Box 4-3 on p 35), as is emphasis on the five factors aggravating atopic dermatitis, particularly secondary bacterial skin infection (see Box 4-2 on p 35). The patient and the parents should be told that the principle underlying good control is the liberal use of lubricants to restore moisture to the skin and protect it from contactants. Using lubricants in this manner avoids the necessity for

high-potency topical glucocorticosteroids and long-term steroid medications. Do not make the patient or parents feel guilty if a flare of the eczema occurs. Reinstitute active treatment immediately. *Therapy is directed at relieving pruritus, not focusing pressure on stopping the child from scratching.*

Follow-up visits

The first follow-up visit should be within 10 to 14 days, so that therapy can be reviewed. It is often helpful at this time to have the parents or child demonstrate how medication is applied and to determine how much was used. Have the medication brought back for each visit so that you can document the quantity used. Evaluation of the response to antihistamines and the need for antibiotics can be completed at the first follow-up visit. Thereafter monthly visits will suffice until the patient is using lubricants only, after which he or she should be reevaluated every 3 to 6 months. Be certain that patients know that you will be available when flares occur, and examine the child for secondary infection at the visit related to the flare-up.

CONTACT DERMATITIS

Contact dermatitis, or dermatitis resulting from substances coming in direct contact with the skin, is divided into two subtypes: primary irritant contact dermatitis and allergic contact dermatitis.

Primary irritant contact dermatitis

Strong chemicals that penetrate the epidermal barrier readily, weaker chemicals that penetrate a faulty epidermal barrier, or substances that remove intercellular lipids produce inflammation of the skin (primary irritant contact dermatitis). The form most commonly seen in pediatrics is diaper dermatitis. Dry skin dermatitis and JPD are other forms commonly seen in children.

Diaper dermatitis

Clinical features The exact incidence of diaper dermatitis is unknown, but roughly 20% of all infants under age 2 years are believed to develop this condition at any time.[23] Four clinical forms are recognized. The most frequently observed is chafing dermatitis, in which involvement of the convex surface of the thighs, buttocks, and waist area is common. Chafing diaper dermatitis most frequently is observed at 7 to 12 months of age, when the baby's urine volume exceeds the absorbing capacity of the diaper, including the superabsorbant diapers (Fig. 4-11). In the second form the dermatitis is limited to the perianal area. This form is particularly observed in newborns or in children who have experienced diarrhea. The third form is characterized by discrete shallow ulcerations scattered throughout the diaper area including the genitalia. In the fourth form, beefy-red confluent erythema involving the inguinal creases and the genitalia with satellite oval lesions about the periphery is seen (Fig. 4-12). This fourth form is observed when secondary invasion with *Candida albicans* occurs. Despite major differences in clinical appearance, all four forms share a similar pathogenesis.

Differential diagnosis   Atopic dermatitis or the other forms of dermatitis may begin in the diaper area. Rarely, psoriasis, Langerhans cell histiocytosis, or the eruptions associated with immunodeficiencies or HIV infection may occur in this area. In perianal forms of diaper dermatitis, perianal cellulitis must be distinguished, and a bacterial culture obtained.[28]

Pathogenesis   Diaper dermatitis is a result of prolonged contact of urine and feces with the perineal skin. Airtight occlusion of feces and urine by diaper covers increases the penetration of these alkaline substances through the epidermal barrier.[24-27] Prolonged contact with water is central to the genesis of the dermatitis. Ammonia by itself is not responsible for the dermatitis. If diaper dermatitis is present for longer than 3 days, there is likely to be secondary *C. albicans* invasion of the inflammatory areas of the skin. *C. albicans* invasion must be suspected in each clinical form of diaper dermatitis.

Treatment   The basis for all treatment programs is to remove the contactants (urine and feces) from the skin surface and eliminate maceration by keeping the diaper area dry. Lubrication of diapered skin with a greasy ointment decreases the severity of diaper dermatitis and may protect the skin from urine and feces. Very frequent diaper changes, followed by application of ointment, limits maceration and decreases recurrences. Diaper changes several hours after the baby goes to sleep for the night and reducing fluids just before bedtime may benefit. Plastic and rubber pants should be avoided when possible. Letting the diaper area skin air dry when practical may be helpful, but avoid moisture and maceration followed by dry air or hot dry air such as a hair dryer. When contamination by urine and feces occurs, the

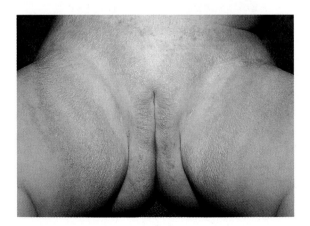

Fig. 4-11
Chafing type of diaper dermatitis

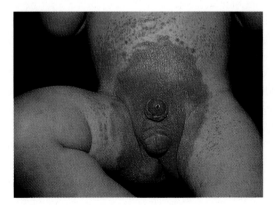

Fig. 4-12
Candidiasis in the diaper area. A positive culture for *Candida* can be obtained from satellite pustules.

skin should be rinsed gently with warm water. A minimum of soap should be used in this area.

Candidiasis in the diaper area requires topical antiyeast therapy such as nystatin. In severe dermatitis hydrocortisone 1% cream twice daily for 1 to 2 days may help to decrease the infant's discomfort. Until toilet training is achieved or diaper care changed, recurrences may be frequent. The incidence of diaper dermatitis decreases with eight or more diaper changes per day.[23]

Patient education Reducing the time of contact of urine and feces with skin is essential. Very frequent diaper changes and lubrication of the skin constitute the best prevention, with careful attention to overnight care. Sleep on a rubber sheet with the baby not wearing a diaper cover may be helpful. Determining the person actually responsible for diaper changes during the daily routine is very helpful in planning a therapy program. In the 7- to 12-month-old, have the parent check the diaper for wetness several hours after bedtime and change the baby if wet. Restriction of fluids in the hour just before bedtime may also be helpful for the toddler.

Follow-up visits The routine visits for pediatric care are sufficient for follow-up, but in severe diaper dermatitis, a revisit in 2 days may be useful.

Dry skin dermatitis

Clinical features A dry, rough skin surface with rectangular scales that have erythema on the scale borders is seen in dermatitis due to dry skin. Horny follicular papules on the proximal extremities and buttocks (keratosis pilaris) are also usually seen. Occasionally the dermatitis will coalesce, and the patient will present with diffuse erythema (Fig. 4-13).

Differential diagnosis The differential diagnosis includes all the other forms of dermatitis, the ichthyoses, and scabies. Children with atopic dermatitis have very dry skin.

Pathogenesis Environmental humidity of less than 30% is the most important factor. Frequent soaping of the skin, removing skin lipids with alcohol or acetone, or the use of drying lotions predisposes to dry skin dermatitis.

Treatment Therapy is designed to restore moisture to the skin by liberal use of water followed by the application of lubricants. Generally, water-in-oil emulsions (see Chapter 22) two or three times a day are sufficient.

Patient education The value of a home humidifier in an area of low environmental humidity and of avoiding frequent soaping of the skin is important to convey to the patient or family. Children with dry skin require daily lubricant therapy.

Follow-up visits One visit in 4 weeks' time to evaluate the therapy program is often sufficient.

Juvenile plantar dermatosis

Clinical features Redness, cracking, and dryness of the weight-bearing surface of the foot are characteristic of JPD. The great toes are often the first area involved. Involvement of the entire forefoot may occur that can mimic tinea pedis (Fig. 4-14). The involvement is usually quite symmetric. Many, but not all, children with JPD may exhibit features of atopic dermatitis.[29]

Differential diagnosis Tinea pedis often mimics JPD. However, JPD is quite common in preadolescence, whereas tinea pedis is uncommon; JPD

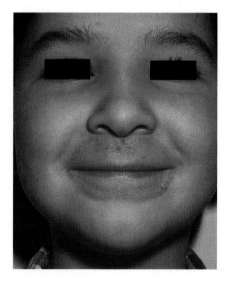

Fig. 4-13
Lip licker dermatitis associated with constant licking of dry lips.

involves weight-bearing areas, whereas tinea pedis involves the instep. Direct microscopic examination of scale with potassium hydroxide (KOH) and fungal culture will help to distinguish the two conditions. Allergic contact dermatitis involves the dorsum of the foot rather than the weight-bearing surface.

Treatment   The use of ointment bases such as Aquaphor or petroleum jelly applied two or three times a day is most useful. The ointment should be

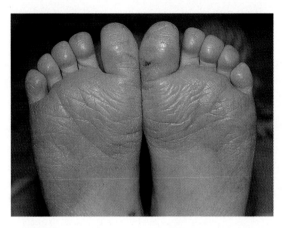

Fig. 4-14
Red, shiny distal sole and toes associated with juvenile plantar dermatosis.

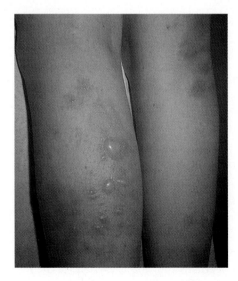

Fig. 4-15
Allergic contact dermatitis due to poison ivy, with blister formation.

applied as soon as shoes are taken off to avoid heat and humidity in a shoe and xerosis in bare feet. Socks may need to remain over lubricated feet to prevent slipping and greasing of floors. Attempts to dry the feet often aggravate the condition as the feet are already dry and chapped. Topical glucocorticosteroid ointments of moderate potency may be required if inflammation is severe.

Patient education   Emphasis that this is neither a fungal infection nor the result of excessive sweating of the foot is important. The patient should recognize that the excessive dryness is similar to chapping of the skin.

Follow-up visits   A visit 2 weeks after therapy is begun is most useful in evaluating compliance and response to therapy.

Allergic contact dermatitis

Clinical features   The exact incidence of allergic contact dermatitis in children is unknown, but some authorities estimate it at 5% to 10% of all dermatitis. In childhood allergic contact dermatitis usually presents as acute dermatitis with erythema, vesiculation, and oozing (Fig. 4-15). The dermatitis is limited to the area of contact with the external substance, such as the stem or leaf of a plant (Fig. 4-16). Less often, children are exposed repeatedly to weaker chemical allergens,

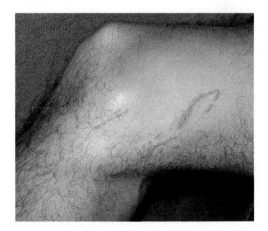

Fig. 4-16
Allergic contact dermatitis on the legs secondary to poison oak; note the linear pattern where the leaf has brushed against the leg.

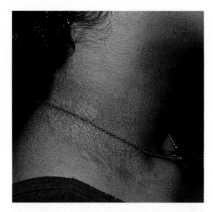

Fig. 4-17
Chronic dermatitis of neck from nickel allergy caused by necklace.

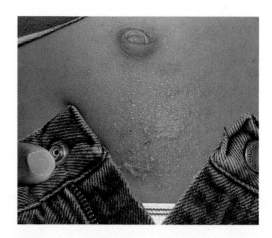

Fig. 4-18
Allergic contact dermatitis to nickel caused by metal snap on blue jeans.

resulting in the development of the features of subacute or chronic dermatitis (Fig. 4-17). Usually the contactant is obvious, although considerable detective work is occasionally required to determine the cause. Once the response occurs and dermatitis is generated, as seen with a strong allergen such as poison ivy, it lasts for 3 weeks, even though the child has not had repeated exposure to the allergen.

Distribution of the dermatitis may provide an important clue to the contact allergen (Fig. 4-18). For example, one may see involvement of the dorsa of the feet in shoe dermatitis; of the earlobes, neck, wrists, and fingers in metal allergy (e.g., due to nickel); of the face and eyelids in cosmetic allergy; of the axilla in deodorant allergy; of the ear canal from medication; of the perioral area from toothpaste or lipstick; or of areas of clothing from exposure to formaldehyde.

Differential diagnosis Although all other forms of dermatitis may mimic allergic contact dermatitis, it is usually localized to one area of skin. A sudden onset of dermatitis limited to the hands or feet in children and adolescents is most likely to be contact dermatitis (Fig. 4-19). Patch testing (described under Follow-up visits) may detect the chemical allergen and help distinguish allergic contact dermatitis from other forms of dermatitis.

Pathogenesis Allergic contact dermatitis is a form of cell-mediated immunity. The process is divid-

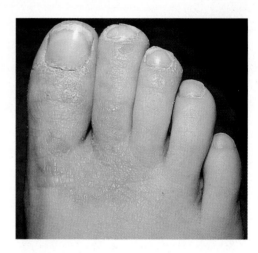

Fig. 4-19
Chronic dermatitis on dorsa of feet and toes due to potassium dichromate allergy from chronic exposure to leather tennis shoes.

ed into two distinct but interrelated phases: the sensitization phase and the elicitation phase. The antigens involved in allergic contact dermatitis are incomplete antigens called haptens (see Box 4-10). The hapten applied to the skin surface penetrates the epidermis, combines with the antigen-binding site of the epidermal Langerhans cell, and is carried via the lymphatics to the regional lymph node. There the antigen is processed by macrophages and presented to T lym-

---

Box 4-10 Characteristics of contact allergens

1. They are haptens.
2. They can penetrate the epidermis.

Box 4-11 Common sources of contact allergens in children

Jewelry, buckles, clothing snaps (nickel)
Shoes (potassium dichromate)
Topical medications, creams, lotions (neomycin, thimerosal, formaldehyde, Quaternium 15, wool alcohol [lanolin])
Perfumes, soaps, cosmetics (balsam of Peru, colophony, "fragrances")
Poison ivy, poison oak, poison sumac, mango rind (urushiol)

Table 4-1.

Most Prevalent Allergens in Children

Allergen	Sensitized (%)
Neomycin	8
Nickel	8
Potassium dichromate	8
Thimerosal	3
Balsam of Peru	2
Formaldehyde	1
Quaternium 15	1
Colophony	1
p-tert-Butylphenol formaldehyde	1
Wool (lanolin) alcohol	1

phocytes. Recognition occurs, as does proliferation of the T lymphocytes specifically programmed to recognize that antigen. These T lymphocytes leave the lymph node and enter the bloodstream, migrating back to the skin. The sensitization phase takes 5 to 7 days to complete in the case of strong chemical allergens; with weak allergens, it may take from weeks to months.

In the elicitation phase, antigen-specific T lymphocytes are present in the skin. The next time the allergen comes in contact with the skin surface and penetrates the epidermis, the T lymphocyte combines with the allergen in the skin and releases inflammatory mediators, causing erythema and the accumulation and activation of mononuclear cells, which results in the dermatitis. This phase begins 6 to 18 hours after the antigen is applied.

A great variety of chemicals are responsible for causing allergic contact dermatitis, varying from the simple metal nickel to complex chemicals such as dinitrochlorobenzene. Common sources of contact aller-

gens in children are listed in Box 4-11. However, they have certain features in common, as seen in Box 4-10.

Treatment Antiinflammatory agents such as glucocorticosteroids are the therapy of choice in allergic contact dermatitis. In localized areas topical glucocorticosteroids of moderate or high potency (see Box 4-8 on p 37 and Chapter 22), applied three times a day may clear the dermatitis and decrease the discomfort.[30] In generalized skin involvement or in acute vesicular involvement, wet dressings and topical glucocorticosteroids for 2 to 3 days give dramatic relief (see Box 4-6 on p 37). This is followed by applications of moderate-potency topical glucocorticosteroids three times a day until the pruritus resolves. When the face or genital area is involved, or when greater than 10% of the skin surface is involved, oral glucocorticosteroids are used, such as prednisone, 1 mg/kg in a single dose every morning for 1 week and then tapered over 7 to 14 days. The popular steroid dose packs do not maintain their antiinflammatory effects for a sufficiently long time and often result in a rebound exacerbation of acute allergic contact dermatitis.

Patient education Knowledge and avoidance of the offending antigen are central to the care of the child with allergic contact dermatitis. Poison ivy/oak dermatitis is the most common allergic contact dermatitis in the United States. Other common contact allergens are listed in Table 4-1.[31, 32] Emphasize that treatment requires 2 or 3 weeks. When exposure to contact aller-

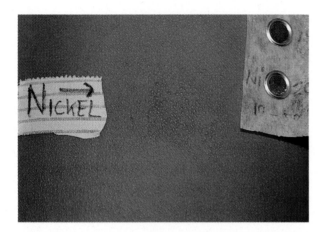

Fig. 4-20
Removal of the patch test after 48 hours in child with positive reaction to nickel.

gens cannot be avoided, barrier preparations such as Stokogard, Hollister Moisture Barrier, or Hydropel may be effective.[33] Immediately washing the exposed skin with soap and water may also be beneficial by decreasing the duration and quantity of exposure.

Follow-up visits   In 3 to 4 weeks, after the allergic dermatitis has subsided, epicutaneous (patch) testing (Fig. 4-20) to identify the offending allergen may be desirable in children in whom the cause is obscure. This is not necessary in acute poison ivy or plant dermatitis. Epicutaneous testing has been standardized and is reliable in detecting the suspected allergen. The test is made on the upper back. The suspected antigens are placed on the chambers, and vertical rows of three to five strips are placed on the upper back and firmly secured with nonirritating occlusive tape. The area is taped securely, so that it is airtight, and the patches are left on for 48 hours without allowing the area to become wet. The patient removes the patches and tape, and the tests are read 72 hours after initial application. Erythema and vesiculation are observed in an allergic reaction, the same clinical and histologic features that are seen in allergic contact dermatitis. In allergic reactions the papules extend beyond the chamber margins, whereas they are limited to the chamber in irritant reactions. The angry back syndrome of hyperreactivity has not been reported in children. Standardized allergens have been developed by the North American Contact Dermatitis Group and may be obtained from the American Academy of Dermatology. Patch testing should be performed by a physician experienced in the interpretation and pitfalls of the procedure.

SEBORRHEIC DERMATITIS

Clinical features

Chronic dermatitis accompanied by overproduction of sebum may occur on the scalp, face, midchest, or perineum in two age groups: the neonate and the adolescent. The scalp appears greasy with accumulation of scales entrapped in the sebum. In some infants it is limited to the scalp, with a greasy accumulation of scales adherent to the scalp (seborrhea capitis). Many infants also have flexural dermatitis as seen in atopic dermatitis. Infants with a tendency to have seborrheic dermatitis may have severe worsening of their dermatitis if they develop persistent diaper dermatitis. In adolescents, erythema and greasy scales in the nasolabial folds and the scalp may be seen. In HIV-infected patients seborrheic dermatitis may be an early sign of aquired immunodeficiency syndrome (AIDS).

Differential diagnosis

Since physiologic overproduction of sebum occurs in many infants during the first 6 months of life, any dermatitis occurring at this age may be mistakenly called seborrheic dermatitis. There is considerable confusion over whether it is necessary to distinguish between atopic dermatitis, contact dermatitis, and seborrheic dermatitis in infants. Most infants with dermatitis eventually demonstrate features consistent with atopic dermatitis, especially if the involvement of the extremities and trunk accompanies the more characteristic lesions of the scalp and face. Scabies may also mimic seborrheic dermatitis in this age group, and identifying mites by scraping unscratched burrows will confirm scabies. Seborrheic dermatitis with petechiae is often seen in Langerhans cell histiocytosis, and this diagnosis may also be excluded by skin biopsy. Immunodeficiency diseases, such as Leiner's disease, severe combined immunodeficiency, and the immunodeficiency that accompanies HIV infection, may be excluded by the history, the presence of signs and symptoms of failure to thrive, severe pulmonary or gastrointestinal infection accompanying the eruption, or the appropriate immunologic or serologic evaluation. Multiple carboxylase deficiency and other biotin-responsive dermatoses also mimic seborrheic dermatitis, and serum biotin levels may be required to confirm the diagnosis.

Seborrheic dermatitis limited to the scalp (seborrhea capitis) must be distinguished from the diffuse form of tinea capitis due to *Trichophyton tonsurans* and from cradle cap. A KOH examination of scalp scrapings plus a fungal culture will distinguish tinea capitis, whereas the absence of redness characterizes cradle cap.

Adolescent seborrheic dermatitis occurs in the nasolabial folds, midface, postauricular area, scalp, and chest. It may be difficult to distinguish from atopic or contact dermatitis, perioral dermatitis, or psoriasis.

Pathogenesis
Although seborrheic dermatitis has been attributed to excessive sebum accumulation on the skin surface, the mechanism is unknown. Similarly, the pathogenesis of the seborrheic-like dermatitis of immunodeficiency or HIV infection is unknown. Although there are many carboxylase enzymes in skin, and biotin may be a cofactor for many skin enzymes, the mechanism of dermatitis is unknown.

Treatment
Topical steroid creams of low potency applied twice daily for several days and then occasionally will often clear the dermatitis and treat recurrences. Keratolytic shampoos on the scalp will be painful if they wash into the infant's eyes, and they may worsen the dermatitis. Tear-free shampoos may be adequate. The shampoo can remain on the scalp for several minutes, while the scalp is lightly scrubbed with a soft brush or toothbrush to remove the scale and crust. The low-potency topical steroid cream can be applied immediately after shampoo. This process can be repeated

daily until adequate improvement or resolution occurs. Oral biotin therapy should be considered if biotin-responsive dermatoses are suspected. On the face, topical steroids should be of low potency and used twice daily for several days and then moisturizers substituted. If perioral dermatitis is suspected, antiacne therapy as outlined in Chapter 3 is used.

Patient education
Patients and parents should be advised that the cause of this disorder is unknown. Although it is tempting to use rigorous methods to remove scale from the scalp, it is unnecessary. Gentle therapy repeated several days in a row is more effective.

Follow-up visits
A visit in 1 week to review diagnostic tests and to evaluate response to therapy is recommended. If the lesions remain thick and crusted, the diagnosis of seborrheic dermatitis is probably incorrect and requires reevaluation of the condition. Thereafter the child should be seen only if the dermatitis does not resolve.

NUMMULAR ECZEMA

Clinical features
Symmetrically distributed areas of dermatitis 1 to 10 cm in diameter are seen primarily on the extremities in this condition (Fig. 4-21). The Latin word *nummulus*, meaning little coin, is used to describe the shape

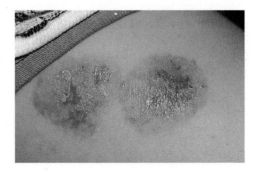

Fig. 4-21
Two oozing coin-shaped areas of dermatitis in nummular eczema.

of the lesions. Two forms occur in children: the wet form, with oozing and crusting (Fig. 4-21), and the dry form, with erythema and scaling. Both forms are persistent, lasting for months if untreated. Most patients volunteer that the lesions are pruritic, and they frequently are scratching the affected skin. Occasionally, a patient will deny touching the lesions.

Differential diagnosis
Nummular eczema is important because it frequently mimics two common pediatric conditions: impetigo and tinea corporis. The wet form is frequently confused with impetigo, and multiple courses of antibiotics are given before the diagnosis is suspected. Biopsy of the lesion readily distinguishes it from impetigo. The dry form can be distinguished from tinea corporis by a KOH examination of skin scrapings or a fungal culture. Some nummular lesions occur in otherwise typical atopic dermatitis or contact dermatitis. Presence of lichenification confirms rubbing and scratching of the lesions when the patient's history suggests absence of trauma to the lesions.

Treatment
The treatment is that which is outlined for atopic dermatitis, although moderate-potency topical steroids are required. Lesions are difficult to resolve, and treatment programs require considerable effort before improvement is seen.

Patient education
Patients should be informed of the chronicity of nummular eczema and its tendency to recur. They should be told the cause is unknown.

Follow-up visits
The child should be seen initially in 2 weeks to evaluate the response to therapy.

KERATOSIS PILARIS, LICHEN SPINULOSUS, FOLLICULAR MUCINOSIS

Clinical features
In keratosis pilaris, prominent follicular plugs are noted over the extensor aspects of the extremities, the buttocks, and the facial cheeks (Figs. 4-22 and 4-23). Individual lesions represent plugs of stratum corneum in individual follicular openings. Dermatitis may surround the plugs. The affected skin surface feels rough and dry. Keratosis pilaris is worsened by drying of skin and is frequently associated with dry skin, ichthyosis vulgaris, and atopic dermatitis. However, some children may present with extensive keratosis

Fig. 4-22
Dry pinpoint red and white discrete papules on the extensor surface of the arm and keratosis pilaris.

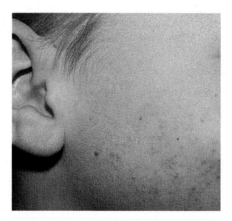

Fig. 4-23
Erythematous papules on the face of a child with keratosis pilaris.

pilaris with no evidence of the other conditions. In these children keratosis pilaris is extensive and often involves the forearms, the lower legs, and much of the face. Keratosis pilaris lesions often improve in a humid climate and become more extensive in a drier climate.

Lichen spinulosus represents grouping of hair follicules with prominent follicular plugs (Fig. 4-24). The lesions are usually hypopigmented and demonstrate fine scale on the intrafollicular skin.

Follicular mucinosis, also called alopecia mucinosis, presents with lesions that appear to be lichen spinulosus but have absent hairs (Fig 4-25). The intrafollicular skin demonstrates scale and may be indurated, giving the appearance of hairless plaques with follicular prominence.

Differential diagnosis

Keratosis pilaris may be confused with microcomedones of acne, molluscum contagiosum, warts, milia, psoriasis, or occasionally folliculitis. Since it is not seen at birth, it should be easily distinguished from neonatal acne and erythema toxicum. Lichen spinulosus may resemble lesions of keratosis pilaris, which group together in one area or several areas. Follicular mucinosis lesions are more indurated and have a more plaquelike appearance.

Pathogenesis

The pathogenesis is unknown. Some authorities regard keratosis pilaris as a disorder of keratinization. They believe that the keratinous plug is produced through abnormal keratinization of the follicular channel. Others believe it is a response to drying of the skin surface, which results in a dry plug of scale lodged in follicular openings. It is more severe in cold, dry climates. Skin biopsy will separate these conditions, as follicular mucinosis will demonstrate mucin in sebaceous glands and the outer root sheaths of affected hair follicles. Follicular mucinosis is occasionally associated with lymphoma in adults, but rarely is it associated with malignancy in children.[34]

Treatment

In the very mild forms of keratosis pilaris, the use of lubricants applied to wet skin may be sufficient to improve the condition, as total resolution is often not possible. In more extensive keratosis pilaris, topical keratolytics may be required, frequently in combination with lubricants. Lactic acid 12% cream (Lac-Hydrin), a urea cream, or a cream with both lactic acid and urea (Eucerin Plus Creme) applied several times a day is frequently beneficial. All treatment strategies require many weeks of therapy to see improvement. Therapy must be continued after

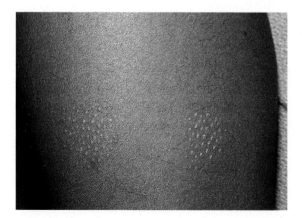

Fig. 4-24
Two areas of lichen spinulosus associated with prominent white follicular plugs.

Fig. 4-25
Hypopigmented plaque of follicular mucinosis with associated follicular plugging and absence of hairs.

improvement is seen. Topical tretinoin (Retin-A) is also effective but may cause significant irritation to the skin, particularly if the child has ichthyosis or associated atopic dermatitis. Often when the child moves to a more humid climate, the condition spontaneously improves.

Lichen spinulosus may require low-potency topical steroids in addition to lubrication for improvement. The plaques of follicular mucinosis require more potent topical steroids and lubrication. Both conditions are difficult to resolve completely.

Patient education

The patient should be informed of the nature of this disease and its likelihood of becoming chronic if untreated and even if treated. They should also be advised of the slow response to therapy and the necessity of long-term treatment and the usual eventual improvement or resolution of these conditions.

Follow-up visits

A follow-up visit in 4 to 8 weeks, to determine response to therapy, is usually indicated. Thereafter, follow-up during routine evaluations is sufficient.

References

1. *Prevalence of dermatologic disease among persons age 1-74: United States,* Washington, DC, 1977, USDHEW Advance Data.
2. Cetta F, Lambert GH, Ros SP: Newborn chemical exposure from over-the-counter skin care products, *Clin Pediatr* 30:286, 1991.
3. Williams HC, Burney PGJ, Hay RJ, et al: The U.K. working party's diagnostic criteria for atopic dermatitis. I. Derivation of a minimum set of discriminators for atopic dermatitis, *Br J Dermatol* 131:383, 1994.
4. Williams HC, Burney PGJ, Strachan D, et al: The U.K. working party's diagnostic criteria for atopic dermatitis. II. Observer variation of clinical diagnosis and signs of atopic dermatitis, *Br J Dermatol* 131:397, 1994.
5. Williams HC, Burney PGJ, Hay RJ, et al: The U.K. working party's diagnostic criteria for atopic dermatitis.

III. Independent hospital validation, *Br J Dermatol* 131:406, 1994.
6. Kay J, Gawkrodger DJ, Marek MD, Jaron AJ: The prevalence of childhood atopic eczema in a general population, *J Am Acad Dermatol* 30:35, 1994.
7. Vickers CFH: The natural history of atopic eczema, *Acta Derm Venereol Suppl (Stockh)* 92:ll3, 1980.
8. Monti JM, Vignale R, Monti D: Sleep and nighttime pruritus in children with atopic dermatitis, *Sleep* 12:309, 1989.
9. Loden M, Olsson H, Axell T, Linde YW: Friction, capacitance and transepidermal water loss (TEWL) in dry atopic and normal skin, *Br J Dermatol* 126:137, 1992.
10. Weston WL: The use and abuse of topical steroids, *Contemp Pediatr* 5:57, 1988
11. Yohn J, Weston WL: Topical glucocorticosteroids, *Curr Probl Dermatol* 2:31, 1990.
12. Burks AW, Mallory SB, Williams LW, Shirrell MA: Atopic dermatitis: clinical relevance of food hypersensitivity reactions, *J Pediatr* 113:447, 1988.
13. Casimir GJA, Duchateau J, Gossart B et al: Atopic dermatitis: role of food and house dust mite allergens, *Pediatrics* 92:251, 1993.
14. Fergusson DM, Horwood J, Shannon FT: Early solid feeding and recurrent childhood eczema: a 10-year longitudinal study, *Pediatrics* 86:541, 1990.
15. Sampson HA, McCaskill CC: Food hypersensitivity and atopic dermatitis: evaluation of 113 patients, *J Pediatr* 107:669, 1985.
16. Sampson HA, Scanlon SM: Natural history of food hypersensitivity in children with atopic dermatitis, *J Pediatr* 115:23, 1989.
17. Sampson HA: The immunopathogenic role of food hypersensitivity in atopic dermatitis, *Acta Derm Venereol (Stockh)* 176:34, 1992.
18. Sigurs N, Hattevig G, Kjellman B: Maternal avoidance of eggs, cow's milk, and fish during lactation: effect on allergic manifestations, skin-prick tests, and specific IgE antibodies in children at age 4 years, *Pediatrics* 89:735, 1992.
19. DeProst YD: Management of severe atopic dermatitis, *Acta Derm Venereol (Stockh)* 176:117, 1992.
20. Hanifin JM, Schneider LC, Leung DYM, et al: Recombinant interferon gamma therapy for atopic dermatitis, *J Am Acad Dermatol* 28:189, 1993.

21. Sheehan MP, Atherton DJ: A controlled trial of traditional Chinese medicinal plants in widespread non-exudative atopic eczema, *Br J Dermatol* 126:179, 1992.

22. Sheehan MP, Atherton DJ, Norris P, Hawk J: Oral psoralen photochemotherapy in severe childhood atopic eczema: an update, *Br J Dermatol* 129:431, 1993.

23. Jordan WE, Lawson KD, Berg RW: Diaper dermatitis: frequency and severity among a general infant population, *Pediatr Dermatol* 3:198, 1986.

24. Weston WL, Lane AT, Weston JA: Diaper dermatitis: current concepts, *Pediatrics* 66:532, 1980.

25. Zimmerer RE, Lawson KD, Calvert CJ: The effects of wearing diapers on skin. *Pediatr Dermatol* 3:95, 1986.

26. Berg RW, Buckingham KW, Stewart RL: Etiologic factors in diaper dermatitis: the role of urine, *Pediatr Dermatol* 3:102, 1986.

27. Buckingham KW, Berg RW: Etiologic factors in diaper dermatitis: the role of feces, *Pediatr Dermatol* 3:107, 1986.

28. Rehder PA, Eliezer ET, Lane AT: Perianal cellulitis. Cutaneous group A streptococcal disease, *Arch Dermatol* 124:702, 1988.

29. Jones SK, English JSC, Forsyth A, Mackie RM: Juvenile plantar dermatosis—an 8-year follow-up of 102 patients, *Clin Exp Dermatol* 12:5, 1987.

30. Vernon HJ, Olsen EA: A controlled trial of clobetasol propionate ointment 0.05% in the treatment of experimentally induced rhus dermatitis, *J Am Acad Dermatol* 23:829, 1990.

31. Weston JA, Hawkins K, Weston WL: Foot dermatitis in children, *Pediatrics* 72:824, 1983.

32. Weston WL, Weston JA, Kinoshita J, et al: Prevalence of positive epicutaneous tests among infants, children and adolescents, *Pediatrics* 78:1070, 1986.

33. Grevelink SA, Murrel DF, Olsen EA: Effectiveness of various barrier preparations in preventing and/or ameliorating experimentally produced Toxicodendron dermatitis, *J Am Acad Dermatol* 27:182, 1992.

34. Gibson LE, Muller SA, Peters MS: Follicular mucinosis of childhood and adolescence, *Pediatr Dermatol* 5:231, 1988.

5

Bacterial Infections (Pyodermas) and Spirochetal Infections of the Skin

Bacteria constantly colonize the skin surface and occasionally invade the epidermal barrier to replicate within the skin. The majority of skin microorganisms in healthy children are nonpathogenic. The two major pathogens found on children's skin are *Staphylococcus aureus* and *Streptococcus pyogenes*.[1,2] The former is found in 5% of children and the latter in 1%. However, during epidemics and in endemic areas, either of these organisms may be recovered from the skin of 50% to 80% of children. In warm, humid climates, and with poor skin hygiene, pyodermas are common in childhood.[1,3] Bacterial toxin–induced syndromes such as scarlet fever, scalded skin syndrome, and toxic shock syndrome (TSS) are uncommon in childhood and result from skin injury by circulating toxins rather than direct bacterial invasion of skin.

IMPETIGO AND ECTHYMA

Clinical features

Erosions covered by moist, honey-colored crusts are suggestive of impetigo (Figs. 5-1 and 5-2).[1-5] Impetigo begins as small (1 to 2 mm) vesicles with a fragile roof that is quickly lost. Multiple lesions are often present, and exposed areas such as the face, nares, and extremities are the most common sites of involvement. The term *bullous impetigo* has been used to describe lesions with a central moist crust and an outer zone of blister formation[2] (Fig. 5-3). The blister is translucent, with a flaccid roof that is easily shed[2] (Fig. 5-4), such that bullous impetigo may be seen as shallow erosions with an outer rim of desquamation.[2] Whether small blisters or large, *impetigo* is the preferred term. Impetigo has a high attack rate and its spread is enhanced by crowding and poor socioeconomic conditions.[1,4] In contrast, ecthyma is characterized by a firm, dry, dark crust with surrounding erythema and induration[2] (Fig. 5-5). Direct pressure on the crust results in the extrusion of purulent material from beneath the crust.

Both ecthyma and impetigo may occur simultaneously in the same patient. The clinical features are so characteristic that bacterial culture is not routinely performed.

Differential diagnosis

Subacute dermatitis, such as nummular dermatitis, herpes simplex infections, and a kerion resulting from

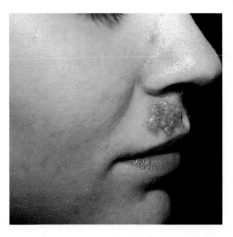

Fig. 5-1
Impetigo. Honey-colored, moist crust just above the upper lip.

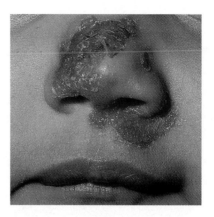

Fig. 5-2
Impetigo. Spread of infection to top of nose from beneath the nose in an infant with impetigo.

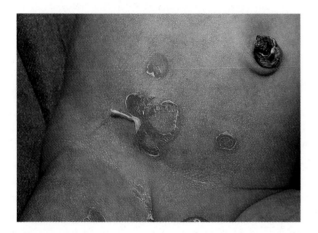

Fig. 5-3
Bullous impetigo. Flaccid blister with thin border of desquamation on the abdomen of an infant.

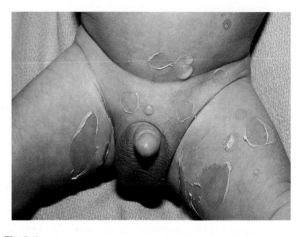

Fig 5-4
Bullous impetigo in a newborn. Multiple areas of flaccid blisters and shallow erosions on a red base.

dermatophyte infections, may have moist crusts and mimic impetigo. Nummular dermatitis has dozens of symmetrically distributed lesions as opposed to impetigo, which has a few nonsymmetric lesions. Herpes simplex is usually a distinct group of lesions that even when crusted demonstrate a group of individual papules or vesicles beneath. Viral culture, fluorescent antibody testing of smears, or examination of Tzanck smear may be required to differentiate. A potassium hydroxide (KOH) examination or fungal culture may be required to distinguish a kerion from impetigo. Bullous impetigo must be differentiated from second-degree burns and from the uncommon immunobullous diseases seen in childhood, such as linear immunoglobulin A (IgA) dermatosis, bullous pemphigoid, and bullous forms of erythema multiforme. A crusted second-degree burn, cutaneous diphtheria, or cutaneous anthrax may be confused with a solitary lesion of ecthyma. Bacterial culture of the purulent material beneath the crust may be required.

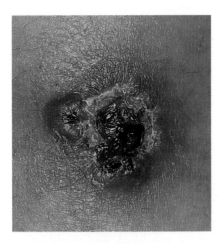

Fig. 5-5
Dry crust with indurated border in a child with ecthyma.

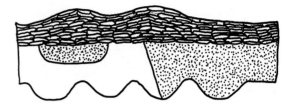

Fig. 5-6
Difference between impetigo and ecthyma. Superficial neutrophilic collection in middermis (*shaded area on left*) in impetigo in contrast to full-thickness involvement (*shaded area on right*) in ecthyma.

Pathogenesis

Invasion of the epidermis by pathogenic *S. aureus* or group A streptococci occurs in impetigo and ecthyma.[1,4] The depth of invasion in impetigo is superficial (into the upper epidermis), whereas the entire epidermis is involved in ecthyma (Fig. 5-6).[2] Microscopic breaks in the epidermal barrier, such as the trauma of scratching dermatitic skin, predispose to impetigo, while staphylococci or streptococci penetrate the lower epidermis in ecthyma after injury to the mid-epidermis and upper epidermis. Often colonization of the skin surface with the two major pathogens occurs several days to a month before the appearance of clinical lesions.[1] It is now recognized that in many areas of North America penicillinase-producing staphylococci are more likely to be responsible for impetigo than streptococci and account for 70% to 80% of childhood impetigo.[2,4-6] For impetigo secondary to an underlying skin disease, such as dermatitis, scabies, psoriasis, or varicella, staphylococci are virtually always responsible.[2,5] Poststreptococcal glomerulonephritis may follow such infections of the skin if nephritogenic strains of streptococci are involved.[6]

Treatment

Systemic antibiotics to eradicate staphylococci and streptococci are the treatment of choice.[2,5] To treat both pathogens, dicloxacillin, 15 to 50 mg/kg/day, cephalexin, 40 mg/kg/day, or cloxacillin, 50 to 100 mg/kg/day orally for a total of 10 days, may be used. Erythromycin, 40 mg/kg/day orally for 10 days, is an alternative, but in many areas of North America, strains of staphylococci resistant to erythromycin have been encountered.[2,5,6] If streptococci are cultured, penicillin V, 125 to 250 mg four times daily for 10 days, may be used. Most topical antibiotics may result in clinical improvement but may prolong the carriage state of the pathogen on the skin.[1,2,5] Topical mupirocin ointment, although as efficacious as oral erythromycin,[2] should be reserved for cutaneous staphylococcal infections such as encountered in immunosuppressed children.[7] Removal of crusts and scrubbing the impetigo skin lesions with antibacterial soaps has not been shown to be effective.[2] Hand washing with a surgical soap and simple measures of good hygiene may reduce the likelihood of spread.

The risk of nephritogenic strains of streptococci varies considerably throughout North America, but an active program in which both patients and contacts are treated will significantly reduce the incidence of acute glomerulonephritis in endemic areas.[2,6]

Patient education

Good hand-washing techniques for the care givers and the infected child, and good general personal hygiene, are useful in preventing further infection of contacts and reducing the chances for future infections. The child should begin treatment with antibiotic therapy before returning to school or day care. The highly contagious nature of these infections should be strongly emphasized, and contacts should be examined if feasible.

Follow-up visits

A visit 10 days to 2 weeks after therapy has begun is useful to determine the therapeutic response and possible spread of the organism to contacts. In recurrent or persistent infections, bacterial culture should be performed to determine if an unusual or antibiotic-resistant organism is present.

CELLULITIS

Clinical features

Tender, warm, erythematous plaques with ill-defined borders are seen in cellulitis.[4,8-11] Occasionally, linear red macules proximal to the large plaque are seen. Regional lymphadenopathy and fever are common findings. A preceding puncture wound or other penetrating trauma to the skin is often noted (Figs. 5-7 and 5-8). Cellulitis of the fingertips in infants is called blistering dactylitis (Fig. 5-9), and several fingers may be involved.[12]

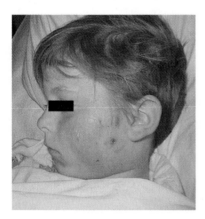

Fig. 5-7
Puncture wound with surrounding cellulitis of the cheek.

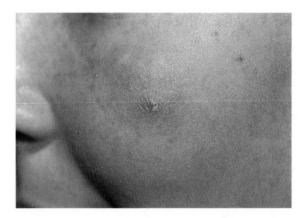

Fig. 5-8
Cellulitis following self-manipulation of acne pustule.

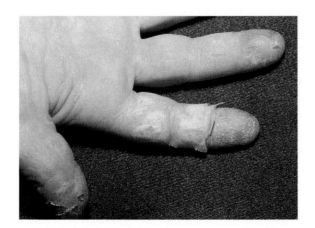

Fig. 5-9
Blistering distal dactylitis.

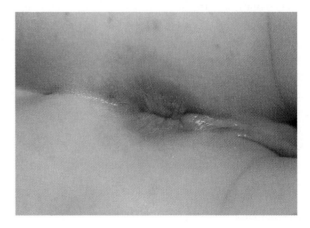

Fig. 5-10
Streptococcal perianal cellulitis. Acutely tender red perianal skin.

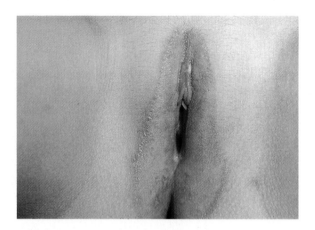

Fig. 5-11
Streptococcal perianal and perivaginal cellulitis.

Perianal cellulitis in infants is increasingly recognized in North America and is characterized by tender perirectal erythema and pain on defecation[13] (Fig. 5-10). Lesions may extend beyond perianal skin and involve perivaginal skin (Fig. 5-11). Infants and toddlers with perianal streptocoocal cellulitis often present with constipation. Perianal cellulitis in infants is virtually always due to streptococci.

Cellulitis over large joints such as the hip, shoulder, or knee may be observed in infants and toddlers.[8-10] Extension into the joint cavity and bone is seen with cellulitis overlying a joint, particularly in infants. A bluish hue within the lesion in infants is particularly seen with *Haemophilus influenzae* cellulitis but is also observed in cellulitis due to other bacteria. Cellulitis of the cheeks or over joints in children aged 3 months to 3 years is predominantly due to *H. influenzae* infection, whereas in older children it may result from streptococci or staphylococci.[6,8-11] Streptococcal cellulitis spreads rapidly, within hours, in contrast to staphylococcal cellulitis.[13] Septicemia *may* follow cellulitis in untreated patients.[6,8-11] Periorbital cellulitis is of great concern because of spread to the brain.[8,10-11]

Differential diagnosis
Erythematous swellings overlying an unrecognized bony fracture may mimic cellulitis, although they may not feel warm. Similarly, pressure erythema, giant urticaria, and contact dermatitis in the early stages may be difficult to distinguish from cellulitis, but they are not tender. The redness and swelling over a septic joint may also mimic cellulitis. Acute cold injury to the fat of the cheeks of infants (popsicle panniculitis) may mimic facial cellulitis. Herpetic whitlow may mimic blistering distal dactylitis and diaper dermatitis, or painful rectal fissures may mimic perianal cellulitis.

Pathogenesis
Invasion of bacteria into the deep dermis and subcutaneous fat, with subsequent spread via the lymphatics, is responsible for the clinical features of cellulitis. Pathogenic streptococci account for most cases of cellulitis; *H. influenzae* and *S. aureus* may also be responsible.[8-11] Blood cultures are most likely to reveal the responsible bacteria.[14] Aspiration of the center or advancing edge of the cellulitis is rarely positive.[14]

Treatment
In an acutely ill child or a child with periorbital cellulitis, hospitalization should be considered. Prompt administration of antibiotics is essential. If a streptococcal infection is suspected, systemic penicillin is given, either as benzathine penicillin, 600,000 to 1,200,000 U intramuscularly, or oral penicillin V, 30 to 60 mg/kg/day for 10 days. In an acutely ill febrile infant or child, hospitalization and intravenous penicillin, up to 2 million U/day, is recommended. If staphylococcal cellulitis is suspected, oral dicloxacillin, 50 to 100 mg/kg/day, is recommended. With *blue* cellulitis suggestive of *H. influenzae*, a blood culture should be obtained before starting antibiotics. Ampicillin, 100 to 200 mg/kg/day, is given intravenously in combination with chloramphenicol, 50 to 85 mg/kg/day. If ampicillin- or chloramphenicol-resistant strains of *H. influenzae* are found in your locale, use of third-generation cephalosporins, such as ceftriaxone, 50 mg/kg intramuscularly every 12 hours, or cefotaxime or cefuroxime, is recommended.

Patient education
The serious and potentially life-threatening nature of cellulitis should be explained. A thorough under-

standing of the portal of entry of bacteria is required. Instructions on the prompt cleansing of wounds should be given.

Follow-up visits

If it is decided not to admit the child to a hospital, a visit within 24 hours is mandatory to assess the response to therapy and observe for signs of toxicity. Daily visits may be required until the child is recovering.

NECROTIZING FASCIITIS (STREPTO-COCCAL GANGRENE)

Clinical features

Diabetic children with ketoacidosis and immunosuppressed children are susceptible to streptococcal gangrene.[15,16] This condition is rare, but public awareness is increasing in North America. Prompt recognition of necrotizing fasciitis may be lifesaving. The lesion begins as cellulitis, with tender erythematous plaques, usually on the leg. Within 2 hours bullae appear on the erythematous surface, accompanied by severe pain. A purulent center develops, followed by the appearance of a black eschar and the subsidence of the acute pain (Fig. 5-12). The decrease in pain correlates well with destruction of the cutaneous nerves as they course through the fascia and subcutaneous tissue. Over the next 2 days frank gangrene may be observed. Usually a clinical diagnosis is sufficient, but when difficulty distinguishing between cellulitis and necrotizing fasciitis occurs, magnetic resonance imaging may be helpful.[17] In newborns the most common location is on the abdominal wall, where the first sign is redness and swelling of the periumbilical skin and the diagnosis of omphalitis is considered. Culture of the deep tissues or blood yields group A streptococci.[15,18]

Pathogenesis

Invasion by group A streptococci through the dermis and subcutaneous fat into the deep fascial compartments occurs because of the faulty host defenses of the immunosuppressed or diabetic patient.[15,16,18] Often

trauma to the skin precedes the appearance of these lesions. Rapid spread and destruction of tissue occur.[18] Compromise of blood flow occurs in deep fascial or muscular compartments, and infarction of large areas of skin and subcutaneous tissue occurs.[15,16]

Differential diagnosis

Cellulitis may mimic necrotizing fasciitis early in the disease, but the rapid evolution of necrotizing fasciitis to form necrotic areas within hours after the onset helps distinguish the two. With the development of gangrene, arterial embolism or thrombosis should be considered. Metastatic calcification with occlusion of major skin vessels may also mimic necrotizing fasciitis, but its slow onset and lack of acute pain are important differentiating features.

Treatment

Prompt surgical debridement down to the fascia is essential and is the most important aspect of therapy.[15,16] Penicillin is the treatment of choice; from 4 to 10 million U/day is given intravenously.[15,18] Correction of the metabolic abnormalities of diabetic ketoacidosis is important. Even with prompt surgical intervention, mortality is high.[15,18]

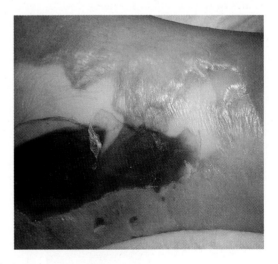

Fig. 5-12
Central black painless necrosis; painful yellow purulent lake and surrounding erythema in necrotizing fasciitis in the leg of a diabetic adolescent.

Patient education

It should be emphasized that good diabetic control and good personal hygiene are essential to prevent such episodes. Prompt cleansing of cuts or skin abrasions and topical antibiotics are suggested, and the patient should be strongly advised to seek prompt medical attention when the early signs of infection appear.

Follow-up visits

After hospitalization a follow-up visit a week later is most helpful to evaluate the patient's progress. Weekly visits may be required to assess healing of the devitalized skin and deeper tissues.

SCARLET FEVER

Clinical features

Scarlet fever occurs most often in children between 2 and 10 years of age. The portal of entry of the streptococci may be either the pharynx or a skin wound. The exanthem appears 24 to 48 hours after infection and consists of erythematous macules and papules, beginning on the neck and spreading downward over the trunk to the extremities[6,15] (Fig. 5-13). In severe

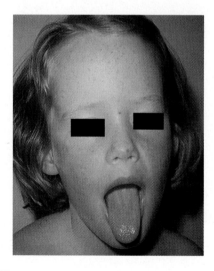

Fig. 5-13
Bright red erythema and strawberry tongue in scarlet fever.

cases the exanthem may be petechial, and a positive tourniquet test is common. Petechiae in a linear pattern are seen along the major skin folds in the axillae and antecubital fossa (Pastia's sign). The palms and soles in scarlet fever are characteristically uninvolved, and a facial flush with circumoral pallor is common. Tongue involvement (a thick white coat with hypertrophied red papillae) is helpful in the differential diagnosis, since "strawberry tongue" is seen with streptococcal but not staphylococcal scarlet fever. Generalized lymphadenopathy is common, with the inguinal lymph nodes particularly enlarged. Desquamation occurs as the eruption fades, progressing in the same manner as it began. In black skin, tiny, slightly erythematous papules resembling gooseflesh are found. Although it is difficult to observe the erythema and the papular nature of the eruption in black children, scarlet fever in these children is identical to that seen in white children.

Recent outbreaks of severe septicemic scarlet fever in North America have been noted.[6,15] Hypotension and a toxic shock–like syndrome are reported. This severe disease is less likely in children than in adults.[6,15,19]

Differential diagnosis

The scarlatiniform eruption is seen in other infectious diseases, such as that appearing in the early stages of viral hepatitis, infectious mononucleosis, mucocutaneous lymph node syndrome, TSS, and rubella. Drug-associated eruptions may also mimic scarlet fever. Drugs that result in scarlatiniform eruptions include the sulfonamides, penicillin, streptomycin, quinine, and atropine. Drug eruptions are more likely to produce mucosal erosions and crusts, which may be a helpful distinguishing sign.

Pathogenesis

Three immunologically distinct scarlet fever–producing toxins have been identified from cultures of *Streptococcus*.[6,15] Toxin release from streptococci is mediated by viral infection of the streptococci. The mechanism of action by the toxin on the skin is felt to depend on receptor-mediated activation of skin cells.

Severe scarlet fever has been associated with the appearance of M type 1 and 3 strains of *Streptococcus* of an increased virulence.[6,15]

Treatment

Penicillin, in the same doses as used for impetigo and streptococcal pharyngitis, is the treatment of choice for scarlet fever.[6,20] Erythromycin is used in penicillin-allergic patients. If staphylococcal scarlet fever is suspected, dicloxacillin, 15 to 50 mg/kg/day orally for 10 days, is recommended. Prompt treatment virtually eliminates the complications of scarlet fever, such as bacteremia, rheumatic fever, pneumonia, and meningitis.

During the later stages of desquamation, bland ointments applied to wet skin will restore the skin surface integrity and reduce cutaneous pain.

Patient education

The association of scarlet fever with rheumatic fever is of great patient concern. It is important to reassure the patient that prompt treatment has virtually eliminated this association. Identification and cultures of patient contacts are essential.

Follow-up visits

Seven to ten days after the first visit, another visit is helpful to observe the response to therapy and to assess further any other sources of streptococcal infection in the household.

FOLLICULITIS, FURUNCULOSIS, AND CUTANEOUS ABSCESSES

Clinical features

The manifestations of infection of the hair follicle vary clinically with the depth of bacterial invasion. Infection at the follicular orifice (superficial folliculitis) appears as tiny pustules, 1 to 2 mm in diameter (Fig. 5-14). Furunculosis (deep folliculitis) appears as a tender erythematous nodule[8,11,21] (Fig. 5-15). Confluence of several adjacent areas of furunculosis produces a tender erythematous tumor that becomes soft and fluctuant after several days. Abscesses are commonly found on the buttocks and trunk but may appear in any location (Fig. 5-16). Other household members may be affected.

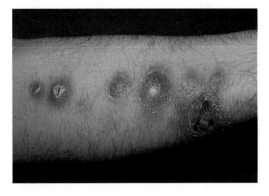

Fig. 5-15
Deep bacterial folliculitis (furunculosis) on arm.

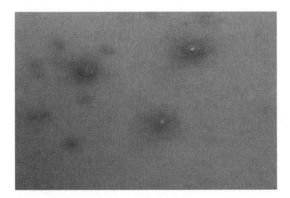

Fig. 5-14
Staphylococcal folliculitis. Multiple pustules on a red base.

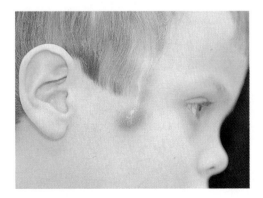

Fig. 5-16
Bacterial abscess. Staphylococcal infection of the cheek of a child.

S. aureus is regularly cultured from furuncles and abscesses, although gram-negative organisms may occasionally be found such as in *Pseudomonas* folliculitis, associated with the use of hot tubs.[22] Superficial folliculitis is often found to contain the normal skin flora. Bacteremia from furunculosis or abscess may occur in an unpredictable fashion, particularly after manipulation of the lesion.[8]

Differential diagnosis

Acne pustules and chemical folliculitis from tars and other compounds contacting the skin may mimic superficial folliculitis. Occasionally, dermatophyte infections due to animal ringworm or *Candida albicans* infections will produce follicular pustules.

Pathogenesis

Invasion of the follicular wall by bacteria is the usual cause of the disease (Fig. 5-17). Obstruction of the follicular orifice is an important factor in the development of the bacterial infection, particularly with staphylococcal folliculitis. Transmission of staphylococci among household members may occur. Occlusion of the skin or prolonged submersion in water contaminated with bacteria also predisposes to folliculitis.[22]

Treatment

Superficial folliculitis may be treated by topical keratolytics, such as the benzoyl peroxide gels, applied

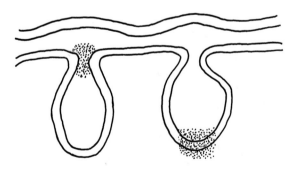

Fig. 5-17
Superficial folliculitis (*left*) with inflammation of the follicular mouth compared with deep folliculitis (*right*) with involvement of the base of the follicle and adjacent deep dermis.

twice daily for 4 to 5 days. Furunculosis and abscesses are best treated by incision and drainage.[8,11] Systemic antistaphylococcal antibiotics, such as dicloxacillin, 15 to 50 mg/kg/day orally, or cephalexin, 40 mg/kg/day for 7 to 10 days, may be required in more severe cases. In chronic recurrent furunculosis, attention to nasal and skin carriers of staphylococci is required. Mupirocin ointment applied to the nares daily and chronic antibiotic treatment with antistaphylococcal drugs or rifampin may be necessary if good household hygiene fails.[8,21]

Patient education

Good personal hygiene is important in preventing follicular skin infections. Thorough hand washing and daily skin cleansing with an antibacterial soap are most useful. It is advisable to instruct all household members in good hand-washing techniques. Avoiding chemicals that have resulted in follicular obstruction is beneficial. In *Pseudomonas* or gram-negative folliculitis resulting from contaminated tubs or pools, proper chlorination or other treatment of the water should be emphasized.[22]

Follow-up visits

Poor personal hygiene is the most likely cause in children with recurrent episodes of furunculosis. Reemphasizing good hygiene for the entire household at the follow-up visit is most important.[21] Evaluation for diabetes mellitus and immunodeficiency is not warranted without recurrent or systemic infection of other organ systems such as the lungs (e. g., pneumonia), central nervous system (CNS) (e.g., encephalitis), or bone.

STAPHYLOCOCCAL SCALDED SKIN SYNDROME

Clinical features

A spectrum of clinical presentations of the staphylococcal scalded skin syndrome (SSSS) is now recognized, ranging from purely localized forms (bullous impetigo) to generalized involvement. Following an

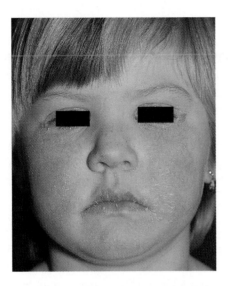

Fig. 5-18
Early SSSS in a toddler with erythema of cheeks.

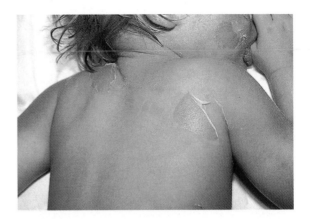

Fig. 5-20
SSSS in a toddler. Erosion with skin separated during examination by pushing on the skin surface.

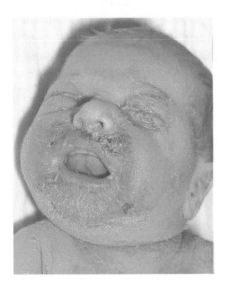

Fig. 5-19
SSSS with periorbital and perioral crusting.

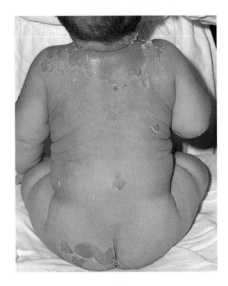

Fig. 5-21
SSSS in an infant. Erythema and shallow erosions with desquamation of the back.

upper respiratory tract infection, a faint erythematous eruption begins on the central face (Fig. 5-18), neck, axillae, and groin.[4,23] The skin rapidly becomes acutely tender, with crusting around the mouth, eyes, and neck (Fig. 5-19). Mild rubbing of the skin results in epidermal separation, leaving a shiny, moist, red surface[23] (Figs. 5-20 and 5-21). In infants and preschool children the lesions are usually limited to the upper body, but in the newborn the entire cutaneous surface may be involved (Ritter's disease)[23] (Fig. 5-22). SSSS is uncommon over 5 years of age.

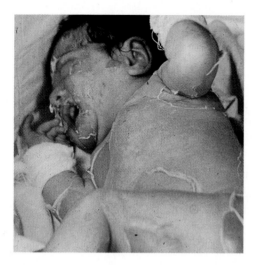

Fig. 5-22
Diffuse erythema and extensive peeling in a newborn with Ritter's disease.

Differential diagnosis

Toxic epidermal necrolysis, which is often drug induced, may be differentiated from SSSS by skin biopsy and by a preceding history of urticarial or target lesions occurring 2 to 3 days before the appearance of bullae.[23] Pathologic examination of tissue from a patient with toxic epidermal necrolysis shows full epidermal necrosis, with a prominent perivascular dermal infiltrate of inflammatory cells. SSSS shows no epidermal necrosis or inflammatory cells on microscopic examination. In the newborn, diffuse cutaneous mastocytosis may mimic Ritter's disease.[24] Occasionally SSSS may resemble exfoliative erythroderma, sunburn, TSS, or streptococcal scarlet fever.

Pathogenesis

S. aureus of phage group II[23,25] elaborates a toxin (*Staphylococcus* exfoliatin A), a serine protease that is carried via the circulation to the skin, where it acts on the cell surface of the epidermal granular cells.[23,25,26] Injury to these cells results in intraepidermal separation of the cells within the granular layer and subsequent shedding of the entire granular layer and stratum corneum when a minor trauma occurs.

Treatment

Oral dicloxacillin, 15 to 50 mg/kg/day, is the treatment of choice. Newborns require intravenous antistaphylococcal antibiotics.[23] The skin should be handled minimally, especially during the first 24 hours. Newborns may require burn therapy protocols with careful attention to fluid and electrolyte losses and prevention of secondary infection of affected skin.[23] During the desquamation stage, bland ointments used twice a day may be helpful in restoring the skin surface and reducing cutaneous pain.

Patient education

It is important to emphasize to the patients that such lesions are not like a burn and that they heal without scarring. In children with normal host defenses, neutralizing antitoxins to the staphylococcal exfoliatin are rapidly formed, and the child recovers promptly. It should also be stressed that only certain staphylococci are capable of producing this condition and that household carriers should be investigated.[23] Asymptomatic carriers may transmit the organism.[27] Nursery outbreaks require prompt investigation and culturing of all those entering the nursery.

Follow-up visits

Routine follow-up care in regular pediatric visits is recommended.

TOXIC SHOCK SYNDROME

Clinical features

A typical presentation of TSS would involve a menstruating adolescent female who presents with a high fever, a scarlatiniform rash, and hypotension, with systolic blood pressure less than 90 mm Hg or orthostatic syncope.[23,28] Prominent desquamation of the palms and soles follows the acute onset of the eruption by 1 to 2 weeks. These four features are the major diagnostic criteria for diagnosis of TSS (see Box 5-1).[4,23,28] Vomiting and diarrhea frequently precede the hypotensive state, and laboratory signs of liver, kidney, or muscle injury may be present.

Box 5-1 Case definition of toxic shock syndrome

Fever (temperature greater than 39.9° C)

Rash (diffuse macular erythroderma)

Desquamation 1 to 2 weeks after the onset of illness, particularly of the palms and soles

Hypotension (systolic blood pressure less than 90 mm Hg for adults or below the fifth percentile for children, or orthostatic syncope)

Involvement of three or more of the following organ systems

Gastrointestinal (vomiting or diarrhea at onset of illness)

Muscular (severe myalgia or creatine phosphokinase level greater than two times normal)

Mucous membrane (hyperemia)

Hepatic (total bilirubin, SGOT, SGPT two times normal)

Hematologic (platelets less than100,000/mm³)

Renal (BUN or creatinine greater than two times normal)

Central nervous system (disorientation or alterations in consciousness without focal neurologic signs when fever and hypotension are absent)

Negative results:

Blood, throat, and cerebrospinal fluid cultures

Serologic tests for Rocky Mountain spotted fever, leptospirosis, or measles

---

BUN, Blood urea nitrogen; *SGOT*, serum glutamate oxaloacetate transaminase; *SGPT*, serum glutamate pyruvate transaminase.

Diffuse redness of the conjunctival, oral, and vaginal mucosa may be present.[23,28] Swelling of the hands and feet may be prominent. Severe myalgias or arthralgias and disorientation, meningismus, seizure, or coma may appear.[23,28] Although the majority of cases have been described in adolescent females, TSS was first noted in infants and children of either sex. In nonmenstrual TSS, pharyngitis or conjunctivitis lasting more than 5 days is observed, and the onset of fever and scarlatiniform rash is early in the course of disease.[23,28] Nonmenstrual TSS has less frequent CNS manifestations, more frequent musculoskeletal involvement, and less anemia than that reported for menstrual TSS.[23,28] The circulatory collapse may be mild or severe, and a fatality rate of 10% has been reported.[28]

Differential diagnosis

Rocky Mountain spotted fever, meningococcemia, and leptospirosis may each present with high fever, dizziness, and a rash. In each, the eruption is acral and purpuric and not scarlet fever–like. Blood cultures and specific serologic tests will help to distinguish these conditions. The SSSS has considerable overlapping cutaneous features with TSS. The presence of skin tenderness and a positive Nikolsky sign favor scalded skin syndrome. Streptococcal TSS may mimic SSSS and can be distinguished by pharyngeal and blood cultures.[23] Kawasaki disease is more likely to occur in patients under age 5, lacks hypotension, and has prominent mucous membrane involvement. The fever in Kawasaki disease lasts for a week or more rather than the 2 or 3 days in TSS. The scarlatiniform skin eruption and desquamation may be the same in both TSS and Kawasaki syndrome.

Pathogenesis

S. aureus infection of the vagina or other tissues, such as the upper respiratory tract and sinuses, initiates the disease.[23,28,29] Prolonged tampon use with positive cultures obtained from tampons in adolescent females is very frequent.[23,28] Blood cultures positive for *S. aureus* may be obtained. Most authorities consider the staphylococcal toxin designated TSS-1 or enterotoxin C as responsible for the skin eruption and the systemic symptoms.[23,28-31] Both of these distinct exotoxins have been implicated, but the precise mechanism of skin injury is unknown.[31]

Treatment

Prompt replacement of fluids to correct the hypotension is recommended, as are other general supportive measures for shock.[23] Treatment with an antistaphylococcal antibiotic, usually given intravenously, is recommended. Bland lubricants may be used on the desquamating skin.

Patient education

It is important to emphasize the conditions that might favor the growth of the pathogenic organism. In adolescent females, discontinuing the use of tampons is advisable. It is unknown whether other antibacterial measures to reduce skin or mucous membrane colonization of staphylococci are useful.

Follow-up visits

The hypotension and acute illness at the onset usually result in hospitalization. Daily examination with documentation of the sequence of events is often necessary to confirm the diagnosis. After discharge, a 1-week follow-up is advisable, as is a visit during the next anticipated menses for follow-up bacterial cultures.

CAT-SCRATCH DISEASE

Clinical features

A primary inoculation papule on skin or mucous membrane 3 to 10 days after the scratch of a cat is found in 58% of patients[32] (Fig. 5-23).

Inoculation of the ocular conjunctivae occurs in 5% of children, which will produce conjunctival granuloma. Persistent tender regional lymphadenitis of the lymph nodes draining the site of the cat scratch is observed in virtually all patients.[32] The lymph nodes become swollen 14 to 50 days after the scratch and remain enlarged for about 3 months, but may be enlarged for up to a year later. About one third of patients will experience a few days of fever, but occasionally fever persists for several weeks. Fatigue, headache, anorexia, vomiting, splenomegaly, sore throat, morbilliform exanthem, purulent conjunctivitis, and parotid swelling are uncommon findings in children with cat-scratch disease.[32] Quite rare are Parinaud's syndrome, encephalitis, and erythema nodosum.

Differential diagnosis

Bacterial lymphadenitis due to *S. aureus*, *S. pyogenes*, atypical mycobacteria, *Francisella tularensis*, or *Brucella* species may mimic cat-scratch disease. Biopsy of a papule or lymph node with Warthin-Starry silver impregnation stain will reveal the cat-scratch bacillus within areas of necrosis or granulomas. Molecular diagnosis by amplifying deoxyribonucleic acid (DNA) obtained from a papule or lymph node by the use of the polymerase chain reaction (PCR) is available in a few centers.[33,34] Other causes of persistent lymphadenopathy in children include lymphomas, cytomegalovirus (CMV), Epstein-Barr virus (EBV), human immunodeficiency virus (HIV), *Toxoplasma*, and deep fungus infection. Kerion caused by dermatophyte infection will produce local lymphadenopathy, but the kerion is much larger than an inoculation papule of cat-scratch disease.

Pathogenesis

The domestic cat is the primary reservoir of cat-scratch disease. A cat scratch (80% of children), bite, or other contact may inoculate the bacteria into the skin.[32] In 4% of cases the contact is a dog. The gram-negative pleomorphic bacillus responsible for cat-

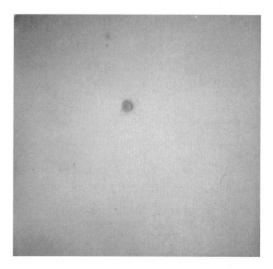

Fig. 5-23
Solitary papule at the site of a cat scratch in cat-scratch disease.

scratch disease is *Rochalimaea henseleae*, and may be detected in the dermis of inoculation papules or the microabscesses of enlarged lymph nodes if obtained within 1 month of the onset of symptoms.[33-35] The host response may obscure the bacillus in long-standing disease. Skin test antigen for cat-scratch disease also contains the organism.[35] This organism is also believed to be responsible for bacillary angiomatosis.[34]

Treatment
In most patients spontaneous resolution of the disease occurs in 2 to 4 months.[32] Antibacterial therapy with ciprofloxacin, gentamicin, rifampin, or trimethoprim-sulfamethoxazole has been reported to be effective.[36] Needle aspiration of a tender lymph node abscess is preferable to incision and drainage. Surgical excision of the lymph node is often done, especially when the diagnosis is in doubt.[32]

Patient education
Disposal of the healthy cat suspected of being the vector is not recommended.[32] About 5% of household contacts may develop cat-scratch disease, usually within 3 weeks of the first case. There is no evidence that the infection can be transmitted from human to human.[32-36]

Follow-up visits
Follow-up 1 week after the first visit is useful to ascertain the growth rate of enlarged nodes or to discuss biopsy results. Further visits are dictated by the child's recovery.

SPIROCHETAL DISEASES

Lyme disease
Clinical features
The earliest feature of Lyme disease is the unique skin eruption called *erythema chronicum migrans* (ECM). ECM begins 4 to 20 days after the bite of a tick, although only one third of patients distinctly recall a tick bite.[37-39] A red papule begins at the site of the tick bite, then slowly enlarges over several weeks to form an annular ring with a flat red border that clears in the center (Fig. 5-24). Sometimes the center remains a red, edematous plaque that feels hot. Fifty percent of patients will develop multiple secondary annular rings, which begin 1 to 6 days after the primary lesion appears.[37-39] Untreated ECM lasts about 3 weeks, then spontaneously resolves but may recur for up to a year or more, accompanied by arthritis or other symptoms.[37-39] Skin lesions are associated with headaches, fatigue, myalgias, and low-grade fever.[38,39] Sometimes nausea, vomiting, sore throat, and lymphadenopathy will accompany ECM. A red nodule may appear on the ear, chest, or axillary fold, which represents borrelial lymphocytoma.[39] Joint, CNS, and cardiac abnormalities begin about 4 weeks after the tick bite, after the ECM has resolved.[37] Fifty percent of untreated Lyme disease patients will develop arthritis.[37,38] The onset of arthritis is abrupt and usually monarticular (knee, shoulder, elbow, temporomandibular, ankle, wrist, or hip), and the affected joint is warm, swollen, and tender, but not red. The first episode lasts 1 week, but up to three recurrences are common. CNS disease occurs in 10% to 15% of untreated patients, with the classic triad of meningitis, cranial nerve palsies, and peripheral radiculoneuropathy.[38,39] The meningitis is characterized by an excruciating headache and stiff neck and may include changes in behavior. The seventh nerve is most frequently involved, with recurrent episodes of facial

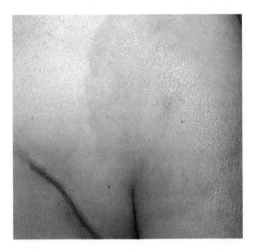

Fig. 5-24
Lyme disease. Annular erythema and central tick bite papule.

palsy. Neuritic pain or focal weakness is seen with the peripheral radiculoneuropathy of Lyme disease. Less than 10% of patients experience cardiac involvement, with atrioventricular block or myopericarditis reported. A great variety of additional neurologic and other organ symptoms are occasionally reported. The erythrocyte sedimentation rate is usually elevated, but other routine laboratory studies are variable.[38,39]

Differential diagnosis

ECM may mimic ringworm or be diagnosed as erythema multiforme or erythema marginatum. ECM evolves slowly, over days; erythema marginatum is transient, often changing hourly. A negative KOH examination and a skin biopsy will help distinguish. In ECM, a dense mononuclear cell accumulation around blood vessels and adnexal structures without epidermal changes is seen. Serologic tests for Lyme disease using enzyme immunoassays for immunoglobulin M (IgM) are useful when noncutaneous symptoms develop. The organism can be cultured on modified Kelly's medium, but yields are too low for practical use.

Pathogenesis

The spirochete *Borrelia burgdorferi* is carried by a variety of ticks, predominantly the deer tick, *Ixodes dammini*. The ticks may be carried by rodents or house pets or attach themselves to grasses or bushes. Humans are incidental hosts. The spirochete has irregular coils, is 10 to 30 μm long, and is found worldwide, although most cases come from northern Europe or the eastern half of the United States.[38-40] Subtypes of *B. burgdorferi* differ in North America and Europe by molecular typing, and this may account for the differences in prevalence.[41] Within a few days after a tick bite, the spirochete migrates within the skin or enters the bloodstream. It appears that all symptoms and signs are directly related to the presence of the spirochete in affected tissues or the immune response to the organism.

Treatment

Some authorities advocate antibiotic treatment at the time of a deer tick bite rather than observation,[40,42] but this recommendation remains controversial.[37,39] For children over 8 years of age, oral tetracycline, 25 to 50 mg/kg/day for 3 weeks, is the treatment of choice.[38,39] Younger children are treated with oral phenoxymethyl penicillin, 50 mg/kg/day. The ECM will disappear within 3 days with successful treatment, and secondary complications are almost always prevented.[43] For mild secondary complications without heart block, oral antibiotics for 4 to 6 weeks are recommended such as amoxicillin, 40 mg/kg/day or doxycycline, 100 mg three times a day for adolescents.[39,41] If CSF pleocytosis or complete heart block is present, intravenous therapy with penicillin G, 250,000 U/kg/day, ceftriaxone, 50 to 100 mg/kg/day, or cefotaxime, 100 to 200 mg/kg/day, for 2 to 4 weeks, may be required.[39]

Patient education

Avoidance of the tick vector is the basis of prevention. Avoidance of high-risk areas, such as wooded, grassy areas during tick season, wearing protective light-colored clothing with long sleeves and caps, using insect repellant, and periodic examination for ticks are required. For children with ECM, parents should be advised about the possibility of secondary complications of arthritis or neurologic disease. The importance of completing the 3 weeks of therapy to avoid complications should be emphasized.

Follow-up visits

After successful treatment, monthly visits for 3 months are useful to observe for late complications. A second antibiotic course may be required should secondary symptoms occur.

Syphilis

Clinical features

Acquired syphilis and congenital syphilis are uncommon yet increasing in industrialized countries, but common in Third World countries.[44-46] Acquired syphilis has three distinct stages.[45] Primary acquired syphilis is characterized by the chancre, a painless, shallow ulcer surrounded by a red indurated border that appears about 3 weeks after exposure (Fig. 5-25).

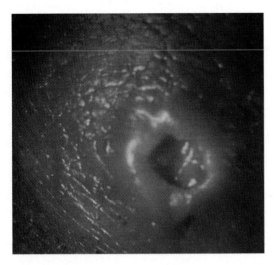

Fig. 5-25
Syphilitic chancre. Painless scrotal ulcer with indurated borders in an 11-year-old boy.

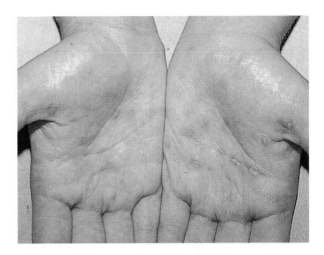

Fig. 5-26
Secondary syphilis. Ham-colored palmar macules on an adolescent with secondary syphilis.

If untreated, the chancre heals spontaneously in 1 to 2 months. Secondary syphilis is usually seen as a morbilliform generalized eruption accompanied by lymphadenopathy, fatigue, headache, and, sometimes, low-grade fever.[45] Involvement of the palms and soles is frequently observed (Fig. 5-26). Nodular, pustular, annular, and papulosquamous lesions are occasionally seen. Mucous patches are seen as weeping erosive areas on oral or genital mucosa. Tertiary stages are rare in childhood.[45]

Congenital syphilis is usually asymptomatic in the newborn period, but may be observed as a persistent rhinorrhea that develops during the newborn period, or in severe cases, as hydrops fetalis.[44-46] The newborn is usually small for gestational age and has mild hepatosplenomegaly.[44,46] Serologic testing of the mother is critical to the diagnosis, as usually the newborn symptoms are so mild as to be overlooked. Signs of late congenital syphilis may be the first clue to maternofetal transmission of syphilis.[45] Late signs begin around 6 years of age and include cloudy corneas (interstitial keratitis) accompanied by photophobia and pain, bilateral eighth nerve deafness, notching of small central and lateral incisors (Hutchinson's teeth), painless swelling of the knees

(Clutton's joint), perforation of the nasal septum leading to a saddle nose deformity and perforated palate, saber tibia, and radial scarring about the mouth (rhagades).

Differential diagnosis

Syphilis is known as the great mimic, and a high index of suspicion for syphilis should be maintained. The primary chancre of acquired syphilis must be distinguished from bacterial ulcers, herpes simplex infections, chancroid, or lymphogranuloma venereum. The absence of pain is a useful distinguishing feature, and identification of *Treponema pallidum* by dark-field microscopic examination of smears of the ulcer base is definitive. Secondary acquired syphilis must be distinguished from pityriasis rosea, infectious mononucleosis, many other viral exanthems, and a number of papulosquamous diseases. Biopsy of a secondary syphilis lesion will reveal numerous plasma cells within a perivascular dermal infiltrate and swelling of the vascular endothelium.[47]

Both a nontreponemal and a treponemal serologic test for syphilis or PCR testing are required.[4,48,49] Nontreponemal tests include the Venereal Disease Research Laboratory (VDRL) test, the rapid plasma reagin (RPR) test, and the automated reagin test (ART). Treponemal tests include the fluorescent treponemal antibody absorption (FTA-ABS) test, the microhemagglutinin for *T. pallidum*, Western immunoblotting for *T. pallidum* antigen, and the *T. pallidum* immobilization test. In congenital syphilis the newborn presents a particularly difficult diagnostic problem because of maternally transferred immunoglobulin G (IgG).[49] In congenital syphilis the maternal syphilis serology should be positive, and the Western IgM immunoblotting test to *T. pallidum* antigen positive in the affected infant.[44] The IgM enzyme-linked immunosorbent assay (ELISA) test and the FTA-ABS should be positive in 80% of the affected babies.[49] HIV testing of the mother should be considered in babies with congenital syphilis.

Hydrops fetalis caused by congenital syphilis must be differentiated from blood group incompatibility, the rhinorrhea from upper respiratory tract bacterial, and viral infections. Hepatosplenomegaly and intrauterine growth failure in newborns must be distinguished from other congenital infections such as herpes simplex, CMV, rubella, and toxoplasmosis.

Pathogenesis
T. pallidum is the spirochete responsible for syphilis. It is spread primarily through sexual contact and invades the bloodstream in the early phase of infection.[45] The incubation period is 10 to 90 days.[4] The chancre of primary syphilis develops at the time the blood-borne infection is maximal; the morbilliform rash of secondary syphilis represents spirochetes that have left the bloodstream and entered the skin.[47] Congenital syphilis represents a more massive infection than acquired syphilis, being blood borne in the fetus from the fourth month of pregnancy onward.[44-46] Rhinorrhea represents tissue infection of the nasopharynx, and late signs of congenital syphilis represent effects on developing tissues or osteomyelitis due to *T. pallidum*.

Treatment
Penicillin is the treatment of choice. Parenteral penicillin given intramuscularly weekly in the form of benzathine penicillin, in doses of 50,000 U/kg/day up to a total of 2.4 million U in a 3-week period, is recommended for children and adolescents with primary or secondary syphilis.[4] If penicillin allergic, tetracycline, 500 mg four times a day, or doxycycline, 100 mg twice daily for 4 weeks, is recommended. Aqueous penicillin G, 100,000 to 150,000 U/kg/day given intravenously every 8 to 12 hours for 10 to 14 days, is recommended for congenital syphilis.[4] If more than 1 day of therapy is missed, the entire course should be repeated. Retreatment is indicated if the clinical signs persist or recur, or if a sustained fourfold increase in a serologic test titer occurs, or if an initial high-titer serologic test fails to show a fourfold decrease within 6 months.[4]

Patient education
Children and adolescents with primary or secondary syphilis should be thoroughly educated on transmission of the disease. All recent sexual contacts of a child or adolescent with acquired syphilis should be identified, examined, serologically tested, and receive treatment if appropriate. Sexual abuse must be suspected in any young child with acquired syphilis. Routine serologic testing for syphilis in early pregnancy, and the importance of prenatal care for prevention, should be emphasized for congenital syphilis.[49] It should be emphasized that untreated syphilis in pregnancy results in death of babies in 40% of cases. Pregnant women at high risk for syphilis should also have serologic testing at 28 weeks of gestation.[4] One should emphasize that in congenital syphilis the long-term prognosis is good with prompt treatment but delayed treatment may result in developmental delays and the complications of late congenital syphilis.

Follow-up visits
Following treatment, children should be seen monthly for 6 months to observe for recurrences and to monitor serologically. In congenital syphilis, serology tests should be obtained at 3, 6, and 12 months of age. Otherwise, follow-up during routine well-child care will suffice.

MYCOBACTERIAL DISEASE

Mycobacterial infections of the skin in children are rare. Of the mycobacterial infections, the one most likely encountered is *Mycobacterium marinum* infection.[50]

Mycobacterium marinum infections
Clinical features

M. marinum produces a chronic granulomatous infection of the skin following direct inoculation through injured skin.[50-53] Contaminated fresh or salt water of warm temperatures (30° to 32° C), such as tropical fish tanks or hot swimming pools, are the usual source of infection in children.[51-53] The first appearance of red papules occurs at the site of abrasion or skin injury within 3 or 4 weeks[50] (Fig. 5-27). The papules may ulcerate, or more likely coalesce to form a red-brown plaque. The surface of the plaque may become verrucous. The plaque may persist for months to years if untreated. The arm and dorsum of the hand account for 80% of lesions, with the remainder on the knee.[51,52] Usually the lesions are solitary, although a pattern of ascending skin nodules on an extremity has been described (sporotrichoid pattern). No lymphadenopathy is found. Adolescents are most commonly infected, but toddlers may also be infected.[52,53]

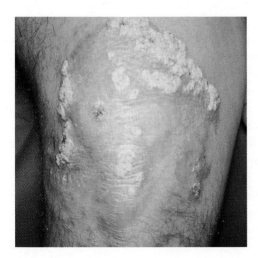

Fig. 5-27
Scaly plaques on the knee of an adolescent male with *M. marinum* infection (swimming pool granuloma).

Differential diagnosis

Verrucous plaques need to be distinguished from warts, psoriasis, or other granulomatous diseases such as sarcoidosis, tuberculosis, or foreign body granulomas. The sporotrichoid pattern must be distinguished from sporotrichosis, and the ulcerative lesions must be distinguished from Langerhans cell histiocytosis and bacterial or fungal ulcers. A skin biopsy stained for acid-fast organisms will help, but culture of the biopsy for atypical mycobacteria and deep fungal organisms will be definitive. History of exposure to a tropical fish tank or swimming in warm waters is helpful.

Pathogenesis

Abrasion or disruption of the skin, plus exposure to warm water containing the organism, is required for infection by the slender, aerobic, acid-fast rod *M. marinum*. The organism induces a granuloma with a mixture of lymphocytes, macrophages, and epithelioid giant cells. The verrucous lesions also feature epithelial hyperplasia.

Treatment

Spontaneous resolution has been reported, but it may require 1 or 2 years, and most authorities recommend antibiotic therapy.[4,51-53] There are no blinded trials of therapy for *M. marinum* cutaneous granulomas. A combination of rifampin and ethambutol for 3 to 6 months has been most successful.[4,51,52] Minocycline, doxycycline, and clarithromycin are alternatives.

Patient education

It should be emphasized that the skin abrasion is crucial to infection, and the child should not swim or immerse their skin in a tropical fish tank when they have a cut or abrasion. Cleaning the fish tank and changing the water may help, but the organism is difficult to remove from contaminated fish tanks.

Follow-up visits

After initiating antibiotic therapy, a follow-up visit at 2 weeks to monitor side effects of the therapy is indicated. If tolerated well, monthly visits until antibiotics are discontinued is indicated. Most authorities recommend continuing treatment for 1 month after the lesion has cleared.[51-53]

References

1. Ferrieri P: The natural history of impetigo, *J Clin Invest* 51:2851, 1972.

2. Dagan R: Impetigo in childhood: changing epidemiology and new treatments, *Pediatr Ann* 22:235, 1993.

3. Taplin D: Prevalence of streptococcal pyoderma in relation to climate and hygiene, *Lancet* i:501, 1973.

4. Report of the Committee on Infectious Disease: *1994 Red Book*, Elk Grove Village, Il, 1994, American Academy of Pediatrics.

5. Schachner L, Gonzalez A: Impetigo: a reassessment of etiology and therapy, *Pediatr Dermatol* 5:139, 1988.

6. Markowitz M: Changing epidemiology of group A streptococcal infections, *Pediatr Infect Dis J* 13:557, 1994.

7. Leyden JJ: Review of mupirocin ointment in the treatment of impetigo, *Clin Pediatr* 31:549, 1992.

8. Ben-Amitai D, Ashkenazi S: Common bacterial skin infections in childhood, *Pediatr Ann* 22:225, 1993.

9. Williams SR, Carruth JA: Orbital infection secondary to sinusitis in children: diagnosis and management, *Clin Otolaryngol* 17:550, 1992.

10. Malinow J, Powell KR: Periorbital cellulitis, *Pediatr Ann* 22:241, 1993.

11. Yagupsky P: Bacteriologic aspects of skin and soft tissue infections, *Pediatr Ann* 22:217, 1993.

12. McCray MK, Esterly NB: Blistering distal dactylitis, *J Amer Acad Dermatol* 5:592, 1981.

13. Rehder PA, Eliezer ET, Lane AT: Perianal cellulitis: cutaneous group A streptococcal disease, *Arch Dermatol* 124:702, 1988.

14. Howe PM: Etiologic diagnosis of cellulitis: comparison of the aspirates obtained from the leading edge and the point of maximal inflammation, *Pediatr Infect Dis J* 6:685, 1987.

15. Rathore MH, Barton LL, Kaplan EL: Suppurative group A beta-hemolytic streptococcal infections in children, *Pediatrics* 89:743, 1992.

16. Zoger S, Harrison MR: Necrotizing fasciitis in two children with acute lymphoblastic leukemia, *J Pediatr Surg* 27:668, 1992.

17. Zittergruen M, Grose C: Magnetic resonance imaging for early diagnosis of necrotizing fasciitis, *Pediatr Emerg Care* 9:26, 1993.

18. Stevens DL: Invasive group A streptococcal infections: the past, present and future, *Pediatr Infect Dis J* 13:561, 1994.

19. Davies HD, Matlow A, Scriver SR, et al: Apparent lower rates of streptococcal toxic shock syndrome and lower mortality in children with invasive group A streptococcal infections compared with adults, *Pediatr Infect Dis J* 13:49, 1994.

20. Shulman ST, Gerber MA, Tanz RR, Markowitz M: Streptococcal pharyngitis: the case for penicillin therapy, *Pediatr Infect Dis J* 13:1, 1994.

21. Zimakoff J, Rodahl VT, Petersen W, Schiebel J: Recurrent staphylococcal furunculosis in families, *Scand J Infect Dis* 20:403, 1988.

22. Trueb RM, Gloor M, Wuthrich B: Recurrent *Pseudomonas* folliculitis, *Pediatr Dermatol* 11:35, 1994.

23. Resnick SD: Staphylococcal toxin-mediated syndromes in childhood, *Semin Dermatol* 11:11, 1992.

24. Orange AP: Diffuse cutaneous mastocytosis mimicking staphylococcal scalded skin syndrome: report of three cases, *Pediatr Dermatol* 8:47, 1991

25. Murono K, Fujita K, Yoshioka H: Microbiologic characteristics of exfoliative toxin-producing *Staphylococcus aureus*, *Pediatr Infect Dis J* 7:313, 1988.

26. Bailey CJ, Smith TP: The reactive serine protease residue of epidermolytic toxin A, *Biochem J* 269:1989, 1991.

27. Hoeger PH, Elsner P: Staphylococcal scalded skin syndrome: transmission of exfoliatin-producing *Staphylococcus aureus* by an asymptomatic carrier, *Pediatr Infect Dis J* 7:340, 1988.

28. Kain KC, Schulzer M, Chow AW: Clinical spectrum of nonmenstrual toxic shock syndrome (TSS): comparison with menstrual TSS by multivariate discriminant analysis, *Clin Infect Dis* 16:100, 1993.

29. Ferguson MA, Todd JK: Toxic shock syndrome associated with *Staphylococcus aureus* sinusitis in children, *J Infect Dis* 161:953, 1990.

30. Rizkallah MF, Tolaymat A, Martinez JS, et al: Toxic shock syndrome caused by a strain of *Staphylococcus aureus* that produces enterotoxin C but not toxic shock syndrome toxin-1, *Am J Dis Child*143:848, 1989.

31. Berkowitz FE: Bacterial exotoxins: how they work, *Pediatr Infect Dis J* 8:42, 1989.

32. Margileth AM: Cat scratch disease, *Adv Pediatr Infect Dis* 8:1, 1993.

33. Koehler JE: *Rochalimaea henseleae* infection: a new zoonoses with domestic cat as reservoir, *JAMA* 271:531, 1994.

34. Waldvogel K, Regnery RL, Anderson BE, et al: Disseminated cat scratch disease: detection of *Rochalimaea henselae* in affected tissue, *Eur J Pediatr* 153:23, 1994.

35. Anderson B, Kelly C, Threlkel R, Edwards K: Detection of *Rochalimaea henselae* in CSD skin test antigens, *J Infect Dis* 168:1034, 1993.

36. Margileth AM: Antibiotic therapy for CSD, *Pediatr Infect Dis J* 11:474, 1992.

37. Steere AM: Current understanding of Lyme disease, *Hosp Pract* 28:37, 1993.

38. Prose NS, Abson KG, Berg D: Lyme disease in children: diagnosis, treatment and prevention, *Semin Dermatol* 11:31, 1992.

39. Melski JW: Primary and secondary erythema migrans in central Wisconsin, *Arch Dermatol* 129:709, 1993.

40. Eppes SC: Physician beliefs, attitudes and approaches toward Lyme disease in an endemic area, *Clin Pediatr* 33:130,1994.

41. Wienecke R, Zochling N, Neubert U, et al: Molecular subtyping of *Borrelia burgdorferi* in erythema migrans and acrodermatitis chronica atrophicans, *J Invest Dermatol* 103:19, 1994.

42. Agre F, Schwartz R: The value of early treatment of deer tick bites for the prevention of Lyme disease, *Am J Dis Child* 147:945, 1993.

43. Salazar JC, Gerber MA, Goff CW: Long-term outcome of Lyme disease in children given early treatment, *J Pediatr* 122:591, 1993.

44. Chhabra RS, Brion LP, Castro M, et al: Comparison of maternal sera, cord blood and neonatal sera for detecting presumptive congenital syphilis: relationship with maternal treatment, *Pediatrics* 91:88, 1993.

45. Lowy G: Sexually transmitted diseases in children, *Pediatr Dermatol* 9:329, 1992.

46. Reyes MP, Hunt N, Ostrea EM Jr, George D: Maternal/congenital syphilis in a large tertiary care urban hospital, *Clin Infect Dis* 17:1041, 1993.

47. Godschalk JC, van der Sluis JJ, Stolz E: The localisation of treponemes and characterization of the inflammatory infiltrate in skin biopsies from patients with primary or secondary syphilis or early infectious yaws, *Genitourin Med* 69:102, 1993.

48. Sanchez PJ, Wendel GD Jr, Grimpel E, et al: Evaluation of molecular methodologies and rabbit infectivity testing for the diagnosis of congenital syphilis and neonatal central nervous system invasion by *Treponema pallidum*, *J Infect Dis* 167:148, 1993.

49. Stoll BJ, Lee FK, Larsen S, et al: Clinical and serologic evaluation of neonates for congenital syphilis: a continuing diagnostic dilemma, *J Infect Dis* 167:1093, 1993.

50. Lotti L, Hautmann G: Atypical mycobacterial infections: a difficult and emerging group of infectious dermatoses, *Int J Dermatol* 32:499, 1993.

51. Iredell J, Whitby M, Blacklock Z: *Mycobacterium marinum* infection: epidemiology and presentation in Queensland 1971-1990, *Med J Aust* 157:596, 1992.

52. Edelestein H: *Mycobacterium marinum* skin infections, *Arch Intern Med* 134:1359, 1994.

53. Kullavanijaya P, Sirimachan S, Bhuddavudhikrai P: *Mycobacterium marinum* cutaneous infections acquired from occupations and hobbies, *Int J Dermatol* 32:504, 1993.

6

Fungal and Yeast Infections of the Skin

DERMATOPHYTES

Dermatophytes are fungi that invade and proliferate in the outer layer of the epidermis (stratum corneum). In addition to invading the stratum corneum, some species may also invade the hair and nails. Dermatophyte infections are common and increase in frequency with increasing age: in hot, humid climates; and in crowded living conditions. For example, tinea capitis is quite prevalent in North America, especially in urban areas.[1,2] In one city in the United States, 4% of asymptomatic children had a positive fungal culture for scalp dermatophytes,[1] and in another, 50% of children with tinea capitis had a household member who was culture positive.[2]

HAIR INFECTIONS (TINEA CAPITIS)

Clinical features

Scalp hair involvement is usually seen in prepubertal children and is largely due to infections with either *Trichophyton tonsurans* or *Microsporum canis*.[3] Each infection has a noninflammatory stage lasting 2 to 8

weeks, followed by an inflammatory stage. Hair loss is a regular feature of tinea capitis. *M. canis* infections are characterized by one or several patches of broken-off hairs that appear thickened and white (Fig. 6-1). The hairs fluoresce yellow-green with Wood's light. In contrast, *T. tonsurans* produces several distinct clinical presentations: a noninflammatory stage in which hairs break off at the follicular orifice in a circumscribed area of the scalp, which leaves small, dark hairs in the follicles, or so-called black-dot ringworm (Fig. 6-2); and three inflammatory stages: (1) diffuse fine scaling of the scalp without obvious broken-off hairs (Fig. 6-3); (2) multiple scaly, pustular bald areas with indistinct margins (Fig. 6-4); or (3) multiple kerions. The widespread inflammatory stages are more commonly seen than the black-dot form and usually are associated with regional lymphadenopathy. The presence of enlarged suboccipital or posterior cervical lymph nodes in association with hair loss should raise suspicions of tinea capitis.

T. tonsurans infections account for 95% of tinea capitis in North America.[1-3]

The diagnosis in the noninflammatory stage should be confirmed by the following three steps: (1)

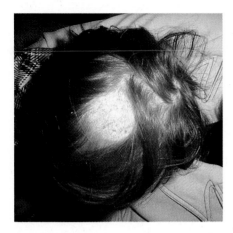

Fig. 6-1
Circumscribed patch of scalp hair loss with thick scales due to *M. canis* infection.

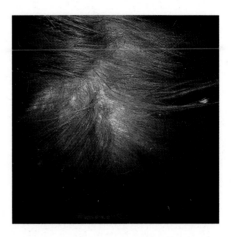

Fig. 6-3
Diffuse scaling in a dandruff-like pattern in *T. tonsurans* infection.

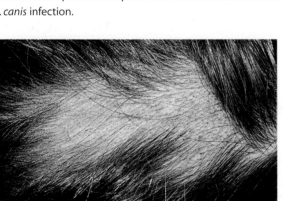

Fig. 6-2
Circumscribed area of hair loss without scalp change and with hairs broken off at the follicular orifice. This is the black-dot pattern of *T. tonsurans* infection.

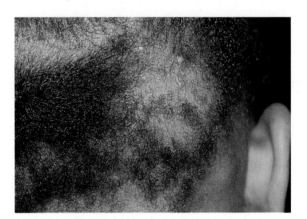

Fig. 6-4
Numerous triangle-shaped patches of hair loss accompanied by pustular kerion formation and enlarged lymph node in *T. tonsurans* infection.

Wood's light examination, (2) potassium hydroxide (KOH) examination, and (3) fungal culture.

1. *Wood's light examination.* Wood's light examination is best performed with a hand-held ultraviolet black lamp with two fluorescent bulbs. The lamp should be held within 6 inches of the scalp to observe for yellow-green fluorescence of the thickened scalp hairs. Lint from clothing fluoresces white from the addition of optical brighteners, and scale entrapped in sebum appears a dull yellow. These may be con-

fused with fungal fluorescence. *M. canis* fluoresces, but the epidemic form of tinea capitis due to *T. tonsurans* does not. The Wood's lamp examination cannot be used to exclude the diagnosis of tinea capitis or for screening children during epidemics.

2. *KOH examination.* KOH examination should be performed in every case of hair loss associated with broken hairs, and in children with diffuse scaling of the scalp. If the hair fluoresces, hold the Wood's lamp in one hand and a curette in the other. Gently

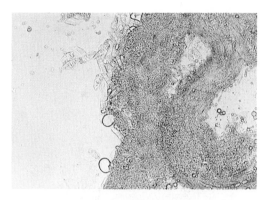

Fig. 6-5
Photomicrograph of hair dissolved in KOH. Mats containing billions of small spores coat the outside of hair, with hyphae seen within the hair shaft in *M. canis* infection.

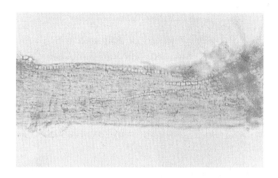

Fig. 6-6
Photomicrograph of hair dissolved in KOH. Hyphae and spores of *T. tonsurans* appear as chains within the hair shaft. There are no spores coating the hair.

remove the fluorescent hairs by scraping the scalp with the curette for KOH examination and culture. The involved hairs are loosened in the follicles and will be included in the scrapings, without pain to the child. If the hair does not fluoresce, use the curette to scrape the follicular openings in the involved area of the scalp hair loss. If a kerion is present, scrape the border of the lesion. The scrapings that include infected hair are placed on a glass microscope slide, partially dissolved in KOH 20%, and placed under a coverslip. Wait 20 to 40 minutes to examine the specimen under the 10× and 40× lenses. In fluorescent hairs the outer surface of the hair is coated with mats containing thousands of tiny spores (Fig. 6-5), and hyphae may be seen within the hair shaft. In nonfluorescent hairs, hyphae and spores are seen within the hair shaft (Fig. 6-6). KOH examinations for dermatophytes are simple procedures that can be performed in the office or clinic, but interpretation may be difficult for the inexperienced.[4]

3. *Fungal culture.* Fungal culture is the most reliable test in the diagnosis of tinea capitis and should be routinely performed in children with suspected tinea capitis. Fungal culture also should be considered for household contacts as 50% of children have a culture-positive household member including adults.[2] A modified Sabouraud dextrose agar (dermatophyte test medium [DTM]) makes this procedure simple. Broken hairs or scrapings obtained by a sterile curette, toothbrush, or moistened gauze are inoculated so as to break the agar surface[5]; the bottle cap is loosely applied, and the culture bottles left at room temperature. If a dermatophyte is present, the agar medium turns from yellow to red in 4 to 5 days. A positive culture can be subcultured on Sabouraud dextrose agar for precise identification.

Inflammatory lesions produce a kerion, which is an erythematous boggy nodule with superficial pustules (Fig. 6-7).[6,7] These lesions are almost completely devoid of hair and will lead to scarring and permanent hair loss if untreated (Fig. 6-8). A kerion will appear 2 to 8 weeks after infection begins and represents an exaggerated host response to the invading fungus. Approximately 40% of untreated tinea capitis caused by *M. canis* or *T. tonsurans* may eventuate in a kerion. Scrapings for KOH examination and fungal culture should be obtained from the edge of lesions, not the inflammatory center.

Differential diagnosis

Alopecia areata and trichotillomania are the major considerations in the differential diagnosis of tinea capitis in children. Alopecia areata may be distinguished by the total absence of hair in a circum-

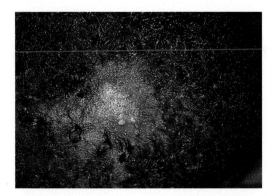

Fig. 6-7
Boggy, red scalp nodule with superficial pustules in kerion.

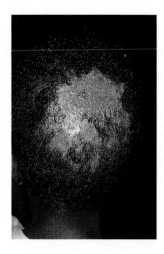

Fig. 6-8
Scarring hair loss in child with previously undiagnosed tinea capitis and kerion.

Table 6-1.
Organisms Responsible for Tinea Capitis

Feature	M. canis	T. tonsurans
Source	Cats and dogs	Other children
Fluorescence	Yellow-green	None
Contagious	No	Yes
Hair loss	Yes	Yes
Kerion	Yes	Yes
Children infected	Rural and suburban	Urban
Clinical patterns	Thickened hairs	Black-dot, dandruff-like, or multiple areas of alopecia

scribed patch, without any associated scalp change. In trichotillomania scalp excoriations, perifollicular petechiae, and hairs broken off at differing lengths are the distinguishing features. Seborrheic dermatitis may mimic the diffuse forms of *T. tonsurans* scalp infection.

In inflammatory tinea capitis (kerion), bacterial pyodermas are often mistaken for kerion. The pustules in kerion are sterile, however, and incision produces only serosanguineous fluid. Bacterial culture of the skin surface may yield *Staphylococcus aureus* and lead to the incorrect diagnosis of pyoderma, but one should recall that *S. aureus* frequently colonizes the skin surface, and such cultures would not detect bacterial invasion.[6] Less commonly, traction alopecia, scleroderma, lichen planus, psoriasis, lupus erythematosus, dandruff, or porokeratosis of Mibelli may be confused with tinea capitis.

Pathogenesis
M. canis is harbored by cats, dogs, and certain rodents, and children handling such animals are susceptible to infection. Humans appear to be a terminal host for *M. canis*, and human-to-human transmission does not occur. When there is delayed hypersensitivity to the organism, a kerion may develop. Histologic study of this lesion shows a mononuclear cell infiltrate consistent with that seen in delayed hypersensitivity reactions. *M. canis* accounts for much of the tinea capitis in suburban and rural areas (Table 6-1).

T. tonsurans is transmitted from human to human and is currently epidemic in North America. It is most prevalent in areas of crowding and accounts for 95% of tinea capitis in inner-city children in North America.[1-3] Transmission is predominantly from sharing hats, caps, combs, or brushes with infected individuals.[1,2]

Treatment
Griseofulvin in a micronized form, 10 to 20 mg/kg/day for a minimum of 6 weeks, is the treatment

of choice.[7,8] Often, treatment for 2 to 3 months is required. Topical antifungal agents cannot reach the hyphae within the hair shaft and are ineffective. In *M. canis,* with successful treatment, the lesions become nonfluorescent 13 days after the administration of griseofulvin is begun. Although griseofulvin has many side effects, including agranulocytosis and aplastic anemia, it is a relatively safe drug in children. Absorption is enhanced by a fatty meal; taking griseofulvin once or twice a day with ice cream or whole milk is a popular prescription. Oral terbinafine has been reported to be equally efficacious to griseofulvin in limited studies.[8] Oral ketoconazole or itraconazole are second alternatives to griseofulvin.[8,9] Side effects with these agents are more frequent than with griseofulvin and these drugs are less efficaceous. They should be used only for resistant cases. In addition to oral griseofulvin, some authorities advocate an antifungal shampoo such as selenium sulfide 2.5% shampoo, applied twice weekly to the scalp, to reduce infectivity and to hasten the child's return to school or child-care setting.[3,7,10]

Kerion responds well to griseofulvin alone. The addition of antibiotics or steroids is not usually required.[7] Some authorities recommend that severely inflamed or long-standing kerions may require a short course of oral steroids to reduce inflammation and prevent scarring alopecia. Prednisone, 1 to 2 mg/kg/day for 5 to 10 days, is recommended.

Patient education

If *M. canis* is found, animal sources should be identified and the animal treated by a veterinarian to prevent infection of other children. In *T. tonsurans,* identification of the likely contacts is necessary. Household contacts should be cultured if possible. Children should not share combs, brushes, or headwear. School and day-care contacts should be referred for evaluation if scaling hair loss is present. Screening of contacts with a Wood's lamp is of no value since the epidemic strains in North America are not fluorescent. Patients should be instructed that hair regrowth is slow, often taking 3 to 6 months. If a kerion is present, some scarring and permanent hair loss may result.

Follow-up visits

A visit in 2 weeks is helpful to ascertain the effectiveness of the griseofulvin therapy. Reexamination for fluorescence and a repeat culture will serve as guidelines for increasing the therapeutic dosage. If the lesions are fluorescence negative, culture negative, or both at 2 weeks, a total of 6 weeks' therapy may be all that is required. Treatment 4 to 6 weeks after the lesions are culture negative is a useful rule of thumb. With the use of an antifungal shampoo such as selenium sulfide 2.5% shampoo plus griseofulvin, the child can usually return to school in 1 week. A follow-up visit every 2 to 4 weeks until hair growth begins is advised. Asymptomatic carriers may be treated with sporicidal shampoos, such as povidone-iodine, econazole, or selenium sulfide,. used twice weekly for 4 weeks.[7,10]

FUNGAL INFECTION INVOLVING THE SKIN ONLY

Tinea corporis
Clinical features
Dermatophyte infections on the body often consist of one or several circular erythematous patches (Fig. 6-9). The patches may have a papular, scaly, annular border and a clear center (Fig. 6-10) or may be inflammatory throughout, with superficial pustules (Fig. 6-11). A most common pattern is a red, scaly

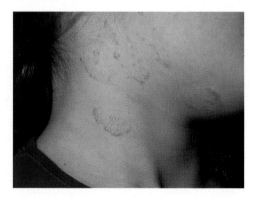

Fig. 6-9
Annular, red, scaly borders with clear center in tinea corporis.

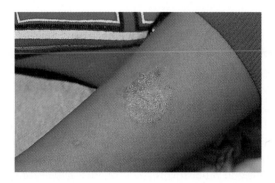

Fig. 6-10
Red, scaly plaque with partial clearing in center in tinea corporis due to *M. canis*.

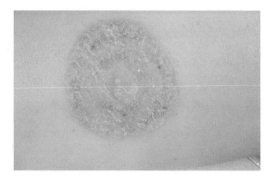

Fig. 6-11
Plaque, red throughout, with prominent pustules, in tinea corporis due to the cattle ringworm, *T. verrucosum*.

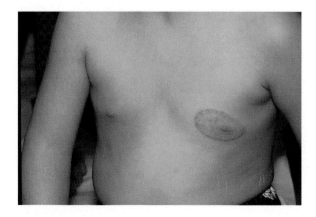

Fig. 6-12
Annular, red, scaly patch, with partial clearing in the center and red follicular papules.

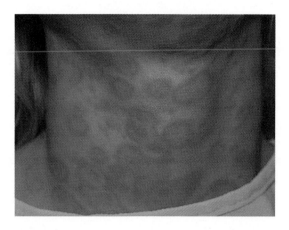

Fig. 6-13
Multiple annular patches on the neck in *M. canis* infection.

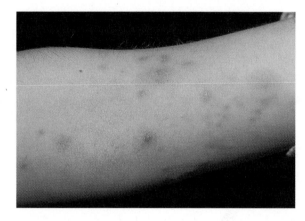

Fig. 6-14
Multiple follicular pustules in a leukemic child with Majocchi's granulomas due to *T. rubrum*.

patch with partial clearing and follicular pustules (Fig. 6-12). Multiple annular lesions may be seen (Fig. 6-13). In immunosuppressed children, including those with cancer, invasion of the follicular orifice by the dermatophytes may predominate. This produces a folliculitis pattern known as Majocchi's granulomas (Fig. 6-14). *M. canis*, *T. mentagrophytes*, *T. tonsurans*, and *T. rubrum* are the most common dermatophytes responsible for tinea corporis.[11] Diagnosis is confirmed by KOH examination of scrapings of thin scales obtained from the border of the lesion. Cultures are not usually done routinely.

Differential diagnosis

Any skin eruption that produces an annular configuration can mimic tinea corporis.[11,12] The herald patch of pityriasis rosea may mimic tinea corporis, as may any of the forms of dermatitis. The herald patch clears in the center but has central scale rather than scale at the edge. It is not unusual to confuse the annular nodules of granuloma annulare for tinea corporis. In granuloma annulare, there is no scale or surface disruption. Psoriasis, parapsoriasis, figurate erythemas, sarcoidosis, secondary syphilis, and lupus erythematosus can also mimic tinea corporis.

Tinea pedis (athlete's foot)

Clinical features

There are three clinical forms of tinea pedis. All are found almost exclusively in the postpubertal adolescent and are uncommon in childhood.[13] The most common form consists of vesicles and erosions on the instep of one or both feet (Figs. 6-15 and 6-16). The dermatophyte may be identified by removing the vesicle roof, scraping the underside of the roof, and examining the scrapings under the microscope for hyphae.

Occasionally, fissuring between the toes, with scaling and erythema in the surrounding skin, is seen. Rarely diffuse scaling of the weight-bearing surface of one or both feet, with exaggerated scaling in the skin creases, the so-called "moccasin foot" tinea pedis, is seen. The most common organisms responsible for tinea pedis are *T. rubrum* and *T. mentagrophytes*.[13]

Differential diagnosis

Atopic dermatitis mimics tinea pedis in prepubertal children. The diagnosis of athlete's foot before adolescence should be viewed with suspicion. Contact dermatitis and other forms of dermatitis may also mimic tinea pedis. Contact dermatitis usually involves the tops of the feet, whereas tinea pedis involves the weight-bearing surface. Juvenile plantar dermatosis (JPD) is characterized by redness, dryness, and fissures of the weight-bearing surface of the foot and may be easily confused with tinea pedis. Fungal scrapings and culture are needed to distinguish tinea pedis from JPD. Scabies, granuloma annulare, and psoriasis may also mimic tinea pedis.

Tinea faciei

Clinical features

Dermatophyte infections on the face occur commonly in children.[11,12] They are erythematous, scaly, and may have a "butterfly" distribution (Fig. 6-17). In other children the lesions may be unilateral (Fig. 6-18). KOH examination of the scaly border will con-

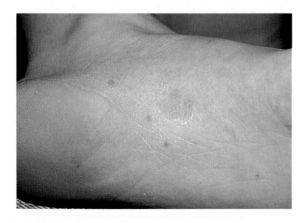

Fig. 6-15
Annular erythema with vesicles on instep of large adolescent male feet. Tinea pedis due to *T. rubrum*.

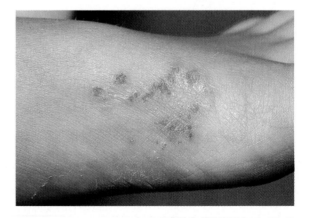

Fig. 6-16
Erosions and blisters on the instep of an adolescent's foot in bullous tinea pedis.

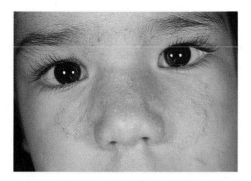

Fig. 6-17
Annular, red, scaly lesions of the nose and malar skin of a girl misdiagnosed as having lupus erythematosus. Tinea faciei due to *M. canis*.

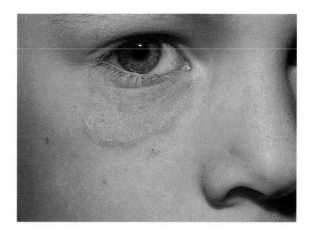

Fig. 6-18
A red, scaly plaque below the eye in tinea faciei caused by *M. canis*.

firm the diagnosis. *M. canis* and the cattle ringworm, *T. verrucosum* are the most commonly involved fungi of tinea faciei in children.

Differential diagnosis

Tinea faciei may mimic lupus erythematosus and other collagen vascular diseases.[12] A KOH examination for hyphae should always be performed in children in whom the butterfly rash of lupus is considered. Atopic dermatitis, contact dermatitis, and seborrheic dermatitis should also be considered.

Tinea cruris
Clinical features

An erythematous, scaly eruption on the inner thighs and inguinal creases characterizes tinea cruris.[11,12] Sometimes an elevated papular, scaly border is present to suggest the diagnosis. KOH examination of the border for hyphae will confirm the diagnosis. Tinea cruris is unusual before adolescence. *T. mentagrophytes* and *Epidermophyton floccosum* are the organisms most often responsible.[11]

Differential diagnosis

Diaper dermatitis and candidiasis may mimic tinea cruris, but these usually occur in infants. Yeast infection in the perineal area may be distinguished by involvement of the scrotum. Several forms of dermatitis also occur in this area. Rarely, erythrasma, a superficial bacterial infection due to *Corynebacterium minutissimum*, will be confused with tinea cruris. Wood's light examination in erythrasma produces a coral-red fluorescence.

Pathogenesis of tinea corporis, pedis, faciei, cruris

Dermatophyte invasion of the stratum corneum, but not the remainder of the epidermis or dermis, is responsible for superficial dermatophyte infections. The exact mechanism of the inflammation is not known, but toxins released by the dermatophyte are thought to be important in initiating the inflammatory response.

Treatment of tinea corporis, pedis, faciei, cruris

Topical therapy is the treatment of choice.[11-13] Terbinafine, ciclopirox, clotrimazole, ketoconazole, oxiconazole, sulconazole, econazole, miconazole, haloprogin, and tolnaftate creams are all efficacious against 90% of dermatophyte species. They are applied twice daily, either as a cream or solution, to the entire area until the lesions have cleared. This often takes 2 to 4 weeks of therapy. Topical terbinafine may produce clinical and mycologic clearing within 1 week.[14,15] Rarely are oral terbinafine, itraconazole, fluconazoles, griseofulvin, or other systemic antifungal agents required.

Patient education for tinea corporis, pedis, faciei, cruris

Knowledge that these fungi are found in soil or animals may help identify the source and prevent other family members from being infected. Be certain to instruct the patient to treat the entire lesion plus about a 1-cm border beyond it. Efforts to keep the affected skin area dry after successful treatment, and changing habits regarding family pets, such as keeping the pets out of the child's room and not allowing the child to carry the pet, may be useful in preventing reinfection, until the pet is cured. When epidemic dermatophytes are involved, examination of contacts and fungal culture of suspicious lesions is recommended.

Follow-up visits for tinea corporis, pedis, faciei, cruris

A visit 2 weeks after therapy is started is helpful to ascertain its efficacy. If no response has occurred, either the diagnosis is incorrect or a resistant dermatophyte has been encountered. At this point it is useful to culture the lesion and perhaps change to a different class of topical antifungal agent. Further follow-up visits may be needed.

INFECTION OF THE NAILS (ONYCHOMYCOSIS, TINEA UNGUIUM)

Clinical features

Distal thickening and yellowing of the nail plate are regular features of onychomycosis (tinea unguium)[11,12] (Fig. 6-19). The yellowing represents separation of the distal nail plate from the nail bed, and entrapment of air between these two structures. Usually only one or two nails, most often the toenails, are involved. It is uncommon to find onychomycosis in childhood; it is almost exclusively limited to adolescence. With toenail involvement a concurrent tinea pedis is usually present.[12,13]

Differential diagnosis

Psoriasis also causes distal yellowing and thickening of the nail, but eventually all 20 nails are involved, and superficial nail pitting is also present.[12] Lichen planus and 20-nail dystrophy also usually involve all 20 nails. Hereditary nail disorders associated with ectodermal defects, such as pachyonychia congenita, are sometimes confused with onychomycosis. Bacterial and candidal nail involvement characteristically result in proximal rather than distal nail plate disease.

Pathogenesis

Dermatophytes may invade nails as well as the stratum corneum.[11,12] They proliferate within the nail plate, destroying its integrity.

Treatment

Successful therapy of onychomycosis is uncommon. Only 17.5% of patients treated responded after 6 to 12 months of griseofulvin therapy.[8,16] One should weigh the consequences of prolonged therapy against the poor success rate.[8,15,16] Oral terbinafine (95%), ketoconazole (80%), and itraconazole (71%) have somewhat higher reported success rates, but they have not been analyzed for long-term relapse rates.[16] Topical agents, with the possible exception of 1% terbinafine generally are not successful unless used in combination with griseofulvin.

Patient education

The difficulty in obtaining a cure with this disease should be thoroughly explained to the patient and the

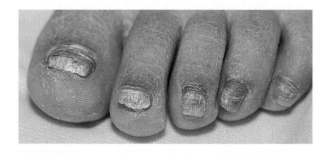

Fig. 6-19
Onychomycosis. Distal thickening and yellowing of four toenails in an adolescent.

parents. They may not desire oral antifungal therapy simply to achieve temporary improvement.

Follow-up visits

Visits at 6-month intervals are useful to follow the course of the illness and observe for the possible involvement of other nails. If oral antifungal agents are used, then evaluation for side effects including laboratory tests at 1-month intervals is recommended.[8]

YEAST INFECTIONS

Tinea versicolor

Clinical features

In tinea versicolor, multiple oval macules with a fine scale are found on the neck, chest, upper back, shoulders, and upper arms of children and adolescents (Fig. 6-20).[17] Occasionally, the lesions are confluent and present as a continuous sheet. Their color depends on the state of pigmentation. In well-tanned or darkly pigmented adolescents, the lesions appear as discrete hypopigmented macules. In the winter months, as normal pigment fades, the lesions may appear as tan or dark-brown macules, hence the term *versicolor* (Fig. 6-21). The infection tends to be persistent. KOH examination of scrapings reveals numerous short curved hyphae and circular spores—the

so-called "spaghetti and meatballs" (Fig. 6-22). Occasionally Wood's light examination reveals an orange fluorescence of the lesions if the patient has not cleansed the affected area recently. Biopsy of these lesions will show periodic acid–Schiff (PAS)–positive hyphae and spores within the stratum corneum.

Differential diagnosis

Seborrheic dermatitis, contact dermatitis, and tinea corporis can mimic tinea versicolor. Vitiligo, pityriasis alba, and other hypopigmented states are also sometimes confused with it. The direct microscopic examination of scales will distinguish.

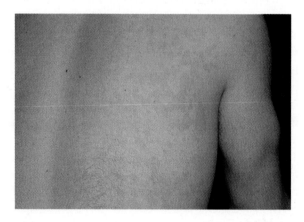

Fig. 6-21
Tan macules of tinea versicolor on a light-skinned child.

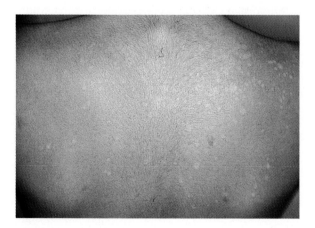

Fig. 6-20
Pink macules with a fine scale over the back of an adolescent with tinea versicolor.

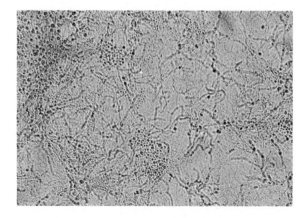

Fig. 6-22
Photomicrograph of KOH examination of tinea versicolor. Multiple short hyphae and spores are seen.

Pathogenesis

The yeastlike organism *Malassezia furfur*, which in its culture phase is called *Pityrosporum orbiculare* or *Pityrosporum ovale*, invades the stratum corneum to produce the lesions of tinea versicolor.[18] The organism thrives in hot, humid climates and commonly colonizes the skin by adolescence.[18] It may colonize the skin of neonates as well.[17,18]

Treatment

Miconazole, ciclopirox, clotrimazole, haloprogin creams, or fluconazole shampoo applied twice daily for 2 to 3 weeks may be efficacious, but all are costly when one considers the amount required to cover the trunk of an child or adolescent.[8] Overnight application of selenium sulfide 2.5% once weekly for 4 weeks is considered the treatment of choice by many.[8,19] Sodium hypochlorite 15% once weekly for 2 months will result in temporary clearing, but the recurrence rate is high.[19] After initial clearing, prevention of recurrence by once-monthly treatment may be considered. Skin irritation is a problem with overnight applications. One may try 10- to 30-minute daily applications for 7 to 14 days as an alternative therapy. In tropical and subtropical climates, oral ketoconazole, fluconazole, or itraconazole given in a single dose once daily for two weeks may be considered in difficult cases.[8] A single oral dose of fluconazole may produce acceptable results.[8]

Patient education

Patients should be instructed that repigmentation of the hypopigmented areas will not occur until they are exposed to the sun, and that a recurrence is likely.

Follow-up visits

A follow-up visit in 1 month's time to evaluate therapy should be considered. If oral therapy is considered, monthly visits to monitor side effects should be instituted.

Candidiasis

Clinical features

In regions of the body where warmth and moisture lead to maceration of the skin or mucous membranes, the tissue is predisposed to invasion by the pathogenic yeast *Candida albicans*. Candidiasis in different body sites has distinct clinical features. In neonates and infants, white plaques on an erythematous base (thrush) are commonly seen on the buccal mucosa and other sites in the oral cavity.[20,21] In this same age group, intertriginous involvement of the body folds is also common, such as in the diaper area.[20] The use of pacifiers in infants may be permissive for oral candidiasis, including involvement of the angles of the lips (angular cheilitis).[20,21]

Fully established diaper candidiasis demonstrates beefy erythema with elevated margins and satellite red plaques (Fig. 6-23). However, erosions, pustules, erythematous papules, and vesicles may also be features of candidiasis of the diaper area. *C. albicans* colonizes the diaper area within 3 days of the development of diaper dermatitis and should always be considered as a secondary infection in long-standing diaper dermatitis.

Intertriginous candidiasis involving the inframammary, axillary, neck, and inguinal body folds may also be seen in obese infants, children, and adolescents.

A rare form of candidiasis (congenital candidiasis) acquired in utero results in generalized erythema of the newborn, with scaling and pustule formation[22,23] (Fig. 6-24). It is particularly observed in very low birth weight infants and acquired from maternal *C. albicans* vulvovaginitis.

Paronychia due to candidiasis is a common result of thumb sucking. The erythema and swelling around the base of the nail are usually not tender (Fig. 6-25).

Vulvovaginal candidiasis appears as a cheesy vaginal discharge, with whitish plaques on erythematous mucous membranes. It is most common in adolescent females.

The rare candidal granulomas are oval red plaques with a thick yellow crust. They are found on the head and neck and other areas of skin in children with defective host defenses.[19,20] In the syndrome of chronic mucocutaneous candidiasis (Fig. 6-26), seen in patients with defective host defenses, persistent thrush with extensive involvement of the tongue and lips and chronic paronychia are present. Severe thrush may be observed in immunodeficient children infected with the human immunodeficiency virus (HIV). Patients on

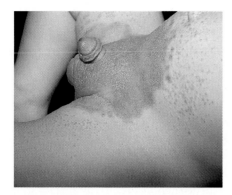

Fig. 6-23
Beefy-red central erythema with satellite pustules in candidiasis of diaper area. Positive cultures can be obtained only from satellite lesions, not from central erythema.

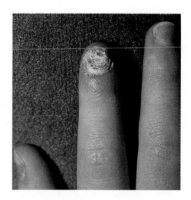

Fig. 6-25
Cuticular nontender swelling and erythema with thickened, disrupted nail surface in paronychia caused by *C. albicans*.

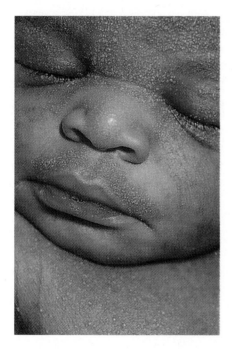

Fig. 6-24
Hundreds of pinpoint pustules with an erythematous base on the face of a newborn with congenital candidiasis.

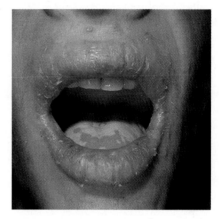

Fig. 6-26
Thick white coating of tongue with scaling and fissuring of lips in chronic mucocutaneous candidiasis.

long-term glucocorticosteroid, antibiotic, or oral contraceptive therapy (in adolescent females) appear unusually susceptible to candidiasis. Similarly, children with diabetes mellitus and reticuloendothelial neoplasms are also predisposed to candidiasis.

The diagnosis can be established by scraping the skin or mucosal lesion and observing the single budding yeast in a KOH preparation under the microscope. *C. albicans* is readily cultured on Sabouraud dextrose agar or cornmeal agar. Interpretation of a positive culture must be made with caution since *C. albicans* may reflect simple colonization.[20]

Differential diagnosis
Herpes simplex, aphthous stomatitis, epidermolysis bullosa, geographic tongue, burns, and erythema multiforme of the oral cavity may mimic thrush.

Diaper dermatitis, bacterial infection of intertriginous areas, Letterer-Siwe disease, linear immunoglobulin A (IgA) dermatosis, and maceration may mimic the intertriginous forms of candidiasis.

Congenital candidiasis may be confused with severe erythema toxicum, miliaria, transient neonatal pustular melanosis, infantile acropustulosis, ichthyosiform erythrodermas, and congenital syphilis or other intrauterine infections.

Paronychia due to *S. aureus* may mimic candidal paronychia, but usually has an acute onset, and the affected nail is tender and fluctuant. Psoriasis, lichen planus, and pachyonychia congenita should also be considered. Gonorrhea, *Trichomonas* infections, and chemical vaginitis may mimic vaginal candidiasis. Psoriasis, impetigo, and deep fungal infections such as sporotrichosis may be similar to candidal granulomas.

Acrodermatitis enteropathica and vitamin deficiency states may be confused with chronic mucocutaneous candidiasis.

Pathogenesis

C. albicans may be considered a part of the normal flora of the skin and mucous surfaces in certain body areas. Colonization of the oral cavity, intestinal tract, and vagina of healthy individuals is common.[19,20] Moisture, warmth, and breaks in the epidermal barrier permit overgrowth and invasion of the epidermis by the organism. It has been demonstrated that *C. albicans* generates inflammation by activation of the complement system within the skin and attraction of neutrophils to skin sites of *Candida* invasion. Keratolytic proteases and other enzymes in *C. albicans* species allow them to penetrate the epidermal barrier more easily than other organisms.[20]

Treatment

Topical therapy with several anticandidal agents is usually efficacious. For infantile thrush the use of nystatin oral suspension four times daily for 5 days is efficacious. In older children with thrush or angular cheilitis, clotrimazole troches may be useful.[20,21] For cutaneous candidosis, nystatin, oxiconazole, ketoconazole, ciclopirox, econazole, haloprogin, miconazole, or clotrimazole in a cream vehicle applied four times daily will result in prompt clearing of the lesions in 3 to 5 days. In the diaper area, application with each diaper change for 2 to 3 days is useful. The antifungal creams may sting or burn if there are breaks in the skin surface. Antiyeast ointments may be substituted.

Correction of the predisposing factors, such as good care of the diaper area, drying of intertriginous areas, and withdrawal of broad-spectrum antibiotics or glucocorticosteroids, is also important in the management of candidiasis. Treatment of candidal vulvovaginitis or candidal infections of the nipples in nursing mothers is valuable in the therapy of thrush.

The following specific treatment protocols may be utilized:

1. *Thrush* Apply nystatin solution topically to the area four times daily for 5 days. With recurrence, a second course of this therapy may be helpful. Simultaneous therapy of *Candida* vulvovaginitis or nipple infection in the mother is most helpful in reducing surface colonization with *C. albicans*. Discarding the infant's pacifier may help.

2. *Diaper candidiasis* Application of nystatin (or one of the other agents listed) in a cream form with each diaper change for 2 to 3 days is most useful if combined with the usual measures to keep the diaper area dry and cool.

3. *Paronychia* Nystatin cream applied nightly under occlusion (a plastic glove covered by a cotton stocking) for 3 to 4 weeks will often clear candidal paronychia. This should be done with caution in infants to be certain they do not aspirate the plastic into their airway.

Patient education

The patient or parents should understand that *C. albicans* is part of the normal skin flora in certain individuals and will reinvade susceptible tissue sites if the predisposing factors favoring overgrowth are not eliminated. Thus careful attention to the treatment of intertrigo and good diaper area care are essential to the long-term satisfactory results. Recurrences should be retreated.

Follow-up visits

An examination 5 to 7 days after initiating therapy is useful to evaluate the therapeutic response and reinforce the measures to diminish warmth and moisture in intertriginous areas. Most therapy failures are due to poor compliance, not host defense defects. Widespread involvement of oral cavity, nails, and skin should trigger a suspicion of immunodeficiency.

References

1. Sharma V, Hall JC, Knapp JF: Scalp colonization by *Trichophyton tonsurans* in an urban pediatric clinic, *Arch Dermatol* 124:1511, 1988.

2. Vargo K, Cohen BA: Prevalence of undetected tinea capitis in household members of children with disease, *Pediatrics* 91:155, 1993.

3. Hebert AA: Tinea capitis. Current concepts, *Arch Dermatol* 124:1554, 1988.

4. Miller MA, Hodgson Y: Sensitivity and specificity of potassium hydroxide smears of skin scrapings for the diagnosis of tinea pedis, *Arch Dermatol* 129:510, 1993.

5. Hubbard TW, De Triquet JM: Brush culture for diagnosing tinea capitis, *Pediatr Infect Dis J* 11:474, 1993.

6. Honig PJ, Caputo GL, Leyden JJ, et al: Microbiology of kerions, *J Pediatr* 123:422, 1993.

7. Honig PJ, Caputo GL, Leyden JJ, et al: Treatment of kerions, *Pediatr Dermatol* 11:69, 1994.

8. Gupta AK, Sauder DN, Shear NH: Antifungal agents. An overview. Part II. *J Am Acad Dermatol* 30:911, 1994.

9. Elewski BE: Tinea capitis: itraconazole in *Trichophyton tonsurans* infection, *J Am Acad Dermatol* 31:65, 1994.

10. Neil G, Hanslo D: Control of the carrier state of scalp dermatophytoses, *Pediatr Infect Dis J* 9:57, 1990.

11. Macura AB: Dermatophyte infections, *Int J Dermatol* 32:313 1993.

12. Goldgeier MH: Fungal infections of the skin, hair and nails, *Pediatr Ann* 22:253, 1993.

13. McBride A, Cohen BA: Tinea pedis in children, *Am J Dis Child* 146:844, 1992.

14. Savin J et al: Efficacy of terbinafine 1% cream in the treatment of moccasin-type tinea pedis, *J Am Acad Dermatol* 30:663, 1994.

15. Evans EGV: A comparison of terbinafine (Lamisil) 1% cream given for one week with clotrimazole (Canesten) 1% cream given for four weeks in the treatment of tinea pedis, *Br J Dermatol* 130(suppl 43):12, 1994.

16. Arikian SR, Einarson TR, Kobelt-Nguyen G, Schubert F: A multinational pharmacoeconomic analysis of oral therapies for onychomycosis, *Br J Dermatol* 139(suppl 43):35, 1994.

17. Nanda A, Kaur S, Bhakoo OK, et al: Pityriasis (tinea) versicolor in infancy, *Pediatr Dermatol* 5:260, 1988.

18. Ashbee HR, Ingham E, Holland KT, Cunliffe WJ: The carriage of *Malassezia furfur* serovars A, B and C in patients with pityriasis versicolor, seborrheic dermatitis and controls.

19. Report of the Committee on Infectious Diseases: *1994 Red Book.* Elk Grove Village, Il, 1994, American Academy of Pediatrics.

20. Thomas I: Superficial and deep candidosis, *Int J Dermatol* 32:778, 1993.

21. Fotos PG, Hellstein JW: *Candida* and candidosis, *Dent Clin North Am* 36:857, 1992.

22. Butler KM, Baker CJ: *Candida:* An increasingly important pathogen in the nursery, *Pediatr Clin North Am* 35:543, 1988.

23. Sahn EE: Widespread erythroderma and desquamation in a neonate, *Arch Dermatol* 129:1189, 1993.

7

Infestations

Arthropods are constantly present in the human environment, and hundreds of species are known to cause skin disease.[1,2] Biting and stinging insects may produce wheals, erythema, and even bullae from contact with the skin.[1,2] The erythematous papule with a central punctum is a common feature of insect bites. In this chapter, scabies, pediculoses, and papular urticaria are discussed in detail, since they are the most common forms of infestations and often require therapeutic intervention. Cutaneous eruptions related to ticks, spiders, mites, and helminths are also considered briefly. Arthropods may be divided into arachnids, which have eight legs (mites, ticks, spiders), and hexapods, with six legs (lice, mosquitoes, fleas, bedbugs, ants, bees, and other insects).

HUMAN MITE INFESTATION

Scabies
Clinical features
Pruritic papules on the abdomen, dorsa of the hands, flexural surface of the wrist, elbows, periaxillary skin, genitalia, and interdigital webs of the hands are seen in scabies[1] (Figs. 7-1 and 7-2). In infants eczematous eruptions of the face and trunk are seen in addition[1,3] (Fig. 7-3). In contrast, the head and neck regions are almost never involved in older children, adolescents, or adults. Most infants have acute dermatitis that is characterized by excoriations, erythematous papules, honey-colored crusts, and pustules. Secondary impetigo is common.

Crusted nodules that may become brown with time may be apparent on the trunk of the infant with scabies[1,3] (Fig. 7-4). When present, S-shaped burrows are diagnostic[1,3] (Fig. 7-5). They are usually found on the wrist, palm, interdigital webs, or genitalia. Nocturnal pruritus is severe. Within one household the disease may vary in severity from asymptomatic infested children to a child with a few nonpruritic papules to hundreds of lesions. Infants are likely to have dozens of lesions, whereas older children and adults may have less than 10 (Fig. 7-6). A high index of suspicion should be maintained in any patient with pruritic skin disease.

Children who are severely retarded and unable to scratch effectively may be infested with thousands of scabies mites, which produce a diffuse hyperkeratosis

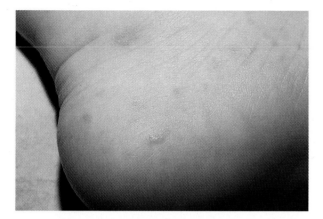

Fig. 7-1
Scabies. Papules and burrows on the foot of an infant.

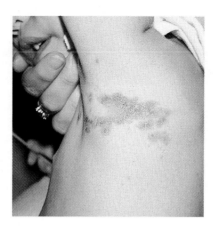

Fig. 7-3
Scabies. Nonspecific eczematous lesions in a child's axilla.

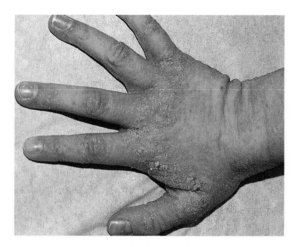

Fig. 7-2
Scabies. Involvement of the dorsa of the hands and interdigital webs in a child.

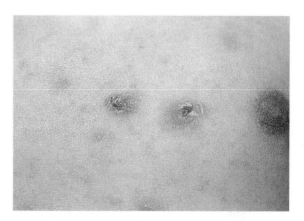

Fig. 7-4
Scabies. Crusted nodules on the trunk of an infant.

of the skin and lichenification that may be confused with ichthyosis.[1,3] Hyperkeratosis and scaling may be particularly prominent on the hands, feet, and genitalia.[1,3] This form of scabies is designated *Norwegian scabies* (Fig. 7-7). Children with malignancies may similarly suffer widespread scabies infestation, with extensive scalp involvement.[4]

Differential diagnosis
The diagnosis is confirmed by scraping an unscratched burrow that is covered with a drop of microscope immersion oil and placing the scrapings on a glass slide. Under the 10× objective of a microscope, the female mite, *Sarcoptes scabiei* (Fig. 7-8), and/or her eggs or feces should be visible (Fig. 7-9). Examination of skin scrapings obtained from the fingerwebs, wrists, or ankles is most likely to be positive.[1,3] Excoriated and crusted lesions are often negative. In children with Norwegian scabies, scraping of the thick scales will often yield several viable mites. Atopic dermatitis, lichen planus, dermatitis herpetiformis, and other severely pruritic skin conditions mimic scabies. Scabies should be suspected in any infant with a sudden onset of severely itchy dermati-

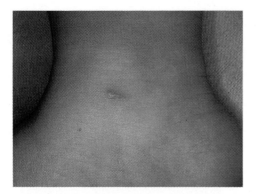

Fig. 7-5
S-shaped burrow diagnostic of scabies. This is the preferred lesion from which to obtain a scraping.

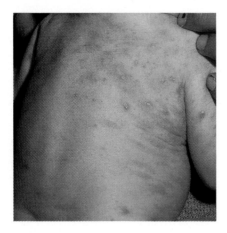

Fig. 7-6
Scabies in an infant. Hundreds of lesions are present.

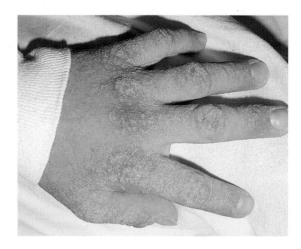

Fig. 7-7
Norwegian scabies. Diffuse scaling of the dorsum of the hand. Scraping of the scales revealed dozens of motile mites.

tis. A careful inspection for burrows, and identification of household members who may have a history of itchy bumps, are necessary. Seborrheic dermatitis of the scalp may mimic scabies seen in children with malignancy.[4]

Pathogenesis

Scabies is caused by the eight-legged human mite, *S. scabiei,* which may be up to 4 mm in length.[1,3] The female mite remains in the stratum corneum, which she traverses at a rate of 0.5 to 5 mm/day. She deposits her eggs during her journey and dies after 30 or 40 days. Her eggs reach maturity in 10 to 14 days,

and a new cycle begins. Transmission of scabies requires human contact, although female mites can survive 2 to 3 days off the human body. A pandemic of scabies has followed each major war of the twentieth century. Human scabies is quite contagious because newly infested individuals may not experience itching for the first 3 weeks of infestation, and only casual contact is required for spread of mites to others.[1,3] Humans are the reservoir for scabies, and infestation of children with animal mites (e.g., dog, cat, chicken) is rare.

Treatment

Application of a scabicide, such as 5% permethrin creme or 1% gamma benzene hexachloride lotion, is curative.[1,3-6] The lotion or cream should be dispensed as the calculated dose needed for therapy. In children and adolescents, application of 5% permethrin creme for 8 to 14 hours produces a 98% cure rate.[1,5,6] One 2-hour application of lindane lotion followed by a bath is curative in approximately 82% of cases; one 6-hour application cures 96% of cases.[3,5] Prolonged contact with the skin may result in significant percutaneous absorption. Gamma benzene hexachloride is concentrated in the central nervous system if absorbed; percutaneous absorp-

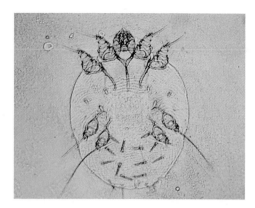

Fig. 7-8
Photomicrograph of female scabies mite recovered from scrapings of burrow.

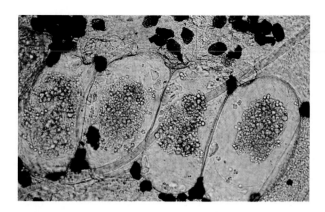

Fig. 7-9
Photomicrograph of oval eggs and dark brown scybala in skin scraping from an infant with scabies.

tion with central nervous system symptoms has been reported in a few infants. Recently some instances of lindane-resistant scabies in North America have been reported.[6] These individuals responded to 5% permethrin creme. In infants under 6 months of age, an alternative scabicide such as sulfur, 6% to 10% ointment twice daily for 3 days, may be substituted. Cautious use of 5% permethrin in infants under 6 months of age may be required. In any infant or toddler, covering the hands with clothing to prevent licking the scabicide from the skin is recommended. For children with only a few lesions, routine retreatment is not necessary.[1] In infants with extensive involvement, several retreatments may occasionally be required. Simultaneous treatment of all household contacts is required.[1,5,6]

Even with the elimination of all viable scabies mites and eggs, itching may persist for 7 to 10 days after successful therapy. Despite the persistence of pruritus, no new lesions should be detected. Treatment failures are often the result of poor compliance or failure to treat an infested household member.

Patient education

One should emphasize the mode of transmission of scabies and identify all household contacts. Instructions on the treatment schedule should be specific; the persistence of itching even after scabicidal therapy and the importance of treating all household contacts should be emphasized.

Follow-up visits

A follow-up visit in 2 weeks is important to ascertain success or failure of therapy. Any new lesions that may have appeared should be rescraped to determine whether infestation has persisted or whether the child is reinfested. If the mite or her products are found, retreatment is suggested. Infants, who tend to have hundreds of lesions, may require several retreatments.

Other mite infestations
Clinical features

Mites from nonhuman sources occasionally infest the skin of children. The canine scabies mite, usually carried on the fur of puppies with mange, may be temporarily transferred to the child.[1] The puppy will have fur loss and crusted lesions. Similarly, harvest mites or chiggers, found in grasses, grains, or overgrowth of bushes, may similarly infest children. Grain mites found in stored seeds and grains and fowl mites found on chickens or domesticated birds, such as canaries, pigeons, or swallows, may also infest children. In each instance the clinical lesions are characterized by urticarial papules, sometimes with hemorrhagic puncta, and, in intense responses, blister formation. Burrows are absent. The distribution on the child's skin depends on the location of the exposed skin. Characteristically, canine scabies produces lesions on the forearms, the abdomen, and the thighs. Harvest mites characteristically produce lesions on the legs and around the beltline. Grain mite lesions occur on the exposed areas of the arms and legs but may be quite generalized. Fowl mites produce lesions on exposed areas of skin.

Differential diagnosis

Scabies and papular urticaria are the most important in the differential diagnosis. A history of exposure to the appropriate source is most significant in the diagnosis of mite infestation. Important historical information includes the new puppy with hair loss and crusts on his skin, exposure to deep grasses and grain or stored grain, and association with birds. Exposed skin infested with fowl mites may mimic a photoeruption.

Pathogenesis

In each case the mites attach themselves to the skin to inject an irritating secretion and then fall off in a few days. Identifying the mites within skin lesions is very difficult. They do not persist on skin, however.

Treatment

Symptomatic relief with topical steroids or oral antihistamines, or both, is useful. Specific scabicides are not required.

Patient education

Prophylaxis is an important part of patient education. Treatment of the infested puppy, the use of good insect repellents (e.g., 6.5% diethyltoluamide [DEET]), and staying away from those areas containing sources that are likely to produce the infestation should be emphasized. Parents and children should know that they cannot pass this eruption to others, and that itching can be quite severe, lasting for several weeks after the initial exposure.

Follow-up visits

A follow-up visit in 2 weeks to ascertain the institution of prophylaxis and the response to therapy is useful.

Ticks
Clinical features

Tick bites are usually painless and inapparent to the child. Usually the tick is noted several days after contact with the skin when pruritus begins. Localized urticarial reactions can be found. A diagnosis is usually made by identifying the presence of the tick in particular cutaneous locations. The most common sites for tick attachment are the occipital scalp (Fig. 7-10), ear canal, axilla, groin, and vulva.[7] Rarely a systemic reaction to a tick bite, characterized by fever, nausea, abdominal cramping, and headache, may occur, as may paralysis similar to Guillain-Barré syndrome, with ascending symmetric paralysis. A persistent, pruritic nodule, sometimes surrounded by hair loss, may be the result of an incompletely removed tick in which mouthparts remain in the skin. Since ticks in certain areas of North America and Europe may carry *Borrelia burgdorferi,* the spirochete responsible for Lyme disease, observation for expanding rings of erythema about the site of the bite is advised for 3 weeks after the bite (see Chapter 5). The potentially severe nature of Lyme disease, and its prominence in the news media, has prompted excessive concern regarding tick bites.[7]

Differential diagnosis

Most tick bite reactions are obvious, since the tick is found attached to the skin. If the mouthparts are left

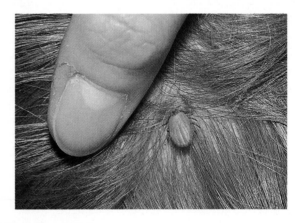

Fig. 7-10
Tick embedded in the occipital scalp of a child.

in and a pruritic nodule remains, the diagnosis may be quite difficult to distinguish from scabies, lichen simplex chronicus, or other infestations. The expanding annular red rings of erythema chronicum migrans may be confused with ringworm, urticaria, or other annular conditions.

Pathogenesis

Tick bites may occur when children play in the woods and when ticks are transferred from dogs or other incidental hosts to children. The tick attaches itself to the skin by its head in an effort to suck blood. The tick cuts the skin surface with chelicerae, introduces its proboscis, and secretes saliva into the wound. The saliva contains a cement substance, anesthetic, and anticoagulant, and may include the neurotoxin responsible for tick paralysis or the spirochete responsible for Lyme disease. The tick engorges with blood from the child, which allows *Borrelia* to proliferate in the tick gut and then reenter the child, after 24 to 48 hours, from the tick saliva.[7] A foreign body granuloma is seen in persistent nodules in the skin where tick head parts remain.

Treatment

Removal of the tick is the treatment of choice. The preferred method of removal is the insertion of a blunt instrument, such as a forceps or tweezers, between the tick head and the child's skin[7] (Fig. 7-11). Gentle outward pressure will cause the tick to

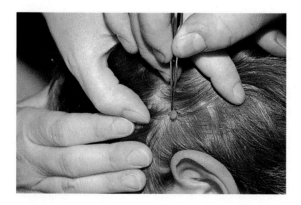

Fig. 7-11
Removal of tick by placing a forceps between the tick and the skin.

back out. This method prevents any injury to the skin and the retention of tick parts within the skin. One should avoid all methods that may injure the skin, such as burning the tick or using noxious substances on the skin. One should not squeeze the body of the tick, and if there is a remnant in the skin, one should consider simple surgical removal. If in an area endemic for Lyme disease, one should save the tick in a glass jar for analysis if the child become ill later. Use of a topical antibiotic, such as tetracycline, after tick removal may prevent Lyme disease.[8]

Patient education

Prevention is the best method for tick bites. Children should try to avoid tick habitats as much as possible, such as dense brush or tall grass, and stay in the center of the path on wooded trails.[7] Children should wear protective clothing, such as long sleeves and caps, preferably of light color so the ticks can be easily seen.[7] They should wear a shirt with a collar to prevent migration and tuck their pants into boots or socks. In endemic areas the regular and careful use of insect repellents, such as 6.5% DEET, during tick season is recommended. Children and their dogs should be routinely inspected for ticks if they have been in wooded areas, and parents advised of the most common locations of tick bites and the preferred method of removal. It should be emphasized that most ticks do not carry Lyme disease.

Follow-up visits

A follow-up visit 2 weeks after a bite to observe for signs of erythema chronicum migrans should be considered in areas endemic for Lyme disease.

Spiders
Clinical features

Hemorrhagic, painful blisters may appear on the skin and evolve over the next few days into a cutaneous infarct with skin necrosis and dry, gangrenous eschar (Fig. 7-12). This reaction usually occurs on exposed areas of skin in a single lesion around the site of a spider bite. The area of skin loss may be large.[2] Systemic reactions, including headache, nausea, vomit-

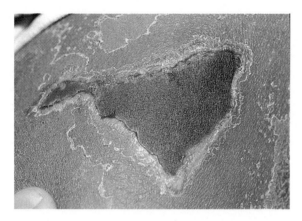

Fig. 7-12.
Spider bite. Central necrosis with eschar and surrounding giant erythema.

ing, chills, malaise, syncope, and coma, may develop.[2] Thrombocytopenia, hemolysis, and hemoglobinuria, which might result in renal failure, have been reported.

Differential diagnosis

Spider bites must be differentiated from other forms of vascular infarction, such as vasculitis. In vasculitis, numerous lesions are present, whereas in spider bites, a single lesion is seen. Other necrotizing infections such as ecthyma gangrenosum, due to *Pseudomonas* infection, and streptococcal gangrene syndrome should be considered in the differential diagnosis. Lesions of herpes zoster, herpes simplex, cutaneous diphtheria, or anthrax may occasionally be confused with spider bite. In children who do not give a definite history of a spider bite, viral and bacterial cultures may be required.

Pathogenesis

Spiders with venom jaws powerful enough to penetrate human skin such as the *Loxosceles* species produce necrotic skin reactions. In North America, the brown recluse spider (*Loxosceles reclusa*) is usually responsible for the lesion.[2] This spider is very prevalent in the midwestern United States but has occasionally been reported over many other areas of North America. The spider is small, 8 to 10 mm in diameter, and bears a violin-shaped band over the dorsal thorax.

It is often found in old buildings. A number of toxins have been found in the venom. Neurotoxins are carried by *Latrodectus* spiders, including black widow spiders. These spiders are responsible for systemic symptoms following a spider bite.

Treatment

High doses of oral corticosteroids may be useful in reducing or preventing the extent of tissue damage in necrotic spider bites. Doses of 2 mg/kg/day of prednisone are usually recommended for a period of 5 days. Surgical removal of the necrotic area has been performed in some instances to prevent spread of the toxin. Hospitalization may be required in severe toxic reactions.

Patient education

One should emphasize that spiders of this type may hide in basements and that recognition of the small, thin-legged spider is important. Children should be kept from abandoned buildings, woodpiles, or other sites favored by spiders.

Follow-up visits

A daily follow-up visit, following initiation of treatment for the spider bite, is necessary to evaluate for the development of systemic symptoms and progression of the individual lesion. The child should be seen until healing is observed.

Pediculoses (louse infestations)
Clinical features

Excoriated papules and pustules on the trunk and perineum are found in children and adolescents with body louse infestations.[1] Often only excoriations or their resultant hyperpigmented or hypopigmented scars are seen on the skin. The louse may be discovered by closely examining the seams of the patient's underwear or the scalp hair. The gelatinous nits of the head louse appear as white, ovoid bodies tightly adherent to the hair shaft[1,9] (Figs. 7-13 and 7-14). Nocturnal pruritus is often severe with all human louse infestations. The prevalence of louse infestations is 34 times higher in whites than in blacks.

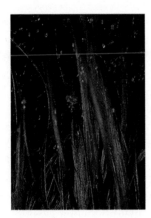

Fig. 7-13
Head lice. Numerous white nits attached to hairs.

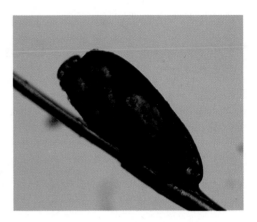

Fig. 7-14
Head lice. Photomicrograph of nit tightly adherent to one side of a hair shaft.

The pubic (crab) louse may be seen crawling among the pubic hairs, or infestation with the pubic louse may present as blue-black crusted macules (maculae ceruleae) in the pubic area.[1] Nits may also be seen attached to pubic hairs. The pubic louse may be seen in the eyelashes or the scalp of newborns.[10] Any "bug" seen crawling from the newborn's eye should be considered a pubic louse unless proved otherwise.

Differential diagnosis

Scabies, dermatitis herpetiformis, neurotic excoriations, and other highly pruritic dermatoses may be confused with pediculoses. Parents with delusions of parasitosis may transfer their delusion to their children. In certain children the retained external hair-root sheath may resemble head louse nits. Retained root sheaths may be easily removed by sliding them distally down the hair shaft, while the nit is tightly adherent to it. The blue-black, crusted macules of pubic lice may be confused with vasculitis, folliculitis, or impetigo.

Pathogenesis

The human louse, a six-legged insect, attaches itself to the skin, ingests blood, and produces skin lesions by mechanical puncture and perhaps by injecting toxic secretions.[1] There are two species of human lice, *Pediculus humanus,* the body louse, which has subspecies *capitis* (head lice) and *humanus* (body lice), and *Pthirus pubis,* the crab louse.[1] The body louse, which is 2 to 4 mm in length, is the longest of the lice that infest humans; the pubic louse is 1 to 2 mm in length. The female produces new offspring every 2 weeks, and each female may produce over 80 offspring during her lifetime. The body louse produces more eggs during her lifetime than the pubic louse. Newly hatched lice mate with old, and hundreds of nits result every 2 weeks. The female louse attaches herself to a hair and slides along it, laying eggs. If hair is not available, clothing fibers are used. Crowded living conditions are most conducive to the spread of lice, which can be transmitted either by person-to-person contact or by fomites, such as hairbrushes, caps, scarves, coats, or carpets. Sharing of clothing is a common source of transmission.[1,9]

Treatment

The application of 1% gamma benzene hexachloride lotion to the affected skin area for 12 to 24 hours is effective in body lice infestation.[1] For head lice or crab lice infestations, 1% gamma benzene hexachloride shampoo, 1% permethrin shampoo, or 0.3% pyrethrin shampoo applied for 10 minutes and then rinsed out results in an 80% cure rate.[9] Shampoo treatments will not, however, remove the gelatinous nits. The use of a warm damp towel for 30 minutes on the scalp will loosen the nits and allow their mechanical removal with a fine-toothed comb (nit comb).[10] Most pediculocide shampoos are supplied with a nit comb. Retreatment in 7 days is recommended. Measuring the distance of the nit closest to the scalp surface will provide a baseline measurement to help determine adequacy of treatment on follow-up. Boiling of clothing, bedding, and other possible fomites is ovicidal and lousicidal and necessary as nits may be attached to clothing.

Patient education

It is tempting for parents to use pediculicides repeatedly in children with lice infestations. One should emphasize the hazards of central nervous system toxicity posed by such usage. All contacts should be identified and treated simultaneously. Students should be readmitted to school the morning after the first treatment. Parents should be advised that mechanical removal of nits is required. Schoolmates should be examined by the school nurse to determine if other children are infested.

Follow-up visits

An office or visiting nurse follow-up to evaluate therapy 1 week after the initial visit is most helpful. If new eggs or nits are seen on the proximal hair shafts, as close or closer to the scalp than the original measurement, then retreatment is necessary. Nits will grow out with the hair shaft and by 7 days after successful treatment should be at least 6 to 7 mm from the scalp margin.

Papular urticaria
Clinical features

Pruritic erythematous papules, with or without an erythematous, urticarial flare, are characteristically arranged in clusters in papular urticaria (Fig. 7-16).[11,12] Such clusters are usually seen over the shoulders, upper arms, and buttocks. Papular urticaria occurs predominantly between the ages of 18 months and 7 years.[12] In intense hypersensitivity, vesicles and bullae may be seen. Recurrent crops of these papules are the rule, with each crop lasting 2 to 10 days (Figs. 7-15 and 7-16). Characteristically the affected child is the only household member involved. The problem may persist from 3 to 9 months and most often begins in spring or summer.

Differential diagnosis

Insect bites, viral exanthems, photoeruptions, acute parapsoriasis, and the early stages of other papu-

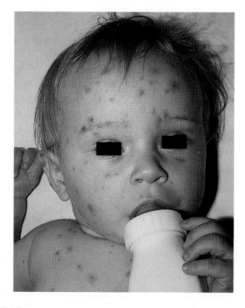

Fig. 7-15.
Papular urticaria. Numerous central papules or edematous papules surrounded by an outer zone of urticaria.

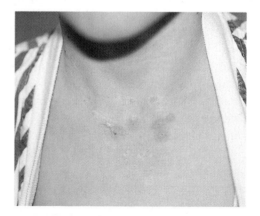

Fig. 7-16.
Papular urticaria. Grouped lesions on the lower neck where a puppy was carried by the child.

losquamous diseases (see Chapter 9) may be confused with papular urticaria.

Pathogenesis

The lesions represent delayed hypersensitivity reactions to a variety of biting or stinging arthropods.[12] Dog and cat fleas are the usual offenders. Less commonly, mosquitoes, lice, scabies, fowl mites, and grain or grass mites are responsible. Epicutaneous testing with homogenized arthropods has reproduced the urticarial papule within 4 to 8 hours. The pathologic features of naturally occurring lesions are similar to those of a delayed-type (tuberculin) skin test.

Treatment

The logical therapy is to remove the offending insect. Dogs or cats should be treated for fleas or mites by a veterinarian. The child should be kept away from the pet. Protective clothing, such as long sleeves, may be useful. The prophylactic use of an oral antihistamine, cetirizine, may reduce the reactions.[13] Use of DEET-containing insect repellents may make the child less attractive to the insect. Caution should be used to not use DEET on large areas of skin or in concentrations greater than 10%.[14] DEET preparations that are 6.5%, such as Skeddaddle, may be used cautiously on the child's skin. Fleas or mites living in carpets or furniture may be eliminated by treatment with a commercial insecticide. Window casings should be treated in the case of bird mites.

Symptomatic relief may sometimes be obtained with topical low-potency glucocorticosteroid creams applied three times daily.

Patient education

When only one member of the household is affected, it is difficult to convince some parents of the cause. The extreme sensitivity of the affected person to the offending arthropod should be explained. Often an obvious source is not evident from the initial history, and a thorough search should be made for the source including inquiries into day care, preschool, and visits to neighbors, friends, and relatives. It is a great relief to both the parents and the child to learn that the sensitivity is transient.

Follow-up visits

A visit within 2 weeks is most useful in reviewing the possible sources and evaluating the response to therapeutic measures. At the follow-up visit it is often easier to convince parents of the cause of the eruption.

HELMINTHS

Cutaneous larva migrans (creeping eruption)

Clinical features

Pruritic, serpiginous, erythematous linear lesions of the skin that advance at the rate of 1 cm/day represent the classic pattern seen in cutaneous larva migrans[15] (Fig. 7-17). Lesions are usually on the feet (Fig. 7-18) and occasionally the arms or legs. Vesicles and bullae may be present along the tract, and pulsatile edema within the erythematous, serpiginous tract may be observed.[15] Some children complain of pain at the site, and edema of the area is noted in about 25%.[15] A history of a child having played along the shorelines of the southeastern or eastern United States is usually obtained. A second clinical form involves strictly the perianal area, buttocks, and thighs, with serpiginous tracts that spread 5 to 10 cm/hr. The child may have peripheral blood eosinophilia, with 10% to 35% eosinophils present.

Differential diagnosis

The annular erythemas, including erythema chronicum migrans, urticaria, and even tinea infections, may be confused with cutaneous larva migrans. The rapid progression and advancement of the border in cutaneous larva migrans and the presence of pulsations within the serpiginous tract are useful differentiating features.

Pathogenesis

Two larvae are responsible for the cutaneous lesions in cutaneous larva migrans found in North America.

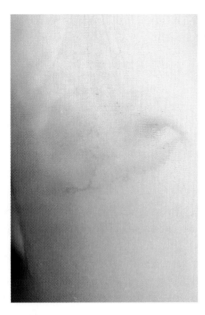

Fig. 7-17
Creeping eruption. Serpiginous red track on the plantar surface of a child with *A. braziliensis* infestation.

Ancylostoma braziliensis is the most common of these larvae and produces the clinical pattern involving the feet.[15] Children playing along the shore of the southern United States are at the greatest risk. *A. braziliensis* is the dog and cat hookworm, and ova of this organism are deposited in the soil or in the sandy beaches from dog and cat excretions and hatch into larvae that will penetrate bare skin.[15] The larvae migrate 1 to 2 cm/day and produce the serpiginous lesions of the skin. Stools are negative for parasite eggs, and identification of the larvae within the tract is quite difficult, since they are often found beyond the area of obvious inflammation. This parasite cannot complete its life cycle in humans, and the larvae disappear within 4 to 6 weeks of their onset. The second form of cutaneous larva migrans is due to the larvae of *Strongyloides stercoralis*. These larvae usually penetrate the skin near the anus and spread onto the buttocks. They are able to leave the skin and may settle in the gastrointestinal tract, and a stool sample examined for ova and parasites will identify the *Strongyloides* larvae or eggs. Larvae from fish or squid nematodes may also produce a creeping eruption.[16]

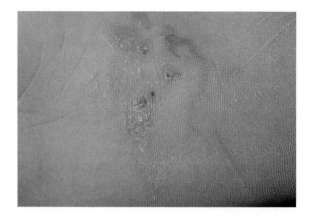

Fig. 7-18
Creeping eruption. Serpiginous tract accompanied by crusted and excoriated lesions from the child's scratching.

Treatment
Topical thiabendazole 15% cream, applied three times a day for 5 to 7 days, is the treatment of choice for creeping eruption due to *A. braziliensis*.[15] Parents should be instructed to treat well beyond the area of obvious skin redness. Oral thiabendazole is also quite effective in a dose of 25 to 50 mg/kg given for 2 to 4 days, and should be used for creeping eruption due to *S. stercoralis*.[15] Oral albendazole and ivermectin have also been shown to be very efficacious.[17]

Patient education
Parents should understand that these infestations may be acquired from sandy beaches or sandboxes, and only in certain regions of North America. Further, they should know that the lesions are not contagious to other children and that usually one treatment protocol is curative.

Follow-up visits
A visit at 4 to 5 days after initiation of therapy is useful to evaluate the response.

Swimmers' itch and seabather's eruption
Clinical features
Pruritic papules appearing in areas not protected by the swimsuit are characteristic of swimmers' eruption, which has occurred in those who swam in freshwater

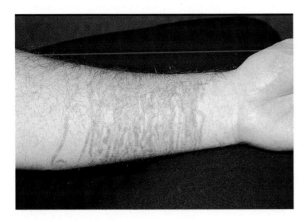

Fig. 7-19
Jellyfish eruption. Multiple linear erythematous areas where jellyfish tentacles contacted the skin.

lakes of the upper Great Lakes region of North America. In seabather's eruption the pruritic papules occur under the swimsuit-covered areas, after swimming in salt waters of the southern United States.[18] At other times jellyfish stings may be linear when the jellyfish tentacles strike the skin (Fig. 7-19). The papules or linear lesions are persistent and may last for at least 2 weeks in both conditions.

Differential diagnosis

Papular urticaria, insect bite reactions, and infestations due to scabies or other mites should be considered in the differential diagnosis. The strong historical and temporal association with swimming is a very useful differentiating point. Linear lesions of jellyfish stings may mimic phytophotodermatitis, where plants such as tall grasses contact the skin and produce linear erythema or vesicles.

Pathogenesis

Parasitic flatworms have been implicated in swimmers' itch. Cercariae are released into the water from infected snails in freshwater lakes of the upper Great Lakes region. The parasites finish their cycle by penetrating the skin of warm-blooded hosts, but do not survive after penetration. The schistosomes usually come from the droppings of infested mammals and waterfowl and are then involved with the snail as

intermediate host. Seabather's eruption is due to cercariae of the *Linuche ungauiculata* jellyfish.[18] When the seawater containing jellyfish larvae flows through the bathing suit, the larvae contact the skin and discharge nematocysts. Linear lesions are the direct result of contact with jellyfish tentacles.

Treatment

Since this is a self-limited disease, no specific anticercaria treatment need be introduced. Symptomatic treatment, such as the use of topical steroid preparations or oral antihistamines, or both, is usually recommended. In severe eruptions oral prednisone for 5 days may be considered.[18]

Patient education

Parents and patients should have an explanation of the source of the itchy eruption and should know that it cannot be transmitted from the infested individual to other humans. They should also be told to recognize that this disease is self-limited and will disappear.

Follow-up visits

Follow-up visits are usually unnecessary.

References

1. Colven RM, Prose NS: Parasitic infestations of the skin, *Pediatr Ann* 23:436, 1994.
2. Warrell DA, Fenner PJ: Venomous bites and stings, *Br Med Bull* 49:423, 1993.
3. Paller AS: Scabies in infants and small children, *Semin Dermatol* 12:3, 1993.
4. Duran C, Tamayo L, de la Luz Orozco M, Ruiz-Maldonado R: Scabies of the scalp mimicking seborrheic dermatitis in immunocompromised patients, *Pediatr Dermatol* 10:136, 1993.
5. Orkin M, Maibach HI: Scabies therapy—1993. *Semin Dermatol* 12:22, 1993.
6. Purvis RS, Tyring SK: An outbreak of lindane-resistant scabies treated successfully with 5% permethrin cream, *J Am Acad Dermatol* 25:1015, 1991.

7. Melski JW: Primary and secondary erythema migrans in central Wisconsin, *Arch Dermatol* 129:709, 1993.

8. Shih C-M, Spielman A: Topical prophylaxis for Lyme disease after tick bite in a rodent model, *J Infect Dis* 168:1042, 1993.

9. Janniger CK, Kuflik AS: *Pediculosis capitis, Cutis* 51:407, 1993.

10. Clore ER, Longyear LA: A comparative study of seven pediculicides and their packaged nit removal combs, *J Pediatr Health Care* 7:55, 1993.

11. Harford-Cross M: Tendency to being bitten by insects among patients with eczema and with other dermatoses, *Br J Gen Pract* 43:339, 1993.

12. Massie FS: Papular urticaria: etiology, diagnosis and management, *Cutis* 13:980, 1974.

13. Reunala T, Brummer-Korvenkontio H, Karppinen A, et al: Treatment of mosquito bites with cetirizine, *Clin Exp Allergy* 23:72, 1993.

14. Couch P, Johnson CE: Prevention of Lyme disease, *Am J Hosp Pharm* 49:1164, 1992.

15. Davies HD, Sakuls P, Keystone JS: Creeping eruption, *Arch Dermatol* 129:588, 1993.

16. Okazaki A, Ida T, Shirai T, et al: Creeping disease due to larva of spiruoid nematoda, *Int J Dermatol* 32:813, 1993.

17. Caumes E, Carriere J, Datry A, et al: A randomized trial of ivermectin versus albendazole for the treatment of cutaneous larva migrans, *Am J Trop Med Hyg* 49:641, 1993.

18. Tomchik RS, Russell MT, Szmant AM: Clinical perspectives on seabather's eruption, also known as "sea lice," *JAMA* 269:1669, 1993.

8

Viral Infections

Viruses may involve the skin by either dissemination to skin during a systemic viral infection accompanied by viral replication in skin (viral exanthem) or by producing a virus-induced skin tumor. A number of viruses are epidermotropic and replicate within keratinocytes.

VIRAL EXANTHEMS

Any cutaneous eruption associated with an acute viral syndrome has been termed a *viral exanthem*. If mucosa is involved, it is termed an *enanthem*. The exact incidence of viral exanthems is unknown, but herpes simplex alone accounts for a yearly incidence of 5.1 children affected per 1000.[1] Most clinicians who care for children report that viral exanthems are common. Enteroviral exanthems are the most frequently encountered in the United States and account for the majority of viral exanthems seen.[1] It should be emphasized that all viruses may cause an exanthem, including those that are rarely associated with an exanthem.[1]

Viral exanthems are seen frequently in general pediatric settings and are considered in the differential diagnosis of drug eruptions. Frequently the clinician will see a child with a generalized eruption who received a medication for the illness. There is no current method to reliably distinguish a viral exanthem from a drug eruption.[1] A variety of different patterns of viral exanthem are seen: a generalized maculopapular eruption that mimics measles (morbilliform), petechial eruptions, vesiculobullous eruptions, scarlet fever–like (scarlatiniform) eruptions, papulonodular eruptions, and oral erosions.[1] Morbilliform eruptions are the most common. It is important to recall that any viral exanthem, including morbilliform eruptions, may have a photodistribution.[1-3] Some exanthems may also be photoactivated by ultraviolet injury.[4] Skin injury by factors other than ultraviolet light may also result in localization of the viral exanthem to the site of injury.[3] Exanthems may also be unilateral as reported in the asymmetric periflexural exanthem[5,6] (Fig. 8-1).

VIRAL EXANTHEMS: THE MORBILLIFORM ERUPTIONS

An eruption that mimics measles (morbilli) is called a morbilliform eruption.[1,7] They are seen as generalized, discrete, red to pink macules. The morbilliform

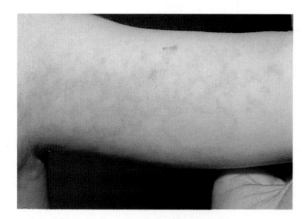

Fig. 8-1
Asymmetric periflexural exanthem. Annular erythema on the inner arm and adjacent axilla in an 8-year-old child.

eruptions include measles, rubella, enteroviral and adenoviral exanthems, roseola, the mononucleosis syndromes, and erythema infectiosum (EI). Many other viruses may occasionally produce a morbilliform eruption (see Box 8-1).

Measles (rubeola)
Clinical features
Classic measles. The features of classic measles include a severe prodrome followed by an exanthematous phase. During the entire course of the illness, the child appears quite ill. After an incubation period of 9 to 14 days, a prodrome of high fever, cough, rhinitis, and conjunctivitis appears.[1,7] The cough is described as "barking," and a diagnosis of bronchitis or croup is usually considered. The prodrome typically includes cervical lymphadenopathy and lasts 3 to 5 days.[1] The preauricular lymph nodes are enlarged. The prodrome is then followed by a cutaneous eruption.

The exanthem begins on the forehead as blotchy erythema and progresses to involve the face, trunk, and extremities with multiple discrete macules and papules (Fig. 8-2). The eruption is preceded by intense erythema of the mucous membranes with focal 1 mm white areas, the so-called Koplik's spots[8] (Fig. 8-3). Bacterial otitis media, bacterial pneumonia, and encephalitis may complicate measles.[1,7] Their exact incidence in

measles is unknown. Severe pneumonia and encephalitis are primary causes of death in measles, and are more likely to complicate measles in young infants, the malnourished or immunodeficient child. Mortality in the United States is estimated at 1 per 1000.[1] Low vitamin A levels, in particular, have been implicated in the severity of measles.[9] Other complications of measles include myocarditis, pericarditis, thrombocytopenia, hepatitis, acute glomerulonephritis, and Stevens-Johnson syndrome.[1]

Atypical measles. In patients who have received killed measles vaccine, or in whom live

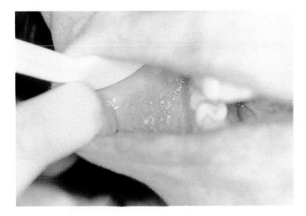

Fig. 8-2
Red macules and conjunctival erythema in a child with rubeola (measles).

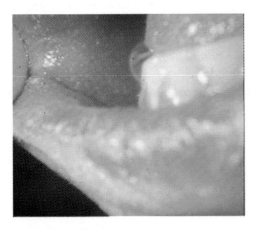

Fig. 8-3
Koplik's spots. Bright erythema of buccal mucosa with pinpoint white macules in rubeola.

Box 8-2   Differential diagnosis of morbilliform eruptions

Common viruses
  Measles
  Rubella
  Roseola
  Erythema infectiosum
  Infectious mononucleosis
  Pityriasis rosea
Common bacteria
  Scarlet fever
Drug eruptions
  Ampicillin
  Penicillin
  Nonsteroidal antiinflammatory drugs
  Salicylic acid
  Barbiturates
  Phenytoins
  Phenothiazines
  Thiazide diuretics
  Isoniazid
Papulosquamous disorders
  Guttate psoriasis
  Graft-vs.-host disease
  Reactive erythemas
  Urticaria
  Papular urticaria
  Erythema multiforme

measles vaccination has failed, a syndrome of high fever, abdominal pain, pulmonary, consolidation, and an acral eruption consisting of vesicular, vesiculopustular, or purpuric lesions may occur (atypical measles)[1] (Fig. 8-4).

Differential diagnosis

Classic measles.   The severity of the prodrome, a high fever, and Koplik's spots in an acutely ill child are the most distinctive features differentiating measles from the other morbilliform eruptions (Boxes 8-1 and 8-2). Viral isolation from mucosa, while difficult, will distinguish measles from other exanthems. Acute and convalescent sera, obtained 1 week and 3 weeks after the onset of the illness, will assist with a retrospective diagnosis.

Atypical measles.   Atypical measles may mimic meningococcemia and Rocky Mountain spotted fever, which are the main considerations in the differential diagnosis. Primarily acral petechiae may be the presenting symptom in echovirus 9 and other enterovirus infections. Other conditions to be considered in the differential diagnosis are listed in Box 8-3.

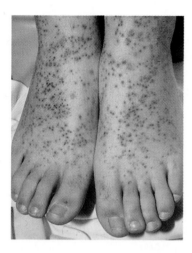

Fig. 8-4
Petechiae and palpable purpura on the feet of an adolescent with atypical measles.

Pathogenesis

Despite the very active measles immunization program in the United States, outbreaks of measles continue to occur.[7,10-12] Measles has not been eradicated because 35% of children are never immunized, and immunization fails in up to 15% of those immunized.[12,13] Reimmunization is now recommended because of the high rate of vaccine failure.[11-13]

The cutaneous eruption is related to the presence of the measles virus within keratinocytes and endothelial cells of the superficial dermal vessels.[1] The clinical lesions are believed to be due to the host response to the virus within the skin. The measles virus, a paramyxovirus, replicates within keratinocytes and induces increased nuclear volume within the epidermal cells, producing multinucleated giant cells (Warthin-Finkeldy cells).

The purpuric cutaneous eruption of atypical measles is thought to be the result of immune complex formation.[14]

Treatment

No specific treatment is available for measles or atypical measles. Symptomatic treatment should be provided and children monitored closely for complications. If secondary bacterial otitis media or bacterial pneumonia occurs, antibiotic therapy should be instituted.

Patient education

The high attack rate of measles should be emphasized, and the patient should be isolated during the contagious period (from the onset of respiratory symptoms through the third day of the cutaneous eruption). Unvaccinated normal infants and children should receive a preventive dose of immune serum globulin, 0.25 ml/kg intramuscularly, as soon as possible after exposure, and 8 weeks later they should be vaccinated with live attenuated measles virus vaccine, provided the child is at least 15 months old.[13] Unvaccinated infants and children with malignancies or immunodeficiencies, or those receiving immunosuppressive therapy, should be given 0.5 ml/kg of immune serum globulin intramuscularly to a maximum dose of 15 ml.[13] Exposure to measles is not a contraindication to vaccination if given within 72 hours of exposure.

Follow-up visits

Close contact should be maintained with the patient with rubeola to watch for bacterial superinfection, the development of severe pneumonia with pulmonary compromise, or encephalitis. A prompt revisit should be scheduled if fever recurs, headache or change in the level of consciousness is observed, or seizures or motor defects are noted. Frequent visits may be required during the course of the illness.

Rubella

Clinical features

Classic rubella. Classic rubella is a mild illness in most children. Rubella acquired postnatally in infants and children usually is accompanied by few or no prodromal symptoms.[1] Up to 50% of rubella infections may be entirely asymptomatic.[1,13] Mild lymphadenopathy may precede the cutaneous eruption by several days. The suboccipital and posterior auricular lymph nodes are usually prominently enlarged. A faint pink, macular eruption appears first on the face and spreads to the trunk and proximal extremities. Within 48 hours, the face and trunk have cleared and the eruption involves the distal extremities.[1,13] The child usually appears well. Rarely, petechiae or purpura may be seen. A monoarthric arthritis may accompany the syndrome, particularly in adolescent girls.[15-17] It may present as the so-called STAR (sore throat, arthritis, rash) complex. In the STAR complex, rubella and human parvovirus B19 are the most likely viruses responsible.[17] The arthritis may persist for several months. Fever is usually absent in young children with rubella, but may be present in older children and adolescents, particularly when arthritis is present.[1,13, 15-17]

Congenital rubella. Rubella acquired during the first trimester of pregnancy may result in rubella embryopathy.[18-20] This may be manifested by neonatal purpura and petechiae due to thrombocytopenia.[19] Of causes of congenital thrombocytopenia, rubella is responsible for 10%.[19] Occasionally jaundice due to rubella hepatitis occurs. Accompanying features include deafness, congenital heart defects, cataract, glaucoma, growth retardation, and psychomotor retardation.[18-20] Any or all of these features may accompany the typical rubella exanthem. Rubella embryopathy can even be found during reinfection of the mother with rubella.[20] The exanthem may recur any time during the first 5 years. In infants with congenital rubella, rubella virus may be recovered from peripheral blood leukocytes, stool, or urine for months to years after birth.[1]

Differential diagnosis

Classic rubella. In distinguishing classic rubella from rubeola, the absence of fever is helpful.[1] Rubella may be difficult to distinguish from enteroviral exanthems, infectious mononucleosis syndromes, or drug eruptions.[1] In the STAR complex, rubella may be indistinguishable from human parvovirus B19 infections or from other viral causes of the exanthem (see Box 8-3).[16,17] Culture of the virus from nasal mucosa will distinguish rubella from other exanthems.

Congenital rubella. Other congenital infections may produce the thrombocytopenia and hepatitis seen with rubella.[19] These include toxoplasmosis, syphilis, cytomegalovirus (CMV), and herpes simplex virus (HSV). Rarely, neonatal lupus, Wiskott-Aldrich syndrome, and hereditary platelet disorders may mimic congenital rubella.[1,19] The presence of cataracts and congenital heart defects should suggest congenital rubella. Viral cultures of urine and throat will distinguish rubella from other congenital infections.

Pathogenesis

Rubella virus, a rubrivirus, is a ribonucleic acid (RNA) virus that enters the bloodstream via the respiratory mucosa. The mechanism of the exanthem is unknown but is believed to be the result of viral dissemination to skin. Rubella virus has been cultured from the synovia in rubella arthritis.[1,20] Rubella embryopathy is still seen because young women are vaccine failures or have not received the vaccine.[21] The exact mechanism of the embryopathy is unknown.

Treatment

There is no specific treatment for rubella. If febrile, fever control measures will suffice. Nonsteroidal anti-inflammatory agents may be required for the arthritis. The management of rubella embryopathy requires a multidisciplinary team to include ophthalmologists, cardiologists, and developmental specialists.

Patient education

Exposure or potential exposure of susceptible women in the first trimester of pregnancy should be determined. If possible, the rubella patient should be kept isolated from pregnant women for 7 days after the rash has appeared.[13] In patients who acquire rubella postnatally, it is contagious from 2 days before the onset of the cutaneous eruption to 7 days after the onset.[1,13] In congenital rubella, virus shedding usually ends by age 6 months, but may continue up to 5 or 6 years.[1,13] The incubation period ranges from 14 to 21 days.[1,13]

When a pregnant woman is exposed to rubella, a serum specimen should be obtained and tested for rubella antibody.[13] If antibody is present, there is no risk of infection. If no rubella antibody is detectable, a second blood specimen should be obtained 3 or 4 weeks later. If antibody is present in the second specimen and not the first, infection is presumed to have occurred, and termination of pregnancy may be considered.[13] If termination of pregnancy is not an option, immune serum globulin should be given, 0.55 ml/kg intramuscularly.[13]

Follow-up visits

Follow-up visits are usually unnecessary in postnatally acquired rubella. In congenital rubella a multidisciplinary approach, such as that offered by a birth defects clinic, is advisable.

Roseola (exanthem subitum, human herpesvirus 6 infection)

Clinical features

Roseola occurs predominantly in infants under 2 years of age.[1, 22,23] It is characterized by 2 or 3 days of sustained fever in an infant who otherwise appears well, following which the temperature falls (often to a subnormal level), and a pink, morbilliform, cutaneous eruption appears transiently and fades within 24 hours (Fig. 8-5). A convulsion at the onset of fever is noted occasionally, but the exact incidence of febrile convulsions is unknown. Mild edema of the eyelids and posterior cervical lymphadenopathy are occasionally seen.[1,22] More frequently, human herpesvirus type 6 (HHV-6) infection produces an illness with cough, fever, and otitis media or a febrile convulsion.[22] An infantile infectious mononucleosis syndrome has also been described.[24,25] HHV-6 infec-

tions are predominantly acute febrile illnesses in infants under 24 months of age.[22-25]

Differential diagnosis

Roseola can be distinguished from other morbilliform eruptions (see Boxes 8-1 and 8-2) by the distinctive history of 3 days of sustained fever in an infant followed by the appearance of a morbilliform eruption after the fever ends. It may be indistinguishable from echovirus 16 infections. Eruptions resulting from treatment with drugs may easily be confused with roseola in infants who received antibiotics for the febrile portion of the illness. The HHV-6 infections that cause otitis media may be difficult to distinguish from bacterial otitis media, and the infectious mononucleosis syndrome mimics illness induced by the Epstein-Barr virus (EBV), CMV, or HHV-7. The febrile convulsion may mimic bacterial or viral meningitis. HHV-6 can be identified by culture of peripheral blood leukocytes,[22] by serodiagnosis,[22,23] or from skin lesions by molecular diagnosis.[26]

Pathogenesis

HHV-6 infection is thought to be the major causative agent for roseola worldwide, whereas in North America, children with echovirus 16 infections probably account for some cases of roseola. HHV-6 is a herpes-group virus that preferentially involves circulating leukocytes.[22,26] It produces predominantly

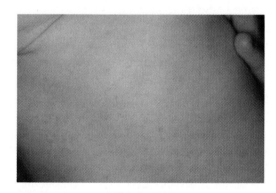

Fig 8-5
Roseola. Faint pink papules on the trunk of an infant with HHV-6 infection.

acute febrile illnesses in infants, and may account for a few cases of infectious mononucleosis, leukemias, or histiocytic syndromes.[22,26]

Treatment

In roseola, fever can be controlled with wet dressings or tepid water sponge baths, supplemental fluids, and antipyretics. HHV-6 is insensitive to current antiviral agents.

Patient education

Parents should be informed of the viral nature of this disorder and told that there is no necessity for antibiotics. If the child is seen during the febrile state, it is worthwhile to document the morbilliform eruption by personally observing it. Parents should be told that the virus responsible for roseola predominantly infects children under 24 months of age, and most older children and adults are immune.

Follow-up visits

To be certain to exclude other infections that may mimic roseola, a follow-up visit 2 days later to ascertain the course of the illness is recommended.

Human parvovirus B19 infection (erythema infectiosum)

Clinical features

The eruptions of erythema infectiosum (EI) (fifth disease) classically begin with an intense, confluent redness of both cheeks, the so-called slapped-cheek appearance (Fig. 8-6), seen in 75% of patients.[1,27] It may then spread to involve the arms (86%), legs (75%), chest (47%), and abdomen (45%), with a lacy, pink to dull-red macular eruption (Fig. 8-7); 25% of patients will have only the lacy eruption on their extremities. The original eruption lasts from 3 to 5 days. Stimulation of cutaneous vasodilation, however, will cause the eruption to "reappear" up to 4 months later.[1] This may result from vigorous exercise, overheating of the skin, or sun exposure. Only 20% of affected children will have mild fever. Occasionally, morbilliform, vesicular, or purpuric skin eruptions are seen. A purpuric hand and foot eruption (purpuric

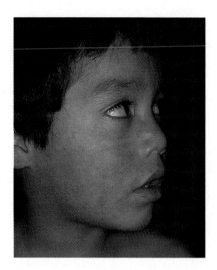

Fig. 8-6
Slapped-cheek appearance of a child with parvovirus B19 infection (erythema infectiosum).

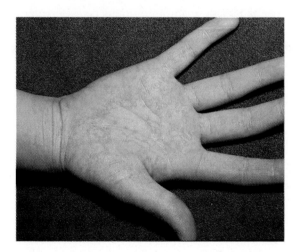

Fig. 8-7
Lacy pink eruption over the thighs in erythema infectiosum.

gloves and socks syndrome) may develop.[1,27] About 20% of infected children and adults are asymptomatic. During some outbreaks of EI, symmetric arthritis of hands, wrists, or knees will be observed.[1,17,27-28] The STAR complex is caused by parvovirus B19 equally as often as by rubella.[17] Joint symptoms usually resolve in 1 to 2 months. In patients with chronic hemolytic anemias, EI may be the cause of transient aplastic crises, and in immunosuppressed children may be responsible for red cell aplasia and severe anemia.[1,27,29] Immunosuppressed patients may be susceptible to persistent infection.[1,27] Conjunctivitis may occasionally be a presenting symptom,[31] and chronic infection has resulted in a picture of systemic necrotizing vasculitis.[32] EI in pregnant women may result in fetal death.[1,27,32,33]

Differential diagnosis

Drug eruptions and the other morbilliform eruptions may be considered in the differential diagnosis, but the lacy, mottled appearance of the EI eruption is characteristic. Occasionally the more violaceous livedo reticularis pattern of skin mottling associated with collagen vascular disease may be confused with EI, especially if associated with arthropathy. The STAR complex can also be caused by rubella and other viruses (see Box 8-3).[17] The petechial or purpuric gloves and socks syndrome should be differentiated from other petechial exanthems, such as enteroviral (see Box 8-4). Diagnosis can be confirmed by analysis of serum obtained within 30 days of the onset of illness for the presence of immunoglobulin M (IgM) B19 antibodies.

Pathogenesis

Human parvovirus B19 is the causative agent of EI.[1,13,27] The virus has been identified within EI skin lesions.[34] The organism replicates in erythroid bone marrow cells, accounting for its role in red cell aplasia of immunodeficiency and transient aplastic crises in children with chronic hemolytic anemias.[1,27-33] Susceptibility to infection has been linked to the presence of the erythrocyte P antigen, which serves as the receptor for parvovirus B19.[35] It is felt that hereditary lack of the receptor is protective against infection. Parvovirus B19 has been implicated in the etiology of Kawasaki disease (see Chapter 11).

Treatment

There is no specific treatment, nor are there any specific control measures, although isolation of patients at risk for complications (pregnant women, immunosuppressed patients, patients with chronic hemolytic anemia) is recommended. Intravenous immunoglob-

---

Box 8-4   Morbilliform viral exanthems with petechiae

Echovirus 9
EBV
Hepatitis
Atypical measles
Echoviruses 4, 7
Coxsackievirus A9
Respiratory syncytial virus
Rubella
Dengue
Parvovirus B19 ("petechial gloves and socks syndrome")

---

ulins may be effective in immunosuppressed children.[13] The disease may no longer be contagious once the skin eruption occurs.

Patient education

The patient or family should be informed of the dangers of parvovirus B19 virus to pregnant women, immunosuppressed patients, and patients with chronic hemolytic anemia (e.g., sickle cell disease). They should be advised to keep the infected child away from these individuals for 2 weeks, and good hand-washing techniques in the affected family should be emphasized.[13] They should also be told of the likely reappearance of the cutaneous eruption for up to 4 months. In children with the STAR complex, the likelihood of persistence of the arthritis should be emphasized.

Follow-up visits

Follow-up visits are unnecessary for the child with normal immunity, unless arthritis or exposure of persons at risk is involved.

Echovirus exanthems
Clinical features

Echovirus exanthems result in morbilliform eruptions associated with two predominant clinical patterns: a roseola-like pattern and the petechial pattern.[1] Infants and toddlers are more likely to have a viral rash with

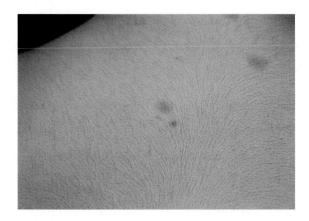

Fig. 8-8
Discrete red macules and a petechia in a child with echovirus infection.

echovirus infections than are older children.[36] Echovirus 16 infection in children is usually seen in epidemic form and may mimic roseola in that the cutaneous eruption may appear after the end of 2 or 3 days of fever.[1] Since its first report, it has been known as the "Boston exanthem," although it is found worldwide.[1] The eruption is characteristically morbilliform, but vesicles or punched-out erosions have occasionally been described. The morbilliform eruption lasts 1 to 5 days. Cervical, suboccipital, and postauricular lymphadenopathy are seen. Aseptic meningitis may occasionally occur, but it is usually seen in children without the cutaneous eruption.

Echovirus 9 results in a morbilliform eruption with acral petechiae (Fig. 8-8). Although a great number of viral infections may present with petechial eruptions (see Box 8-4), echovirus 9 accounts for most epidemics of petechial eruptions.[1,36] Echovirus 9 infects preschool children primarily, and they present with a syndrome of fever, sore throat, abdominal pain, and vomiting. Echoviruses 2, 4, 6, 11, 25 and 30 produce similar symptoms.[1] Aseptic meningitis is common.[36] The petechial eruption lasts 2 to 7 days. Some coxsackieviruses produce similar clinical patterns. Complete recovery follows.

Differential diagnosis

Roseola due to HHV-6 should be considered in the differential diagnosis of echovirus morbilliform eruptions (see Boxes 8-1 and 8-2). Roseola may mimic the Boston exanthem, but the fever and eruption in the latter often overlap. The identification of echovirus 16 in stools or throat washings helps to distinguish between these two disorders. Atypical measles, Rocky Mountain spotted fever, and meningococcemia are the major considerations of serious diseases in the differential diagnosis of echovirus 9 infections (Box 8-4). Other echoviruses, streptococcal infections, EBV, hepatitis, rubella, coxsackieviruses, dengue, and typhus may also be considered.

Pathogenesis

Echoviruses are small RNA viruses of the picornavirus group, which have been found worldwide.[1,36] There are 31 known types. The viruses are characteristically "summer" viruses and produce epidemics particularly in crowded living conditions.[1] The incubation period is 3 to 5 days when the virus is spread by the enteric route.[36] The viruses use decay-accelerating factor (CD55) as a receptor.[37] Despite enteric replication of the echovirus, gastrointestinal symptoms are uncommon. It is not known whether the virus appears within the cutaneous eruption. The mechanism that produces the cutaneous eruption is also unknown.

Treatment

There is no specific treatment. Symptomatic fever control is useful.

Patient education

The contagious nature of the disease should be emphasized.

Follow-up visits

Follow-up visits are unnecessary.

Infectious mononucleosis (human herpesvirus 4, 5, 6, and 7 infections)
Clinical features

The annual incidence of infectious mononucleosis is estimated at 50 per 100,000 children, with the highest incidence found among adolescents and young adults.[1] As opposed to acute viral infections, the onset

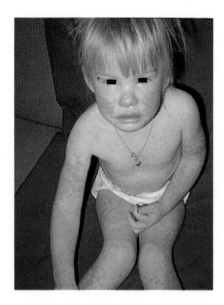

Fig. 8-9
Child with bright red morbilliform eruption due to infectious mononucleosis plus ampicillin.

is often insidious. The usual presenting symptoms and signs are fatigue (100%), fever (in 85%), generalized lymphadenopathy (85%), sore throat with exudative tonsillitis (70%), headache occurs in 45% of patients, and splenomegaly occurs in 45%.[1,38] Jaundice and hepatomegaly occur in up to 30% of patients. A pink, fleeting morbilliform eruption occurs in 15% of patients and may last 1 to 5 days. Treatment of children with infectious mononucleosis with ampicillin or penicillin for the sore throat results in an increase in incidence of morbilliform eruption in up to 80%. With antibiotic use, the eruption becomes bright red and more papular and may persist for 7 to 10 days (Fig. 8-9). The morbilliform eruption is the most characteristic seen with infectious mononucleosis, but occasionally other cutaneous eruptions may occur.[1,38] Urticaria has been described as a prominent presenting feature, and petechial eruptions associated with thrombocytopenia may be seen occasionally. Palmar erythema has also been reported as a presenting symptom of infectious mononucleosis. Neurologic symptoms such as spatial and visual distortion or signs of encephalitis, meningitis, neuritis, or

Guillain-Barré syndrome may accompany the cutaneous eruption.[1]

The acute phase with fever and sore throat lasts 2 to 3 weeks. Extreme fatigue and lethargy may persist for 3 months, however.[1,38] Rare complications include splenic rupture, thrombocytopenia, agranulocytosis, hemolytic anemia, orchitis, and cardiac involvement.[1] Blood transfusions may precede the onset of mononucleosis as the viral agents are carried in leukocytes.[1,39,40] In children infected with the human immunodeficiency virus (HIV), EBV infections are commonly seen.[41]

Differential diagnosis

Laboratory studies are most useful in aiding with the diagnosis, with the detection of heterophil antibodies by Paul-Bunnell test as the most important diagnostic criterion.[1] The laboratory findings most often encountered and their frequencies are as follows:

Finding	*Patients (%)*
Epstein-Barr virus antibody IgG or IgM	85
Lymphocytosis	92
Atypical mononuclear cells in peripheral blood film	92
Liver enzyme abnormalities	80
Hypergammaglobulinemia	80
Heterophil antibodies	75
Indirect Coombs' test	50
Thrombocytopenia	50
Hyperbilirubinemia	40

During the early phase of infectious mononucleosis, the possibility of streptococcal pharyngitis is usually considered, as are other causes of pharyngitis. Infectious mononucleosis can be distinguished from the other morbilliform eruptions (see Boxes 8-1 and 8-2) by its prolonged course, the prominent symptom of excessive fatigue, and the laboratory findings. If arthritis occurs, it must be differentiated from rubella or parvovirus B19 as causes of the STAR complex[17] (see Box 8-3). The petechial eruption must be differentiated from other causes of thrombocytopenic pur-

Box 8-5 Viruses responsible for infectious mononucleosis

EBV
CMV
HHV-6
HHV-7
Rubella
Human parvovirus B19

pura in children, such as idiopathic thrombocytopenic purpura, lupus erythematosus, and malignancies. A similar syndrome may be produced by CMV, HHV-6 and HHV-7, rubella, and parvovirus B19, but exudative tonsillitis and heterophil antibodies are not present[1,38] (see Box 8-5). EBV mononucleosis is most prevalent in the adolescent, whereas CMV and others are most prevalent in infantile and childhood mononucleosis.[38] Isolation of EBV from oropharyngeal secretions will distinguish.[1,38-40]

Pathogenesis

It is now accepted that EBV (HHV-4) is responsible for most cases (85%) of infectious mononucleosis.[1,38,40] The incubation period is 4 to 8 weeks in adolescents but is usually shorter in prepubertal children. The period of communicability is uncertain, since most patients with infectious mononucleosis excrete small amounts of virus for months after the onset of symptoms, and there are asymptomatic carriers of EBV. In crowded conditions, intrafamilial spread of EBV is common, and infants may be infected. HHV-5 (CMV), HHV-6 and HHV-7, and parvovirus B19 may be responsible for the infectious mononucleosis syndrome, particularly in infants and toddlers.[38,39]

Treatment

In mild cases no treatment is required.[1,13] In hemolytic anemia, thrombocytopenic purpura, airway interference, neurologic involvement, or in selected patients with toxemia and prolonged fever, systemic glucocorticosteroids may be given.[1,13,38] Prednisone, 2 or 3 mg/kg/day for 3 days, is recommended for adolescents. Ampicillin or penicillin should not be administered in routine cases, because of the high frequency of drug rashes. Acyclovir has yet to be convincingly demonstrated to be efficacious in infectious mononucleosis, but the drug is active against EBV in vitro.

Patient education

Concern that the spleen may rupture, which occurs in 0.5% of patients, should prompt avoidance of contact sports or other vigorous activity in which abdominal injury is likely.[1] Neurologic complications occur in 1.5%, and patients should be warned about mental symptoms.[1,38] They should also be apprised of the prolonged convalescence from this disorder and of the need to increase activities in a stepwise fashion.

Follow-up visits

Weekly visits should be scheduled in patients with mild to moderate disease to ascertain the course of the disease and observe complications. In severe disease daily visits or hospitalization may be necessary.

Hepatitis viruses A and E
Clinical features

Although viral hepatitis is usually not associated with exanthems, it is a disease that should not be overlooked when searching for the cause of a viral exanthem. Exanthems associated with hepatitis viruses A and E are primarily morbilliform, but urticarial and scarlatiniform eruptions have been described.[1,42-44] Children infected with hepatitis A often have nonspecific symptoms of low-grade fever, irritability, and upper respiratory tract symptoms without cutaneous involvement or mild jaundice.[42-44] Subclinical hepatitis is more likely to occur by 10:1.[42] The morbilliform eruption of hepatitis A and hepatitis E (Fig. 8-10) characteristically precedes the icteric stage by 1 to 10 days.[42-44] The entire disease may last 3 to 4 weeks. Hepatitis A and hepatitis E are primarily waterborne enterically transmitted infections, with hepatitis A producing local outbreaks, whereas hepatitis E has

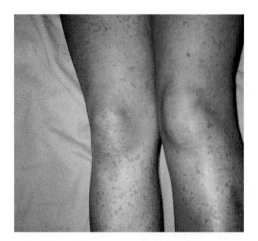

Fig. 8-10
Morbilliform eruption of the legs in an adolescent with pre-icteric hepatitis.

produced large epidemics in the Indian subcontinent and Southeast Asia.[1]

Differential diagnosis
The other viral exanthems, particularly rubella and parvovirus B19, should be considered (see Boxes 8-1 and 8-2) during the prodromal phase of morbilliform and urticarial eruptions. Urticaria due to other causes may be impossible to distinguish. The serum aminotransferase levels will be elevated markedly early in hepatitis, and be a important distinguishing test.[42-44] The eventual development of icterus, hepatic tenderness, and hepatic enlargement will allow a retrospective diagnosis of hepatitis. Pruritus may be severe during the icteric phase, particularly in hepatitis E. Diagnosis is usually made by the serologic test for IgM antihepatitis A or IgM antihepatitis E by enzyme-linked immunosorbent assay (ELISA) or radioimmunoassay.[43]

Pathogenesis
Hepatitis A and hepatitis E are single-stranded RNA viruses that replicate in the liver but not the bowel. Virus shedding into the bowel occurs during the prodromal phase and may last throughout the remainder of the illness. A viremic phase may occur that is believed to be responsible for the cutaneous eruptions. The usual source of infection is human feces through contaminated water supplies and food, particularly shellfish.

Treatment
Symptomatic treatment only is usually given. Bed rest and adequate diet are supportive measures. For exposed individuals, human immune serum globulin, 0.02 ml/kg, is given as soon as possible after exposure.[13] Hepatitis A vaccines may be licensed soon in the United States.[13]

Patient education
It should be emphasized that hepatitis A and hepatitis E are transmitted by the enteric route and possibly the oral route. Contaminated food or water sources should be sought. The importance of personal hygienic measures, such as hand washing, in preventing spread should be emphasized.

Follow-up visits
Patients should be seen weekly until the jaundice has disappeared. Although the course is benign in 95% of children, hepatitis is variable and may progress to liver failure.[1,42-44]

Hepatitis B, C, and D infections, including papular acrodermatitis (Gianotti-Crosti syndrome)
Clinical features
Urticarial and serum-sickness–like eruptions are the most common skin eruptions seen with hepatitis B,[1,45-47] but a distinct eruption called papular acrodermatitis (Gianotti-Crosti disease) has been associated with hepatitis B.[1,48,49] Groups of large, flat-topped, nonpruritic papules appear in acral areas in papular acrodermatitis.[1] They involve the cheeks (Fig. 8-11), buttocks, and limbs, and are particularly prominent over the hands (Fig. 8-12), elbows, and knees (Fig. 8-13). The skin lesions are often preceded by low-grade fever and mild upper respiratory tract symptoms. Of children described as having this syndrome, 85% are less than 3 years of age, although

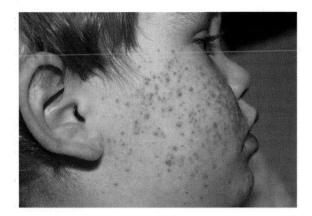

Fig. 8-11
Gianotti-Crosti syndrome. Multiple discrete papules on the cheek.

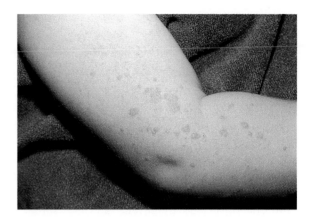

Fig. 8-13
Gianotti-Crosti syndrome. Grouped papules on the proximal extremities.

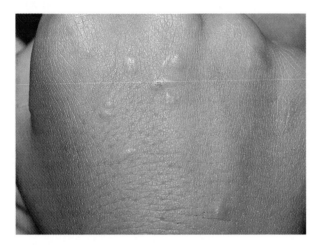

Fig. 8-12
Gianotti-Crosti syndrome. Skin-colored papules on top of the hand.

Box 8-6   Viruses responsible for papular acrodermatitis (Gianotti-Crosti syndrome)

EBV
CMV
Hepatitis B
Coxsackievirus A16

---

it may occur in school-age children.[48] The eruption persists unchanged for 2 to 8 weeks and may be recurrent.[49] Generalized lymphadenopathy and hepatosplenomegaly develop in some children along with the cutaneous eruption. In such children, atypical lymphocytes are seen in peripheral blood films, and liver enzyme levels, especially serum aminotransferases, are elevated. Hepatitis-associated antigen may be detected in these children 10 days after the eruption appears. Icterus usually does not devel-

op. It is evident that only a portion of children with papular acrodermatitis have hepatitis B, and it is less likely in the United States than in Europe or Japan.[1,48] EBV has recently been associated with outbreaks of papular acrodermatitis,[50,51] and other viruses such as CMV and coxsackievirus A16 may be involved[51] (see Box 8-6).

If a child is infected with both hepatitis B and hepatitis D, a fulminant picture of severe jaundice with encephalopathy, bleeding, and fluid and electrolyte imbalance may ensue.[1]

The urticarial or serum-sickness–like eruption of hepatitis B and hepatitis C is characterized by joint swelling and fixed urticaria.[1, 45-47] It lasts 7 to 10 days and resolves with the onset of hepatic symptoms. Anaphylactoid purpura with purpuric papules on the distal extremities and a periarteritis nodosa pattern are rarely associated with hepatitis B infection.[1]

Differential diagnosis

In irritant contact dermatitis, atopic dermatitis, and lichen planus, flat-topped acral papules that mimic papular acrodermatitis may be seen, but they are usually associated with severe pruritus and disruption of the skin surface. A serum-sickness reaction resulting from drugs or serum products or from rubella or parvovirus B19 infections may mimic the prodrome of hepatitis. In hepatitis, however, the joint swelling is usually symmetric, in contrast to rubella, in which it is often monoarthritic. In the United States, children with Gianotti-Crosti syndrome are not routinely screened for hepatitis B.

Pathogenesis

In the majority of infants with papular acrodermatitis in the United States, no associated virus has been identified, but in a few, EBV, CMV, or coxsackievirus A16 has been associated.[50,51] In Europe 30 % of patients with papular acrodermatitis have mild viral hepatitis B[48]; hepatitis B surface antigen (HBsAg) has been demonstrated in the lymph nodes in such children, with liver biopsy findings consistent with acute viral hepatitis. HBsAg antigenemia persists for 2 months in affected children and may last for several years. Hepatitis B virus has been identified as a double-stranded DNA virus that replicates via reverse transcriptase. It produces complete virus particles as well as capsids that circulate in the blood and can be detected ultrastructurally or by antibody testing.[1] Hepatitis C is a single-stranded RNA virus.[1,45-47] Hepatitis D is a unique single-stranded RNA virus that cannot enter the hepatocytes unless accompanied by the hepatitis B virus.[1] The morbilliform eruption is associated with HBsAg-positive hepatitis. Hepatitis antigen-antibody immune complexes have been identified in the sera and skin of patients with eruptions of the urticarial, anaphylactoid purpura, and periarteritis nodosa types.

Treatment

No treatment is needed for Gianotti-Crosti syndrome. Individual lesions are not responsive to topical steroids.[1] If children with Gianotti-Crosti syndrome are hepatitis B positive, it is important to prevent them from donating blood or blood products and to protect laboratory personnel. Enteric transmission of hepatitis can occur, and contact with patients' blood should be avoided. Isolating the patients from contact with persons at risk for severe hepatitis may be important. Exposed persons may be given large doses of hepatitis B immunoglobulin (HBIG), 0.06 ml/kg of body weight, within 24 hours of exposure, and 1.0 ml of hepatitis B vaccine given intramuscularly within 7 days of exposure. The vaccine should be repeated 1 and 6 months afterward. For perinatal exposure, 0.5 ml of HBIG should be administered within 12 hours of birth, with 0.5 ml of vaccine given within 7 days and at 1 and 6 months. The incubation period for hepatitis B and hepatitis C is 6 weeks to 6 months.[1,45-47]

Patient education

The prolonged nature of the Gianotti-Crosti syndrome eruption should be emphasized. The importance of evaluating contacts, if hepatitis B is found, should be emphasized. It should be emphasized that many virus agents may be responsible for papular acrodermatitis, and its significance is the prolonged course.

Follow-up visits

A visit 2 weeks after the initial visit to determine whether the signs and symptoms of hepatitis B have developed is recommended. If the child is hepatitis B positive, sera should be retested for HBsAg and antibodies to HBsAg 3 months later to detect possible chronic carriers.

VIRAL EXANTHEMS: VESICULOBULLOUS ERUPTIONS

After dissemination to skin during a viremic phase, there may be productive viral infection of keratinocytes, with ballooning degeneration of cells resulting in vesicle formation. This is particularly characteristic of the herpes group of viruses.

Herpes simplex (human herpesvirus 1 and 2 infections)

Clinical features

Grouped vesicles on an erythematous base are the characteristic lesions of herpes simplex in the skin, regardless of the location.[1] On mucous membranes the blister roof is easily shed, and the blister base (erosion) is seen. Herpesvirus infections may be primary or recurrent.[1,52] Recurrent infections represent reactivation of latent HSV. In the immunosuppressed child the erythematous base may be lost or large erosions seen.[1,13] Several distinct clinical patterns are seen.

Gingivostomatitis. In infants and children 60% of herpes simplex infections appear as a gingivostomatitis (Figs. 8-14 and 8-15), almost always due to HSV type 1 (HSV-1).[1,52] It primarily appears in infants less than 6 months of age, with pain in the mouth and throat on attempted swallowing, accompanied by fever and irritability. Erosions are extensive throughout the oral cavity, with moist crusts and foul breath. The child often is unable to eat. It lasts 7 to 14 days. Many infants are asymptomatic or suffer a mild pharyngitis on their first encounter with HSV-1.

Recurrent herpes simplex virus infection. HSV after initial exposure may persist in nerve ganglia and be reactivated by a number of factors, including fever, ultraviolet light, trauma, and the menses.[2,52,53] The mechanism of this reactivation of latent virus and its subsequent replication within epidermal cells are unknown.[1,13] Nonetheless, once recurrent skin involvement appears, the disease is contagious and can be transmitted to other areas of skin or to other persons.

Sites of involvement vary, but the most common are the lips, eyes, cheeks, and hands.[1,52,53] When specific skin locations are involved, the clinical appearance may vary. In all forms, however, grouped vesicles on an erythematous base are present. Regional lymphadenopathy may occur in all forms of herpes simplex.[1]

Herpes labialis. Recurrent herpes simplex infection of the lip occurs in 20% of all infants and children infected with HSV, and accounts for the majority of all recurrent infections.[1,52] It appears as

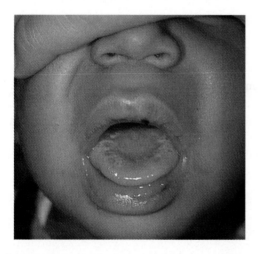

Fig. 8-14
Infant with primary herpes gingivostomatitis.

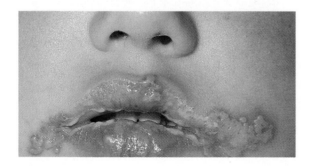

Fig. 8-15
Primary HSV-1 gingivostomatitis in an infant.

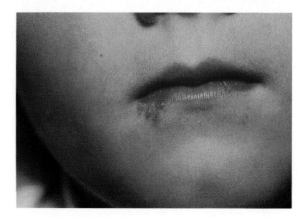

Fig. 8-16
Recurrent herpes labialis of the lower lip and adjacent skin in an adolescent.

grouped vesicles on one portion of the lip, usually the lower lip, and typically follows an acute febrile illness or intense sun exposure (Fig. 8-16). The period from the appearance of the vesicles until complete healing averages 8 days. HSV-1 can be recovered from the vesicles during the first 24 hours after onset. A prodrome of severe pain accompanies the lesions in 85% of patients.[1,52]

Herpes keratitis. Although the cornea is involved in only 8% to 10% of children infected with HSV-1, this is a serious infection, potentially leading to scarring and loss of vision.[1,52] Any herpes simplex infection on the skin around the eye, whether accompanied by a red eye, should prompt a search for herpes keratitis (Fig. 8-17). Dendritic ulceration of the cornea may be present and is an important characteristic. Ophthalmologic consultation should be obtained.

Herpes hand and finger infections. HSV-1 infection of the hand and finger occurs in 10% of infants and children, with perhaps a predilection for thumbsuckers[1] (Fig. 8-18). Because it causes pain and erythema, it is often initially considered a pyoderma or cellulitis. A careful history will elicit the prodrome of pain, and careful examination will reveal thick-roofed blisters. Since the stratum corneum is

thick on the palms and fingers, the vesicles appear deceptively deeper in the skin than in their epidermal location.

Herpes facialis. Recurrent episodes of grouped vesicles on the cheek or forehead are less common than other forms of HSV of the head and neck, but frequently they are confused with impetigo[1,52] (Fig. 8-19).

Herpes progenitalis. Herpes progenitalis, predominantly due to HSV type 2 (HSV-2) infection, occurs almost exclusively in adolescents and young adults.[1,54] Just as in HSV-1 gingivostomatitis, the symptoms may vary from none to severe widespread erosions, accompanied by fever, lymphadenopathy, severe pain, and lassitude. Recurrent herpes progenitalis characteristically presents with a prodrome of pain followed by the appearance of grouped vesicles on an erythematous base in a localized area of the genitalia. It is important to bear in mind that recurrent genital herpes is contagious and sexually transmitted.[54] It is a common venereal disease among adolescents and young adults.

Neonatal herpes simplex. Neonatal herpes simplex may develop in approximately 10% of infants born of parents with active HSV-2 infection.[54,55] In natally acquired herpes simplex, 67% is due to HHV-

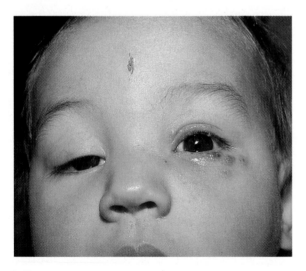

Fig. 8-17
Herpetic keratitis. Involvement of eyelid and conjunctiva in a child.

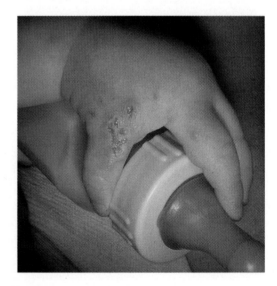

Fig. 8-18
Herpetic whitlow of the thumb of baby who is a thumb sucker.

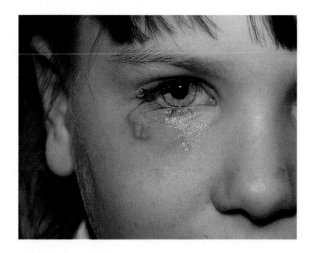

Fig. 8-19
Recurrent eruption of cheek in a child with herpes facialis.

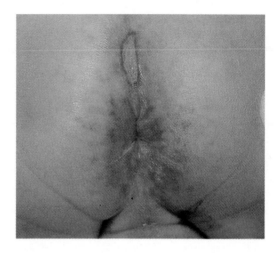

Fig. 8-21
Perianal erosions in a newborn with HHV-2 infection.

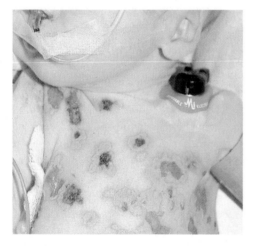

Fig. 8-20
Widespread blisters on the trunk in neonatal herpes.

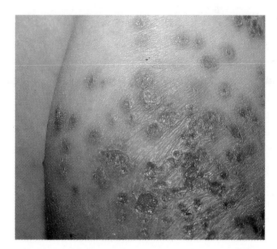

Fig. 8-22
Discrete ulcers and hundreds of erosions associated with dermatitis in an infant with atopic dermatitis and widespread herpes simplex infection (Kaposi's varicelliform eruption, eczema herpeticum).

2, 33% to HHV-1.[55] Signs may be present at birth, but grouped vesicles on an erythematous base may appear up to 7 days after birth (Figs. 8-20 and 8-21). The disease may be mild, with primarily cutaneous manifestations, but central nervous system function may ultimately be impaired.[55] More usual is a systemic illness with jaundice, progressive hepatosplenomegaly, dyspnea, hypothermia, and central nervous system symptoms. A severe encephalitis ensues, and death occurs in 48 to 96 hours.[1,55]

Herpes simplex virus infections in immunodeficiency states. In infants or children with genetic immunodeficiency, those receiving immunosuppressive drugs, with severe protein-calorie malnutrition, or with cancer-associated immunodeficiency, atypical forms of HSV infection occur.[1] Grouped vesicles often become large bullae and may lack an erythematous border. Deep erosions may occur even in the absence

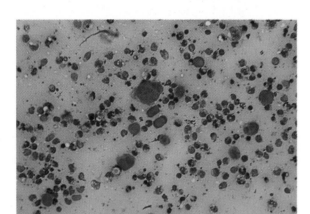

Fig. 8-23
Photomicrograph of smear of blister contents shows giant cells in herpes simplex infection. (Tzanck smear.)

Box 8-7   Vesiculobullous virus infections

Common
  Herpes simplex
  Varicella-zoster
  Hand-foot-and-mouth disease
    (coxsackievirus A16)
Uncommon
  Orf
  Influenza
  Coxsackieviruses A5, 9, 10
  Echoviruses 4, 9, 11, 17, 25
  Variola
  Vaccinia (cowpox)

---

of inflammation.[1] Purpura or hemorrhage appears within the bullous lesions. After 24 to 48 hours of local skin involvement, generalized skin involvement and visceral involvement may ensue. Herpes encephalitis or pneumonia may result in death.

Kaposi's varicelliform eruption (eczema herpeticum).   Infants and children with atopic dermatitis, burns, and other conditions that disrupt the epidermal barrier are susceptible to the development of generalized HSV infection characterized by high fever, lassitude, hundreds of skin vesicles, and sometimes death.[1] Severe infections may develop in these patients, even when their dermatitis is inactive (Fig. 8-22).

Differential diagnosis
A rapid clinical clue to HSV (or varicella-zoster virus [VZV]) infection is the finding of epidermal giant cells on a Tzanck preparation (Fig. 8-23; see Chapter 2 for technique). Rapid diagnostic tests using fluorescent- / or dye-labeled antibodies are available to stain smears and appear to be 90% or more reliable.[56] Isolation of HHV-1 or HHV-2 is the diagnostic gold standard, but requires at least 24 hours. Molecular diagnosis using the polymerase chain reaction techniques can be done in less than 24 hours, but is not widely available.

Other virus infections to be considered in the differential diagnosis of herpes simplex are listed in Box 8-7.

Gingivostomatitis.   Gingivostomatitis must be differentiated from aphthous ulcers, which are shallow, irregular, ragged, recurrent ulcerations on the oral mucosa. In erythema multiforme, in contrast to HSV gingivostomatitis, symmetric iris and target lesions are present on the skin. In herpangina, which is caused by enteroviruses, ulcers are limited to the anterior tonsillar pillars and have a linear arrangement; isolation of coxsackievirus A confirms the diagnosis.

Recurrent herpes simplex virus infection. Recurrent skin infection due to HSV must be differentiated from herpes zoster. Since both infections demonstrate epidermal giant cells on Tzanck smear, antibody testing or viral culture is the preferred method for differentiating the two on first infection. The history of recurrent lesions in the same skin area suggests HSV rather than varicella-zoster virus. VZV infections often have three or more groups of vesicles, HSV one or two.

Herpes labialis.   Impetigo may mimic herpes labialis. Gram stain and bacterial culture of the lesions will help distinguish the two.

Herpes keratitis.   Herpes keratitis should be differentiated from bacterial conjunctivitis and epidemic adenovirus keratoconjunctivitis. The characteristic grouped vesicles on an erythematous base in periocular skin will help distinguish HSV from these infections. Furthermore, HSV is usually unilateral, whereas bacterial and adenovirus infections, although initially unilateral, often become bilateral.

Herpes hand and finger infections. HSV hand and finger infections are often confused with bacterial cellulitis. A Tzanck smear of the vesicle base is a rapid method of distinguishing HSV from bacterial infection.

Herpes facialis. Impetigo may mimic facial herpes on the cheek or forehead. A Tzanck smear, HSV antibody test, or bacterial and viral culture will often distinguish the two.

Herpes progenitalis. Herpes progenitalis may mimic other venereal diseases. Also, it is not unusual to note more than one venereal disease simultaneously in the sexually active person. A smear and culture for gonorrhea and a serologic test for syphilis are most helpful in such cases.

Neonatal herpes simplex. Other congenital infections (e.g., *t*oxoplasmosis, *o*ther [congenital syphilis and viruses], *r*ubella, *C*MV, and *h*erpes simplex virus, the so-called TORCH complex) may mimic neonatal HSV. Vesicular skin lesions are not present in any of these, however. In neonatal bacterial sepsis, isolated vesicular or pustulovesicular lesions may occur. They are not grouped as in HSV infection, and Gram stain and bacterial culture will distinguish them from herpes simplex.

Pathogenesis

HHV-1 and HHV-2 are complex DNA viruses with an incubation period of 2 to 12 days. They are epidermotropic viruses, and productive viral infection occurs within keratinocytes. Active infection occurs despite high titers of specific antibody. This no doubt reflects the intracellular infection characteristic of these viruses in which antibody cannot interact with the active virus, which is transferred from cell to cell. There are two possible outcomes of epidermal cellular infection: productive and nonproductive infection. Productive infection is characterized by the biosyn-

thesis of infectious progeny and epidermal cell death, producing the intraepidermal vesicle. Nonproductive infection results in the perpetuation of all or part of the viral genome and survival of the epidermal cell, producing epidermal giant cells. It is uncertain whether fusion of several epidermal cells or nuclear division without cytoplasmic division is responsible for the epidermal giant cells seen on Tzanck smear.

Treatment

Oral acyclovir or famciclovir capsules are the specific therapy for localized cutaneous herpes simplex infections.[1,57] Oral acyclovir has been safe and effective in children. In severe primary herpes simplex infections, such as herpes gingivostomatitis or Kaposi's varicelliform eruption, acyclovir may be very useful, especially if initiated within 72 hours of the onset, in doses of 20 to 40 mg/kg/day. In localized forms of herpes simplex, such as those limited to a certain small area of skin, systemic therapy is usually not required. Neither topical nor systemic antiviral agents, however, will prevent recurrences of herpes simplex, although they may prevent transfection of the virus to adjacent skin sites or to family members or playmates if given prophylactically.[1,57] In patients experiencing frequent, severe recurrences, 6 months of acyclovir prophylaxis may be considered.

In herpes keratitis, topical 5-iodo-2-deoxyuridine ophthalmic ointment may be most efficacious.[1] Similarly, topical adenine arabinoside (Vira-A) is also useful for herpes simplex keratitis.[1] Before initiation of treatment, consultation with an ophthalmologist is recommended.

In neonatal herpes simplex infections, and in Kaposi's varicelliform eruption, intravenous acyclovir and adenine arabinoside have proved equally effective.[1,55] Supportive measures, such as fever control, maintenance of fluid and electrolyte balance, and thermal regulation, are necessary. Infected patients shed virus and should be isolated.

Patient education

Patients with local cutaneous infection should be informed of the contagious nature of the disease.

Avoidance of precipitating factors may be most useful (e.g., avoiding sun exposure or using sunscreens in sun-activated recurrent herpes simplex and discontinuing sexual activity in herpes progenitalis). In patients with atopic dermatitis or other skin diseases susceptible to disseminated HSV infections, optimal treatment of the underlying skin disease and consistency of care may be useful in preventing future episodes.

Follow-up visits

Careful ophthalmologic follow-up (every 1 to 2 days) is required in herpes keratitis. Disseminated infections often require hospitalization and intensive supportive therapy. Neonatal HSV requires careful developmental and neurologic examinations at 3-month intervals. Cutaneous herpes lesions may recur throughout childhood following neonatal herpes simplex.

Chickenpox and zoster (human herpesvirus 3 infections)

Clinical features

Varicella (chickenpox). Varicella is characterized by the abrupt onset of crops of skin lesions.[1,58,59] Individual lesions begin as faint erythematous macules that progress to edematous papules and then to vesicles during 24 to 48 hours (Fig. 8-24). The vesicles then develop moist crusts that dry and are shed,

leaving a shallow erosion. Successive crops of lesions appear during the next 2 to 5 days, so that at any one time several stages of skin lesions can be observed concomitantly: macules, papules, vesicles, and crusted lesions (Fig. 8-25). Skin lesions may appear in sites of skin injury[3] or be localized to areas of sun exposure.[2] Lesions frequently involve mucous membranes, and isolated erosions may be seen in the conjunctiva, oral cavity, or nasal mucosa.[1,58] Fever is usually low grade, and associated symptoms are mild. In a single family varicella lesions may vary from fewer than 10 in one child to hundreds in another.[1] The total duration is 7 to 10 days, but frequently children stay home 14 days due to school or other contagion-restriction policy.[60] The disease is highly contagious from 1 to 2 days before the onset of the skin eruption to 5 to 6 days afterward.[1,13,58]

Secondary bacterial infection of one to three of the many varicella skin lesions is common (1% to 4%), producing the so-called bullous varicella.[61] Often this

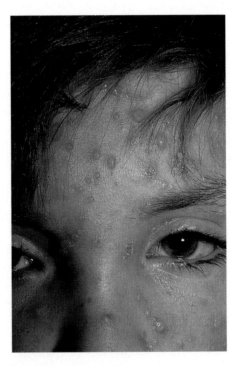

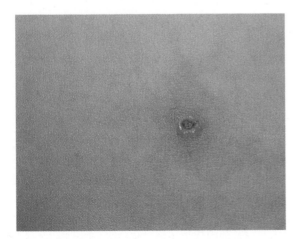

Fig. 8-24
Varicella. Umbilicated vesicles on a red base.

Fig. 8-25
Blisters, papules, and crusted lesion in a child with varicella.

is the result of *Staphylococcus aureus* infection. Pneumonia may complicate varicella in some children, and rarely, Reye's syndrome, acute cerebellar ataxia, or encephalitis may ensue.[61] Severe generalized HHV-3 infections may develop in immunosuppressed persons, with high fever, encephalitis, pneumonia, hepatitis, or disseminated intravascular coagulation.[58]

Herpes zoster. In children who have previously had varicella, recurrent infection results in herpes zoster.[58] Two to three groups of lesions appear within several adjacent dermatomes (Fig. 8-26). They begin as macules and edematous papules and progress to grouped vesicles on an erythematous base. Rarely, dermatomal pain may precede the eruption in children, and postzoster neuralgia may also occur, but rarely. Almost all children, however, have a mild illness lasting 7 to 10 days. Pruritus may be severe. The thoracic segments are involved in 60% of children with herpes zoster, with the childhood distribution depicted in Figure 8-27. If the nose is involved, herpes zoster ker-

atitis is likely to occur, and it may be as severe as HSV keratitis. Ophthalmic zoster is also more likely to be associated with severe pain than is zoster of other skin regions in children. Herpes zoster involving skin around the eyes, nose, and forehead requires a careful

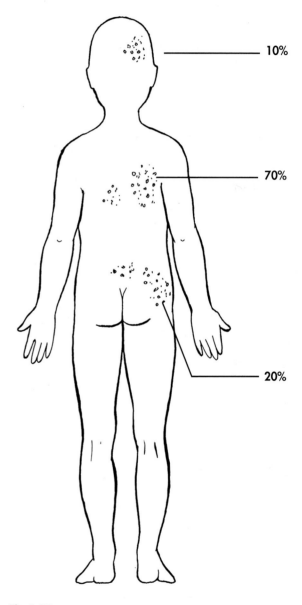

Fig. 8-27
Common distribution of herpes zoster in childhood: 10% cranial nerve involvement, 70% thoracic dermatome, 20% lumbosacral involvement.

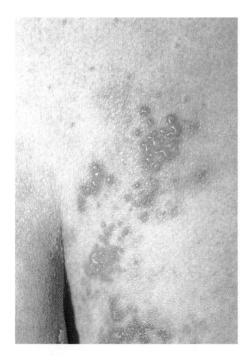

Fig. 8-26
Several groups of blisters occurring over adjacent thoracic dermatomes in a child with herpes zoster.

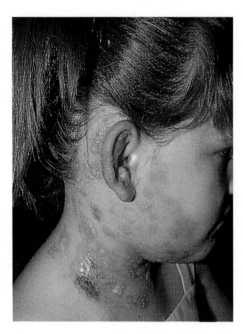

Fig. 8-28
Involvement of the ear and adjacent skin associated with facial palsy in herpes zoster of geniculate ganglion (Hunt syndrome).

ophthalmologic examination. Herpes zoster may be the initial finding in acquired immune deficiency syndrome (AIDS), but it is rarely the presenting finding in childhood cancer. In immunosuppressed children disseminated herpes zoster occurs 1 to 5 days after the dermatome infection begins. Even immunosuppressed children with disseminated herpes zoster recover without sequelae, but visceral involvement can occur. Involvement of the geniculate ganglion results in pain in the ear, vesicles on the pinnae, and facial palsy (Ramsay Hunt syndrome) (Fig. 8-28). Motor paralysis of other nerves may follow herpes zoster.

Differential diagnosis

Varicella. Typical varicella is seldom confused with other illnesses (Box 8-4). In hand-foot-and-mouth disease, vesicles are limited to acral areas, and vesicular forms of insect bite reactions (papular urticaria) usually have a typical history of bites. Acute parapsoriasis may mimic varicella in that it produces crops of lesions in different stages. True vesicles are less

common in parapsoriasis, and papules with central purpura are more common. Rickettsialpox and dermatitis herpetiformis are rare in children, but may mimic varicella. A Tzanck smear of the vesicle base will differentiate varicella from these vesicular diseases. Occasionally, disseminated HSV infection will mimic varicella. Viral cultures may be necessary to distinguish between herpes simplex and varicella.

Herpes zoster. Local cutaneous HSV infections may also mimic herpes zoster in children. Usually HSV involves one group of vesicles, and herpes zoster involves three to four clusters of grouped vesicles. Viral culture may be required to distinguish the two. Impetigo is sometimes confused with herpes zoster, but honey-colored crusts, Gram stain of lesions, and bacterial cultures will help distinguish it from herpes zoster.

Pathogenesis

HHV-3 is a complex herpes-group DNA virus that infects in much the same way as herpes simplex (see Herpes Simplex, Pathogenesis). The incubation period ranges from 10 to 27 days and averages 14 days. Productive infection occurs within keratinocytes, producing ballooning degeneration of cells and an intraepidermal blister.

Treatment

In the healthy child varicella does not require specific therapy.[62] Wet dressings, soothing baths, and oral antihistamines will give symptomatic relief of the pruritus in children. Zoster immune globulin, if given within 72 hours after exposure of an immunosuppressed host, may modify varicella. Secondary bacterial infection of varicella lesions should be treated with antistaphylococcal drugs, such as dicloxacillin, 12.5 to 25.0 mg/kg/day in four divided oral doses for 7 to 10 days.

Systemic antiviral agents, such as intravenous or oral acyclovir, have been used for childhood HHV-3 infections with success. It is recommended that it not be given to otherwise healthy children, but be considered in those likely to have complcations, such as adolescents and children with chronic pulmonary disease—especially if they are taking inhaled or systemic steroids—or children receiving chronic salicylate therapy.[62] In immunosuppressed children, children with ophthalmic zoster, or children with Ramsay Hunt syndrome, acyclovir, 20 mg/kg/dose in four doses, may be a valuable therapeutic strategy.[62] The role of varicella vaccine, although efficacious in preventing or attenuating varicella, is controversial.[63]

Patient education

The highly contagious nature of varicella should be emphasized, and the child should be isolated until all lesions are crusted, which usually occurs 5 to 6 days after eruption of the lesions. Contact with the elderly, neonates, and immunocompromised children should be avoided.

Postvaricella scarring is always a concern for parents. What appear to be highly vascular purple-red scars return to normal skin color in 6 to 12 months and often leave little evidence of scarring. Patients should be advised to wait at least 1 year before seeking help for postvaricella scars.

Follow-up visits

A visit in 48 hours to assess the development of secondary bacterial infection is useful in children with varicella. Children with disseminated zoster, ophthalmic zoster, or Ramsay Hunt syndrome should be seen daily until symptoms improve.

Hand-foot-and-mouth disease (coxsackievirus infection)

An abrupt onset of scattered papules that progress to oval or linear vesicles in an acral distribution should suggest hand-foot-and-mouth disease.[1] The individual lesions are seen on the palms, fingertips, interdigital webs, and soles of the feet, and are few in number (Figs. 8-29 and 8-30). Discrete oral lesions may also be seen (Fig. 8-31). Such children are not ill and characteristically are afebrile. During epidemics, incomplete forms may be seen.[1] In some epidemics skin lesions may be more numerous and involve both proximal and distal extremities. Oral lesions appear as discrete, shallow, oval erosions.

Differential diagnosis

In the early nonvesicular stage, rubella and the other morbilliform lesions must be considered (see Box 8-4), but the sparsity of lesions and the lack of truncal involvement make those diagnoses unlikely. In the vesicular stage, the disease may be confused with varicella, but the acral distribution of the lesions, the lack of pru-

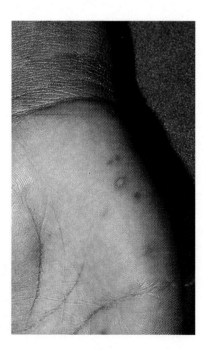

Fig. 8-29
Oval blisters of the palms in child with hand-foot-and-mouth disease (coxsackie virus A16 infection).

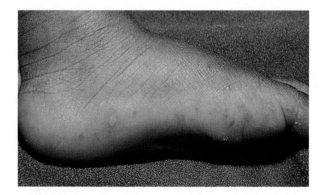

Fig. 8-30
Oval blisters on the feet of a child with hand-foot-and-mouth syndrome.

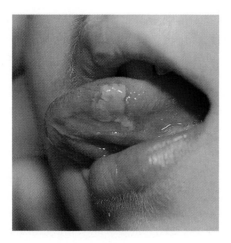

Fig. 8-31
Erosion of the tongue in a child with hand-foot-and-mouth syndrome.

ritus, and the oval to linear nature of the individual vesicles will help differentiate hand-foot-and-mouth disease from varicella. Insect bites may also mimic hand-foot-and-mouth disease, particularly if they occur on acral-exposed skin. Isolation of coxsackievirus from throat washings or serologic evidence will distinguish.

Pathogenesis

Several coxsackievirus group A enteroviruses have been found to be responsible for hand-foot-and-mouth disease. The epidemic form is almost always due to coxsackievirus A16, but coxsackieviruses A2, A5, and A10 have also been associated.[1] Recent molecular analysis reveals homology among coxsackievirus A16, A2, and enterovirus 71.[64] The incubation period is 3 to 5 days, and the virus enters by the enteric route, with the eruption reflecting a viremic phase. The disease is contagious from 2 days before to 2 days after the onset of the eruption, but virus excretion in feces may persist for 2 weeks.[1]

Treatment

No treatment is necessary.

Human immunodeficiency virus infections
Clinical features

The cutaneous manifestations of HIV-1 disease in children are predominantly the result of bacterial,

fungal, and viral infections.[65-67] Clinical findings of perinatally acquired HIV infection are usually noted at about 4 months of age, but may be first manifested as early as 3 months or as late as 21 months.[65-67] The initial features are usually lymphadenopathy, persistent diarrhea, hepatosplenomegaly, and failure to thrive. As HIV infection progresses to AIDS, more features of opportunistic infections appear.[65-67] AIDS has many features that mimic congenital immunodeficiency diseases, such as severe combined immunodeficiency (SCID). Often the first sign of AIDS is persistent thrush, recalcitrant to antiyeast therapy. The failure to clear thrush should be distinguished from the infant who gets thrush, clears with therapy, and then has a recurrence off therapy. AIDS infants with thrush also will have failure to thrive, lymphadenopathy, hepatosplenomegaly, and esophageal involvement. Chronic cough, clubbing of the fingers, and hypoxemia are the features of *Pneumocystis carinii* pneumonia, the most common infection of children with AIDS.[65-67]

A dermatitis that mimics "seborrheic" dermatitis is observed in half the children who have HIV infection.[65,66] It is not specific. Severe herpes gingivostomatitis or zoster (Fig. 8-32) may be the presenting finding. Children with HIV infection may exhibit hundreds of molluscum contagiosum lesions, and giant molluscum lesions may be seen. Recurrent pyodermas with *S. aureus* are frequent, and cellulitis or septicemia may develop from cutaneous infections that otherwise should be well localized to the epidermis. Unusual dermatophyte infections in children, such as onychomycosis and widespread tinea faciei, may be found. Severe crusted scabies with hundreds of live mites, the so-called Norwegian scabies, may occur. Purpura is common and may be the result of thrombocytopenia or severe viral or bacterial infections. A persistent folliculitis called *eosinophilic folliculitis* may be seen.[66,67]

Drug eruptions are far more common than predicted, particularly morbilliform and toxic epidermal necrolysis reactions with trimethoprim-sulfamethoxazole.[65-67] A picture that mimics acrodermatitis enteropathica may accompany the failure to thrive and result from nutritional zinc deficiency. Kaposi's

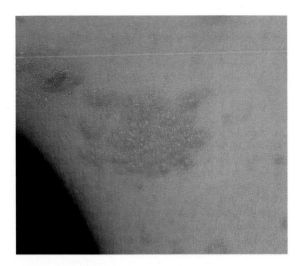

Fig. 8-32
Herpes zoster in a 12-year-old boy who is HIV positive.

sarcoma of skin has not been reported in children with HIV infection.

Differential diagnosis
Virtually every known skin infection will mimic some infection seen in the infant or child with AIDS. Severe malnutrition states and congenital immunodeficiencies may display the same findings. An HIV serology confirmed by Western immunoblotting techniques is the most sensitive to distinguish HIV infection, and it should be done on every infant or child suspected of having HIV.[68] In HIV-1–exposed infants, it may be difficult using serologic tests alone to establish the diagnosis.[68]

Pathogenesis
The agent responsible for AIDS is HIV-1, a retrovirus that selectively infects T lymphocytes, including those that are epidermotropic.[69] It can be isolated from blood leukocytes and also found in small amounts in tears, semen, saliva, vaginal secretions, cerebrospinal fluid, and breast milk. Eighty percent of affected infants in the United States are infected by transplacental passage of HIV from the mother.[67-69] Older children are infected by sexual contact and from blood products prior to 1985. In sexually active adolescents, seroprevalence is 0.2%.[70] If the infant's mother was a prostitute or intravenous drug user, the likelihood of infant infection is quite high.[67,68] Once T lymphocytes are infected by HIV, it relentlessly destroys the child's cell-mediated immunity, leaving the child at the mercy of a huge variety of opportunistic infectious agents.

Treatment
Children are best managed at large medical centers experienced in the care of AIDS patients. Infectious disease experts should be involved in their care. Treatment is directed at the specific opportunistic infection and the antimicrobial selected directed by culture and sensitivities. Several antiretroviral drugs, including zidovudine and didanosine, may suppress the disease.[71] Viral resistance to zidovudine may be overcome with dual-drug strategies using both effective agents.[72]

Patient education
Information about the transmission of HIV and support groups for AIDS families are essential.[70,73] Preventive measures such as sex education for adolescents and treatment of HIV-positive mothers with antiretroviral agents may reduce the disease.[70,73] It should be emphasized that many unusual infections may be encountered, and vigilance for early signs and symptoms of infection must be encouraged. There is currently no effective vaccine.

Follow-up visits
Frequent visits are required, and establishing a close relationship with an AIDS clinic is advisable.

VIRUS-INDUCED TUMORS

Certain viruses do not destroy keratinocytes but induce proliferation, resulting in benign tumors of skin.

Warts (human papillomavirus infection)
Clinical features
Human papillomavirus (HPV)–induced epithelial tumors produce a variety of clinical lesions known

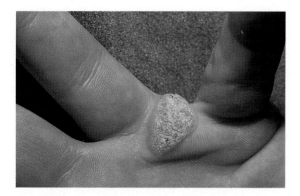

Fig. 8-33
Common wart on the hand.

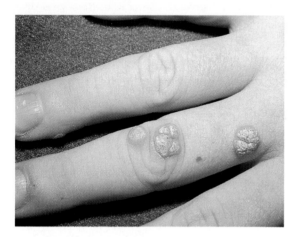

Fig. 8-34
Common warts on a child's fingers.

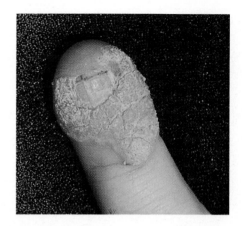

Fig. 8-35
Periungual warts.

Table 8-1.

Clinical Warts and Associated Human Papillomavirus Type

Clinical wart	HPV type
Common wart	HPV-2a,b,c,d,e; some HPV-4
Plantar (weight-bearing) wart	HPV-1a,b,c; HPV-4, 60, 63, 65
Flat warts	HPV-3a,b; HPV-10a,b
Condyloma acuminata	HPV-6a,b,c,d,e,f; HPV-11a,b; HPV-16

collectively as *warts*.[74] Different HPVs are associated with specific clinical patterns. Table 8-1 lists the clinical types of warts and the HPV type responsible. Warts are very commonly seen in children. By age 11, 4% of children in the United Kingdom had warts.[75]

The common wart (verruca vulgaris) appears as a solitary papule, with an irregular, rough surface (Figs. 8-33 and 8-34). They are usually found on the extremities, but they may be found anywhere on skin, including the scalp and genitalia.

Periungual warts occur (Fig. 8-35) around the cuticles of fingers or toes and are spread by trauma.

Filiform warts appear as spiny projections from the skin surface with a narrow stalk (Fig. 8-36). In children they are usually seen on the lips, nose, or eyelids.

Flat warts have a flat-topped, smooth surface. They tend to be multiple and skin-colored to light tan (Fig. 8-37). They are grouped, will appear within sites of skin trauma, and are usually observed on the face or extremities.

Plantar (weight-bearing) warts appear as rough papules that disrupt the dermal ridges (Fig. 8-38). They are frequently painful when the child is walking. They may be grouped together to produce "mosaic" warts. Discrete rough papules less than 5 mm that preserve the dermal ridges and are called "ridged warts" may be seen on plantar or palmar surfaces.[74]

Venereal warts (condylomata acuminata) are multiple discrete or confluent papules with a rough surface that appear on the genital mucosa, adjacent dry

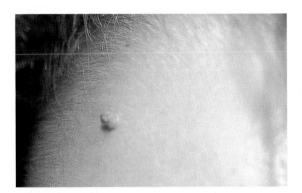

Fig. 8-36
Filiform wart.

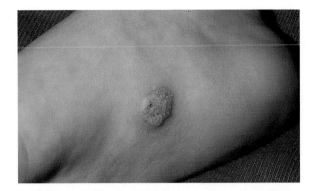

Fig. 8-38
Plantar (weight-bearing) wart.

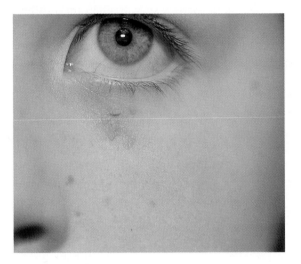

Fig. 8-37
Multiple flat warts (verruca plana) of the eyelid and cheek.

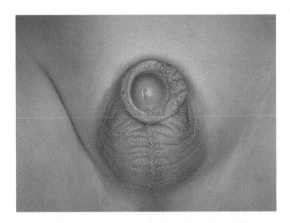

Fig. 8-39
Venereal warts (condyloma acuminata) of the foreskin in a male infant.

skin, or both (Figs. 8-39 and 8-40). Common warts also appear on genital or perigenital skin, particularly in toddlers.[77-79]

The natural history of warts is variable, and the incubation period is unknown, but transmission from child to child, adult to child, and mother to newborn is well documented.[75-77] Most warts spontaneously resolve in 12 to 24 months, but may persist for longer periods in some children. Warts in the immunosuppressed child are very persistent. Most warts are asymptomatic, except weight-bearing warts, although large warts anywhere may develop painful fissures.

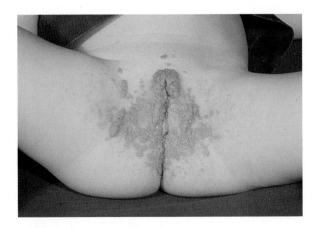

Fig. 8-40
Venereal warts in a female infant.

Differential diagnosis

Common warts and filiform warts are so characteristic that they present no diagnostic problem. Plantar warts must be differentiated from calluses, which have a smooth, rather than irregular surface and preserve the dermal ridges. The so-called ridged wart may be impossible to distinguish from calluses. Condylomata acuminata must be distinguished from the moist smooth papules of secondary syphilis (condylomata lata), which appear as moist papules in genital areas. A serologic test for syphilis will readily distinguish the two. Flat warts are often overlooked and may be misdiagnosed as lichen planus, lichen nitidus, seborrheic keratosis, or birthmarks. The linear or grouped arrangement of flat warts is helpful in dsiagnosis, as is their occurrence along areas of skin trauma. Diagnosis can be established by biopsy and HPV molecular typing, but these procedures are rarely required, and warts remain a clinical diagnosis.

Pathogenesis

Immunity to warts is not well understood, but inducing inflammation around a single wart may result in regression of all others. The HPV is located within the epidermal cell nucleus, which may be an immunologic privileged site where viral antigen has little opportunity to interact with antibody or white blood cells.[80] HPV induces vacuolated epidermal cells with eosinophilic inclusions.[74] The HPV induces keratinocyte proliferation with relatively normal differentiation, giving rise to a benign epithelial tumor.

Treatment

Most wart therapy is designed to be cytodestructive—that is, to destroy all the epidermal cells within the wart tumor, and, hopefully, all the HPV as well. The recurrence rate for all wart treatment strategies is high, and it is unlikely the wart will resolve with a single treatment. Cryotherapy usually has the smallest recurrence rate from a single treatment. Table 8-2 summarizes usual treatments for wart types.

Cryotherapy. A cryosurgery probe, spray unit, or copper bar cooled in liquid nitrogen may be used for cryotherapy but a cotton swab with a loose, pointed tip is most commonly used. The cotton swab is dipped in a thermos containing liquid nitrogen ($-195°$ C), and the saturated swab is applied to the center of the wart until a white "ice ball" extending 1 to 3 mm beyond the margin of the wart is formed. The freeze is maintained 10 to 30 seconds. Warts greater than 7 mm in diameter should not be frozen, because scarring is likely to result. In 1 to 2 days a blister, sometimes hemorrhagic, forms. Removing the blister roof in 1 week and refreezing may be necessary. Cryotherapy is best for common warts but should not generally be used on periungual or plantar warts. Freezing a forceps in liquid nitrogen and grasping the narrow stalk of a filiform wart for 30 to 45 seconds is effective.

Salicylic acid plasters. Cotton plasters impregnated with 40% salicylic acid can be used on plantar and periungual warts. The plaster is cut to size, the paper backing removed, and the gummed side placed against the wart. It should be secured by trainer's tape so the plaster does not move for 3 to 5 days. Sweating mobilizes the salicylic acid out of the plaster so that it may enter the skin. When the plaster is removed, the patient should soak the wart in water for 45 minutes, then rub off the "dead, white wart." A new plaster is taped in place, and the process is repeated for two more changes.

Salicylic acid paints. Prescriptions for salicylic acid–containing solutions can be provided for home use. The solutions should be applied with a toothpick by microdrops. They should be applied once or twice a day for 4 to 6 weeks. This method will not work on warts over 5 mm. Redness around the base of the wart and itching may herald the onset of wart regression. These preparations should be used for periungual warts or small common warts.

Retinoic acid. Retinoic acid in a 0.025% cream or 0.05% cream may be used for flat warts and applied once or twice daily for 4 to 6 weeks. It is ineffective in common, plantar, or periungual warts.

Cantharidin. Currently unavailable in the United States, this vesicant can be quite effective in periungual warts. It should be applied carefully with

Table 8-2.
Treatment of Viral Warts

| Type of wart | Treatment | | Response rate (%) |
	First choice	Alternative	
Common	Cryotherapy	Salicylic acid paint	80-90
Periungual	Cantharidin	Salicylic acid paint or plaster	60
Flat	Retinoic acid	Salicylic acid paint	50
Filiform	Surgery	Cryotherapy with forceps	50
Plantar	Salicylic acid plaster	Salicylic acid paint	60
Venereal	Podophyllum or Condylox	Cryotherapy	90

a toothpick to cover the size of the wart. It produces a tender blister beneath the wart 2 or 3 days after application, and the wart is eventually sloughed off. It is difficult to regulate the size of the blister, and the response may vary from application to application. Cantharidin should never be used in intertriginous areas.

Podophyllum. Podophyllum, a plant extract, is a microtubule inhibitor that blocks cell division. It can be effective against genital warts and common warts. It is applied by the health care provider in a 25% alcohol solution and applied with a toothpick to the warts. It should be washed off in 4 hours. It is an irritating substance, and application to perianal skin often induces defecation. A purified podophyllotoxin is now available for use by the patient (podofilox [Condylox]). It is applied carefully with a toothpick twice daily for 3 days, then 4 days later reapplied for 3 days if the warts remain. Podophyllum in excessive doses is a neurotoxin causing an areflexic coma.

Surgery. The recurrence rate after surgical excision of a wart approaches 100%, presumably because of transfection of HPV at the time of surgery. Removing a filiform wart by cutting its narrow base is one exception. Some authorities recommend the use of a sharp curette on the remaining wart after 3 or 4 weeks of salicylic acid plasters.

CO_2 lasers, electrodesiccation, and x rays. These therapies always result in scarring and other undesirable side effects, with a high recurrence rates. They are not recommended. The pulsed-dye laser will not scar, but it is not particularly effective.

Cimetidine. Some authorities have used 3 months of oral cimetidine, a H_2 blocking agent, to nonspecifically improve immunity to the HPV.[81] This is usually used in conjunction with another strategy and should be reserved for resistant warts.

Patient education
It should be emphasized from the initial visit that one treatment is unlikely to cure the wart, and many treatments may be necessary. A careful explanation of the poor host immunity to the HPV is helpful. For genital warts in infants and toddlers, the possibility of sexual abuse should be considered. However, it is well established that vertical transmission of genital warts from an infected mother can occur, and many genital warts are of common HPV types with a parent, sibling, or care giver having common warts of the same type.[77-79] This makes it impossible to diagnose sexual abuse by the presence of genital warts alone. The clinician should carefully examine the child for other forms of physical or sexual abuse, including the oral cavity as well as genitalia. A history of unusual behavior in the child, such as withdrawal, sleep disturbances, phobias, or new onset of enuresis or encopresis, should be solicited. If suspicious history or physical findings other than the genital warts are obtained, reporting to the appropriate social agencies is recommended.[78,79]

Follow-up visits
A visit 2 weeks after initiating therapy is needed to ascertain the need for retreatment.

Molluscum contagiosum
Clinical features

White or yellow-white 1- to 6-mm discrete papules with a central umbilication are seen in molluscum contagiosum[1,82] (Figs. 8-41 and 8-42). Occasionally, large lesions of 15 mm will be found. A dermatitis often surrounds larger lesions (Fig. 8-43). Some lesions may extrude keratinous contents from the central umbilication (Fig. 8-44). In infants and toddlers, lesions are usually observed around the eyes, axilla, and proximal extremities, but lesions can be found in other locations.[1] In the child with atopic dermatitis, dozens to hundreds of lesions can be seen. Genital grouped lesions can be found in sexually active adolescents.[1,82] Hundreds of lesions in the older child should raise the suspicion of AIDS.

Differential diagnosis

Warts, closed comedones, and tiny epidermal cysts may mimic molluscum contagiosum. Careful inspection, however, will reveal the central umbilication characteristic of molluscum contagiosum, and micro-

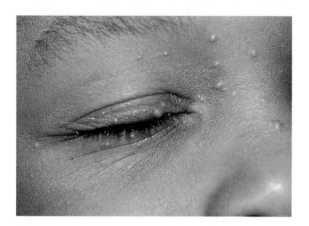

Fig. 8-41
Multiple molluscum papules on an infant's face.

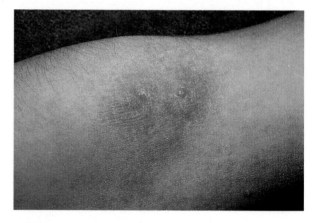

Fig. 8-43
Erythema and scaling surround resolving lesions of molluscum contagiosum (molluscum dermatitis).

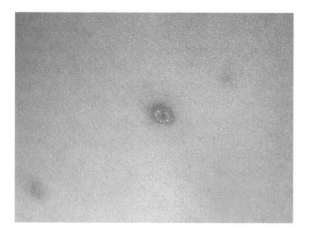

Fig. 8-42
Umbilicated dome-shaped papule characteristic of molluscum contagiosum.

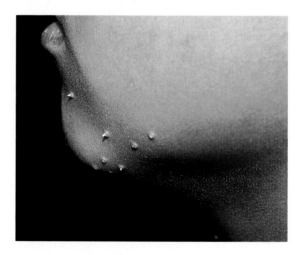

Fig. 8-44
Molluscum extruding their contents.

scopic examination will differentiate the disease from other skin papules. At first glance, molluscum may appear to be blisters, but palpation and careful inspection will reveal their solid nature. Extrusion of the papule contents onto a glass slide and Wright's stain will reveal the characteristic viral inclusions.

Pathogenesis

Molluscum contagiosum is caused by a poxvirus that induces epidermal cell proliferation.[82,83] Three types are recognized by restriction endonuclease analysis of viral DNA.[83] Molluscum type 1 is believed to be responsible for common lesions on the extremities, head, and neck. Types 2 and 3 are most often associated with genital lesions in the adolescent or young adult. The incubation period is 2 to 7 weeks, and the child is contagious as long as active lesions are present.

Treatment

Removal of a papule is curative. In older children the use of a sharp dermal curette to remove the entire papule is the treatment of choice. Some clinicans prefer to empty the contents with a needle. In infants and young children this method is frightening and painful. In such children a drop of cantharidin or podophyllum, applied to the central umbilication with a wooden toothpick, is less traumatic than excision. Recurrences are common, since it is often difficult to detect the pinpoint early lesions of molluscum.

Patient education

The highly contagious nature of molluscum contagiosum should be emphasized. The lesions are benign, and patients should not be unduly concerned.

Follow-up visits

A visit 1 to 2 weeks after initial therapy is advisable to determine the need for retreatment.

References

1. Hogan PA, Morelli JG, Weston WL: Viral exanthems, *Curr Probl Dermatol* 4:35, 94 1992.

2. Norval M, El-Ghorr A, Garssen J, et al: The effects of ultraviolet light irradiation on viral infections, *Br J Dermatol* 130:693, 1994.

3. Belhorn TH, Lucky AW: Atypical varicella exanthems associated with skin trauma, *Pediatr Dermatol* 11:129, 1994.

4. Jones VF, Badgett JT, Marshall GS: Repeated photoreactivation of herpes simplex virus type I in an extrafacial dermatomal distribution, *Pediatr Inf Dis J* 13:238-239, 1994.

5. Bodemer C, de Prost Y: Unilateral laterothoracic exanthem in children: a new disease? *J Am Acad Dermatol* 27:693, 1992.

6. Gelmetti C, Grimalt R, Cambiaghi S, et al: Asymmetric periflexural exanthem of childhood: report of two new cases, *Pediatr Dermatol* 11:42, 1994.

7. McGrath D, Swanson R, Weems S, et al: Analysis of a measles outbreak in Kent County, Michigan in 1990, *Pediatr Infect Dis J* 11:385, 1992.

8. Koplik H: The diagnosis of the invasion of measles from a study of the exanthema as it appears on the buccal mucous membrane, *Arch Pediatr* 13:918, 1896.

9. Arrieta AC, Zaleska M, Stutman HR: Vitamin A levels in children with measles in Long Beach, California, *J Pediatr* 121:75, 1992.

10. Darmstadt GL, Halsey NA: Measles, in mother-infant pairs, *Pediatr Infect Dis J* 11:492, 1992.

11. Pabst HF, Sprady DW, Marusyk RG, et al: Reduced measles immunity in infants in a well vaccinated population, *Pediatr Infect Dis J* 11:525, 1992.

12. Centers for Disease Control and Prevention. Reported Vaccine-preventable diseases—United States 1993, and the childhood immunization initiative, *JAMA* 271:651, 1994.

13. Report of the Committee on Infectious Diseases: Elk Grove Village, Il, 1994. *1994 Red Book*. American Academy of Pediatrics.

14. Fulginiti VA, Eller JJ, Downie AW: Altered reactivity to measles virus; Atypical measles in children previously immunized with inactivated measles virus vaccine, *JAMA* 202:1075, 1967.

15. Ueno Y: Rubella arthritis. An outbreak in Kyoto, *J Rheumatol* 21:874, 1994.

16. Mangi RJ: Viral arthritis—the great masquerader, *Bull Rheum Dis*, 43:5, 1994.

17. Jundt JW, Creager AH: STAR complexes: febrile illness associated with sore throat, arthritis and rash, *South Med J* 86:521, 1993.

18. Arnold JJ et al: A fifty year follow-up of ocular defects in congential rubella: late ocular manifestations, *Aust N Z J Ophthalmol* 22:1, 1994.

19. Hohfield P, Forestier F, Kaplan C, et al: Fetal thrombocytopenia: a retrospective survey of 5,194 fetal blood samplings, *Blood* 84:1851, 1994.

20. Paludetto R, Van den Heuvel J, Stagni A, et al: Rubella embryopathy after maternal reinfection, *Biol Neonate* 65:340, 1994.

21. Lawman S, Morton K, Best JM: Reasons for rubella susceptibility among pregnant women in West Lambeth, *J R Soc Med* 87:263, 1994.

22. Hall CB, Long CE, Schnabel KC, et al: Human herpesvirus-6 infection in children, *N Engl J Med* 331:432, 1994.

23. Pruksananonda P, Hall CB, Insel RA, et al: Primary human herpesvirus-6 infection in young children, *N Engl J Med* 326:1445, 1992.

24. Hanukoglu A, Somekh E: Infectious mononucleosis-like illness in an infant with acute herepesvirus-6 infection, *Pediatr Infect Dis J* 13:750, 1994.

25. Leach CT, Sumaya CV, Brown NA, et al: Human herpesvirus-6: Clinical implications of a recently discovered ubiquitous agent, *J Pediatr* 121:173, 1992.

26. Leahy ML, Friednash M, Krejci S, et al: HHV-6 in Langerhans cell histiocytosis as detected by the polymerase chain reaction, *J Invest Dermatol* 101:642, 1993.

27. Brown KE, Young NS, Liu JM: Molecular cellular and clinical aspects of parvovirus B 19 infection, *Crit Rev Oncol Hematol* 16:1, 1994.

28. Marshall JB, McMurray R: Acute polyarthritis. Fifth disease passed from child to adult, *Postgrad Med* 95:165, 1994.

29. Brown KE, Green SW, Antonez de Mayolo J, et al: Congenital anaemia after transplacental B19 parvovirus infection, *Lancet* 343:895, 1994.

30. Yoshida M, Tezuka T: Conjunctivitis caused by parvovirus B19 infection, *Ophthalmologica* 208:161, 1994.

31. Finkel TH, Torok TJ, Ferguson PJ, et al: Chronic parvovirus B19 infection and systemic necrotizing vasculitis: opportunistic infection or causative agent? *Lancet* 343:1255, 1994.

32. Kerr JR, O'Neill HJ, Coyle PV, et al: An outbreak of parvovirus B19 infection; a study of clinical manifestations and the incidence of fetal loss, *Ir J Med Sci* 163:65, 1994.

33. Guidozzi F, Ballot D, Rothberg AD: Human B19 parvovirus infection in an obstetric population. A prospective study determining fetal outcome, *J Reprod Med* 39:36, 1994.

34. Schwartz TF, Wierbitzky S, Pambor M: Case report: detection of parvovirus B19 in a skin biopsy of a patient with erythema infectiosum. *J Med Virol* 43:171, 1995.

35. Brown KE, Hibbs JR, Gallinella G, et al: Resistance to parvovirus B19 infection due to a lack of virus receptor (erythrocyte p antigen), *N Engl J Med* 330:1192, 1994.

36. Sawyer MH, Holland D, Aintablian N, et al: Diagnosis of enteroviral central nervous system infection by polymerase chain reaction during a large community outbreak, *Pediatr Infect Dis J* 13:177, 1994.

37. Bergelson JM, Chan M, Solomon KR, et al: Decay-accelerating factor (CD55), a glycosylphosphatidylinositol-anchored complement regulatory protein, is a receptor for several echoviruses, *Proc Nat Acad Sci U S A* 91:6245, 1994.

38. Lajo A, Borque C, Del Castillo F, et al: Mononucleosis caused by Epstein-Barr virus and cytomegalovirus in children: a comparative study of 124 cases, *Pediatr Infect Dis J* 13:56, 1994.

39. Sayers AH: Transfusion transmitted viral infections other than hepatitis and human immunodeficiency virus infection. Cytomegalovirus, Epstein-Barr virus, human herpesvirus 6 and human parvovirus B19, *Arch Pathol Lab Med* 118:346, 1994.

40. Sixbey JW, Shirley P, Chesney PJ, et al: Detection of a second widespread strain of Epstein-Barr virus, *Lancet* 2:761, 1989.

41. Cohen JI: Epstein-Barr virus lymphoproliferative disease associated with acquired immunodeficiency, *Medicine* (Baltimore) 70:137, 1991.

42. Wright R: Viral hepatitis. Comparative epidemiology, *Br Med Bull* 46:548, 1990.

43. McIntyre N: Clinical presentation of acute viral hepatitis, *Br Med Bull* 46:533, 1990.

44. Dollberg S, Berkun Y, Gross-Kieselstein E, et al: Urticaria in patients with hepatitis A virus infection, *Pediatr Infect Dis J* 10:702, 1991.

45. Reichel M, Mauro TM: Urticaria and hepatitis C, *Lancet* 336:822, 1990.

46. Stremmel W, Schwarzenrube J, Niedrau C, et al: Epidemiology, clinical course and treatment of chronic viral hepatitis, *Hepatogastroenterology* 38:22, 1991.

47. Chang M-W, Ni Y-H, Hwang L-H, et al: Long term clinical and virologic outcome of primary hepatitis C virus infection in children: a prospective study, *Pediatr Infect Dis J* 13:769, 1994.

48. Caputo R, Gelmetti C, Ermacora E, et al: Gianotti-Crosti syndrome: a retrospective analysis of 308 cases, *J Am Acad Dermatol* 26:207, 1992.

49. Patrizi A, Di Lernia V, Neri I, et al: An unusual case of recurrent Gianotti-Crosti syndrome, *Pediatr Dermatol* 11:283, 1994.

50. Lowe L, Hevert AA, Duvic M: Gianotti-Crosti syndrome associated with Epstein-Barr virus infection, *J Am Acad Dermatol* 20:336, 1989.

51. Baldari U, Monti A, Righini MG: An epidemic of infantile papular acrodermatitis (Gianotti-Crosti syndrome) due to Epstein-Barr virus, *Dermatology* 188:203, 1994.

52. Spruance SL: The natural history of recurrent oral-facial herpes simplex virus infection, *Semin Dermatol* 11:200, 1992.

53. Jones VF, Badgett JT, Marshall GS: Repeated photoreactivation of herpes simplex virus type 1 in an extrafacial dermatomal distribution, *Pediatr Infect Dis J* 13:238, 1994.

54. Prober CG: The management of pregnancies complicated by genital infections with herpes simplex virus, *Clin Infect Dis* 15:1031, 1993.

55. Overall JC Jr.: Herpes simplex virus infection of the fetus and newborn, *Pediatr Ann* 23:131, 1994.

56. Goodyear HM: Rapid diagnosis of cutaneous herpes simplex infections using specific monoclonal antibodies, *Clin Exper Dermatol* 19:294, 1994.

57. Kuzushima K, Kudo T, Kimura H et al: Prophylactic oral acyclovir in outbreaks of primary herpes simplex virus type 1 infection in a closed community, *Pediatrics* 89:379, 1992.

58. Tyring SK: Natural history of varicella-zoster virus, *Semin Dermatol* 11:211, 1992.

59. Drwal-Klein LA: Varicella in pediatric patients, *Ann Pharmacotherapy* 27:938, 1993.

60. Lieu TA, Black SB, Rieser N, et al: The cost of childhood chickenpox: parent's perspective, *Pediatr Infect Dis J* 13:173, 1994.

61. Jackson MA, Bury VF, Olson LC: Complications of varicella requiring hospitalization in previously healthy children, *Pediatr Infect Dis J* 11:941, 1992.

62. American Academy of Pediatrics Committee on Infectious Disease. The use of oral acyclovir in otherwise healthy children with varicella, *Pediatrics* 91:858, 1993.

63. Bernstein HH, Rothstein EP, Watson BM, et al: Clinical survey of natural varicella compared with breakthrough varicella after immunization with live attenuated Oka/Merck varicella vaccine, *Pediatrics* 92:833, 1993.

64. Poyry T, Hyypia T, Horsnell C, et al: Molecular analysis of coxsackievirus A 16 reveals a new genetic group of enteroviruses, *Virology* 202:982, 1994.

65. Prose NS, Mendez H, Menikoff H, et al: Pediatric human immunodeficiency virus infection and its cutaneous manifestatons, *Pediatr Dermatol* 4:67, 1987.

66. Keredl FA, Pennys NS: Cutaneous manifestations of AIDS in adults and children, *Curr Probl Dermatol* 1:101, 1989.

67. Smith KJ, Skelton HG, Yeager J, et al: Cutaneous findings in HIV-1 positive patients: a 42 month prospective study, *J Am Acad Dermatol* 31:746, 1994.

68. Simpson BJ Andiman WA Difficulties in assigning Human Immunodeficiency virus-1 infection and seroconversion status in a cohort of HIV-exposed in children using serologic criteria established by the Centers for Disease Control and Prevention. *Pediatrics* 93:840, 1994.

69. Bryant ML, Ratner L: Biology and molecular biology of human immunodeficiency virus, *Pediatr Infect Dis J* 11:390, 1992.

70. Lindegren ML, Hanson C, Miller K, et al: Epidemiology of human immunodeficiency virus infection in adolescents, United States, *Pediatr Infect Dis J* 13:525, 1994.

71. Ogino MT, Dankner WM, Spector SA: Development and significance of zidovudine resistance in children infected with human immunodeficiency virus, *J Pediatr* 123:9, 1993.

72. Husson RN, Mueller BU, Farley M, et al: Zidovudine and didanosine combination therapy in children with human immunodeficiency virus infection, *Pediatrics* 93:316, 1994.

73. Wilfert CM, Pizzo PA: A blueprint for care, treatment and prevention of HIV/AIDS, *Pediatr Inf Dis J* 13:920, 1994.

74. Beutner KR: Cutaneous viral infections, *Pediatr Ann* 22:247, 1993.

75. Williams H, Pottier A, Strachan D: The descriptive epidemiology of warts in British schoolchildren, *Br J Dermatol* 128:504, 1993.

76. Bender ME: The protean manifestations of human papillomavirus infection, *Arch Dermatol* 130:1429, 1994.

77. Gutman LT: Transmission of human genital papillomavirus disease: Comparison data for adults and children, *Pediatrics* 91:31, 1993.

78. Handley JM, Maw RD, Bingham EA, et al: Anogenital warts in children, *Clin Exp Dermatol* 18:241, 1993.

79. Hurwitz S: Anogenital warts and sexual abuse in children: a perspective. *Fitzpatrick's J Clin Derm* Mar/Apr: 38, 1994.

80. Androphy EJ: Molecular biology of human papillomavirus infection and oncogenesis, *J Invest Dermatol* 103:248, 1994.

81. Orlow SJ, Paller A: Cimetidine therapy for multiple viral warts in children, *J Am Acad Dermatol* 28:794, 1993.

82. Highet AS: Molluscum contagiosum, *Arch Dis Child* 67:1248, 1992.

83. Porter CD, Archard LC: Characterization by restriction mapping of three subtypes of molluscum contagiosum virus, *J Med Virol* 38:1, 1992.

9

Papulosquamous Disorders

Children affected with papulosquamous disorders have skin lesions characterized by red or violaceous macules that progress to papules and develop scales. The exact prevalence of this group of diseases is unknown.[1] However, psoriasis alone has a yearly prevalence of 3.1 per 1000 U.S. children. Pityriasis rosea accounts for a further increase in the prevalence of papulosquamous eruptions in childhood. Thus papulosquamous disorders are common in children and should be readily recognized by those caring for them. The clinician should recognize that this group of diseases is chronic, lasting months to years. It is important for the clinician to distinguish these diseases with raised lesions from flat scaly conditions, such as the ichthyoses or the various forms of desquamation.

PSORIASIS

Clinical features

Psoriasis is thought to be a hereditary disorder that requires an interplay of genetic and environmental factors for full clinical expression.[2,3] Childhood-onset psoriasis is more likely to demonstrate an affected family member than late-onset psoriasis.[2,4] Psoriasis is a clinical diagnosis, based on the presence of thick silvery scales on at least some lesions, the characteristic distribution, nail involvement, and the presence of the isomorphic phenomenon. The eruption consists of erythematous macular or papular lesions that develop a thick, silvery scale (Fig. 9-1). Discrete scaly papules (guttate lesions) may be seen, or groups of papules may coalesce to form raised, sharply marginated erythematous plaques. The sites of predilection for psoriasis include the scalp, ears, eyebrows, elbows, knees, gluteal crease (Fig. 9-2), genitalia, and nails. Complete examination of the entire cutaneous surface is necessary because lesions may be few in number. The most common clinical picture of psoriasis in childhood is involvement of the elbows, knees, and scalp by a few plaques (Figs. 9-3 and 9-4). Sixty-six percent of children have this form.[1,4]

Guttate psoriasis, the term given to the form of psoriasis with multiple discrete papules, begins on the trunk as multiple erythematous macules that mimic a viral exanthem (Fig. 9-5). Guttate psoriasis was the form of psoriasis seen in 34% of children in one study.[4] As noted, the lesions progress to papules that

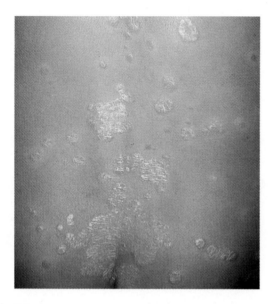

Fig. 9-1
Papules and plaques, some of which are covered with thick, silvery scales over the back of a child with psoriasis.

develop a silvery scale (Fig. 9-6). These droplike papules (guttata is the Latin word for "drop") are seen predominantly on the trunk and proximal extremities. Guttate psoriasis may follow a sore throat, particularly streptococcal pharyngitis, by 2 to 3 weeks.[5] Follicular accentuation of the skin lesions may be seen. Children with guttate psoriasis should be evaluated for pharyngeal[5] or rectal[6] streptococcal infection. Children with an episode of guttate psoriasis are likely to develop psoriasis vulgaris within 5 years.[1]

The isomorphic (Koebner) phenomenon, in which psoriatic lesions develop in sites of skin trauma several days after the traumatic event, is a useful diagnostic feature of psoriasis.[1] It occurs in a linear fashion along a scratch, but may also be precipitated by lacerations, abrasions, sunburn, insect bites, or pressure (Fig. 9-7). In some children it may appear in a nevoid distribution and mimic epidermal nevi.[7]

Scalp involvement with psoriasis results in accumulation of thick scales throughout the scalp, with thickened scales along the frontal hairline and behind the ears (Fig. 9-8). The scalp is involved in 82% of children with psoriasis. Hair loss does not occur.

Involvement of the palms and soles is uncommon in children, but psoriasis may appear as fissured, painful, symmetric plaques (Fig. 9-9) or as multiple small, sterile pustules.[8] Pustular lesions on the palms and soles may be associated with common plaques of psoriasis elsewhere.[8]

Genital involvement (perineal area, penis, inguinal folds, labia) occurs in 44% of children with psoriasis.[4] Gluteal cleft involvement is common (Fig. 9-2), as is involvement of the penis (Fig. 9-10).

Nail signs in psoriasis (see Box 9-1) include the following: multiple tiny pits on the surface of the nails (pitting); yellowing of the distal nail owing to separation of the nail plate from the nail bed (onycholysis); thickening of the distal nail (distal hyperkeratosis); or thickening, crumbling, and destruction of the entire nail (Fig. 9-11). All 20 nails may be involved, and

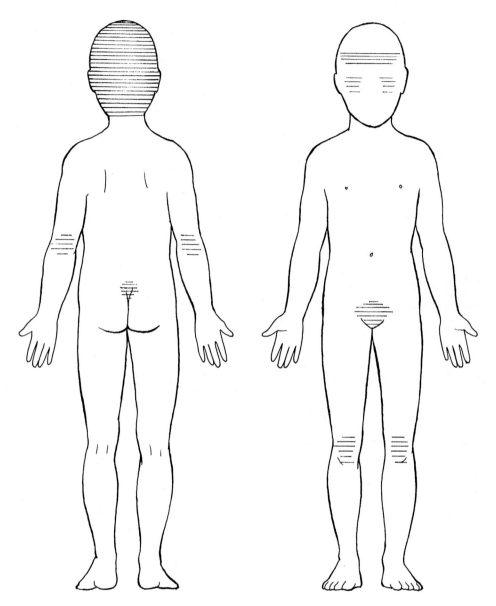

Fig. 9-2
The distribution of childhood psoriasis vulgaris.

rarely, nail changes may be the presenting feature of psoriasis in children. Nail changes are seen in 15% of children[1,4,9] with psoriasis, but absence of nail involvement does not exclude the diagnosis of psoriasis.

Erythroderma with thousands of pinpoint pustules, which eventuates in sheets of desquamation, is called *pustular psoriasis* and is quite rare in childhood,

but may result from treatment of psoriasis with systemic steroids[10] (Figs. 9-12 and 9-13). Pustular psoriasis may be accompanied by lytic bone lesions.[11]

Itching is a variable feature in psoriasis; most children do not complain of it. Scratching of lesions or picking off the scales may induce the isomorphic phenomenon and make individual lesions worse.

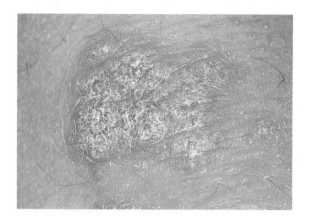

Fig. 9-3
Plaque of psoriasis with silvery scale on the leg of a child.

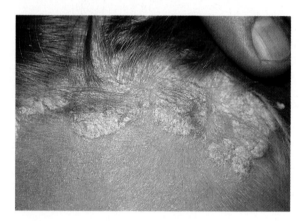

Fig. 9-4
Scaly plaques of the scalp in psoriasis.

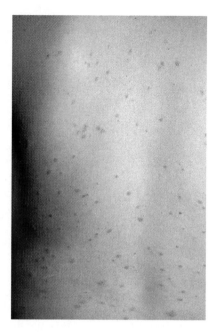

Fig. 9-5
Dozens of discrete, red papules scattered on the back of a child with acute guttate psoriasis following a streptococcal throat infection.

Arthritis is seldom seen in 1% of children with psoriasis.[12] Arthritis may precede or follow psoriasis and involves the metacarpophalangeal joints, proximal interphalangeal joints, or the axial skeleton[12,13] (Fig. 9-14). Juvenile psoriatic arthritis can only be diagnosed by the simultaneous presence of joint and characteristic skin changes of psoriasis.[12]

Differential diagnosis
Conditions to be considered in the differential diagnosis of papulosquamous disorders are listed in Box 9-2. Lichen planus with involvement of the elbows and knees can mimic psoriasis. However, the silvery scale and red color of psoriatic plaques distinguish them from the purple papules of lichen planus. Whitish plaques of the oral mucosa are seen in lichen planus, but not in psoriasis. The isomorphic phenomenon is also seen in lichen planus, but the papules are purple. In contrast to psoriasis, linear epidermal nevi are present from birth. Flat warts occurring along a line of skin trauma do not have a scaly surface. Lichen striatus appears as a solitary lesion progressing down an extremity. Scaly macules on the elbows and knees seen in childhood dermatomyositis may be confused with psoriasis. The presence of a malar photoeruption and muscle weakness and pain will help distinguish dermatomyositis. Hypertrophic cutaneous lupus lesions may mimic psoriasis, but the scale is thin, not thick, and central atrophy is present. Guttate psoriasis is most often confused with pityriasis rosea. The large "herald patch" of pityriasis rosea is lacking in guttate psoriasis, and the overlying scale in pityriasis rosea is thin and central, rather than thick and diffuse, as in psoriasis. Early guttate lesions are not scaly and may be confused with a morbilliform viral exanthem, urticaria, drug eruption, or secondary syphilis.

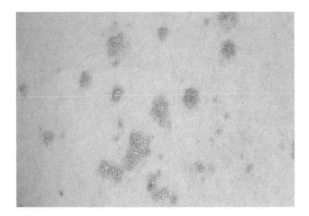

Fig. 9-6
Guttate papules on the back of a child with streptococcal perianal cellulitis.

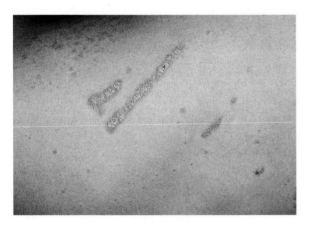

Fig. 9-7
Psoriasis appearing within the line of a previous scratch demonstrating the isomorphic (Koebner) phenomenon.

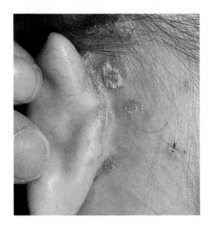

Fig. 9-8
Scaly papules behind the ear and in the scalp.

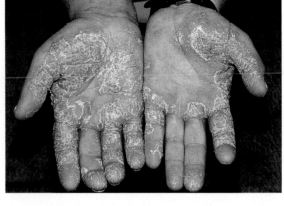

Fig. 9-9
Scaly fissured psoriasis plaques on a child's palms.

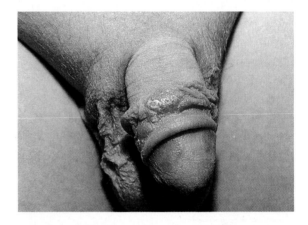

Fig. 9-10
Scaly plaque on foreskin and red plaque on glans penis in child with psoriasis.

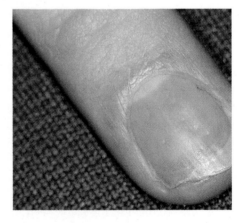

Fig. 9-11
Nail pitting in a child with psoriasis.

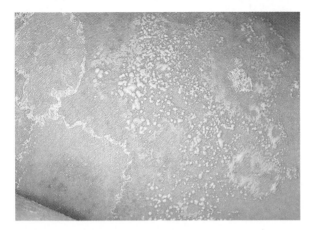

Fig. 9-12
Pinpoint pustules, erythema, and sheets of desquamation in a child with pustular psoriasis.

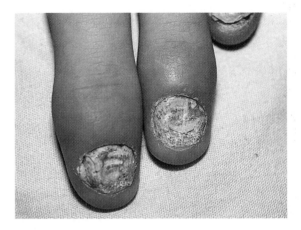

Fig. 9-14
Childhood psoriatic arthritis. Erythema and swelling of the distal interphalangeal joints with total nail dystrophy.

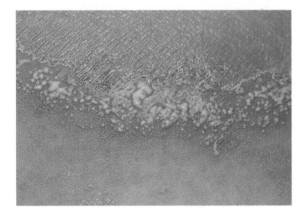

Fig. 9-13
Pinpoint pustules at border of childhood pustular psoriasis.

Scaling in the scalp in psoriasis is nongreasy, in contrast to the seborrheic dermatitis of adolescents. In atopic dermatitis of the scalp, the scales are mild, thin, and dry in contrast to the thick scales of psoriasis.

Nail pitting occurs in alopecia areata, but the pits are broader, more shallow, and fewer in number than in psoriasis. Onycholysis and hyperkeratosis of the nails occur in lichen planus, but synechiae from the cuticle to the fingertip and narrowing of the nail are seen. Fungal involvement of the nail is seen rarely in childhood, and usually only one or two nails are involved in contrast to psoriasis. Twenty-nail dystro-phy may be difficult to distinguish from psoriasis, although onycholysis and "oil spots" are found in psoriasis, but usually not in 20-nail dystrophy. In the absence of classical psoriasis skin lesions elsewhere, it requires following the child over many months to finally distinguish the two. All 20 nails are affected in ectodermal dysplasia and its variants, but alopecia, dental disorders, and other features are usually present to distinguish them from psoriasis.

Genital psoriasis must be differentiated from candidal intertriginous infections by potassium hydroxide (KOH) examination and fungal culture.

Pathogenesis

In most families with juvenile-onset (type 1) psoriasis, inheritance is apparently autosomal dominant, but environmental factors influence the expression of psoriasis significantly.[1,3] The histocompatibility antigens HLA-Cw6 and HLA-DR7 are increased in psoriasis, but apparently are not closely linked to the genes responsible for psoriasis.[1,3] Preliminary studies indicate a psoriasis susceptibility gene on chromosome 17q.[14] Genomic imprinting may occur in psoriasis, as there is increased likelihood of childhood psoriasis if the father had psoriasis.[3]

The classic pathologic features of psoriasis seen on skin biopsy denote inflammation associated with features of epidermal proliferation. The epidermis is thickened, with elongation of the rete ridges to the same level (regular acanthosis), increased epidermal mitosis, parakeratosis (nuclei retained in the stratum corneum), thinning of the granular layer, and microabscesses of neutrophils within the epidermis and stratum corneum. In the dermis the dermal papillae are clubbed, and there is vasodilation of dermal blood vessels and a lymphocytic infiltrate around them.[15] The lymphocytic infiltrate in both early and well-established lesions demonstrates activated lymphocytes with CD4+ cells early on.[15] Increased numbers of epidermal cells enter the mitotic cellular pool; the epidermal turnover time in psoriasis is three to four times faster than that of normal skin.

The factors responsible for increased epidermal turnover are unknown. In many ways the psoriatic epidermis mimics skin healing from a wound. In children the association with streptococcal infection is intriguing, and there is some experimental evidence to suggest that psoriasis patients, particularly children with guttate psoriasis, have greater lymphocyte activation by specific streptococcal antigens than do children without psoriasis.[5,6] Infection of the throat or perianal skin with streptococci may precipitate acute guttate psoriasis.[5,6] Studies on the inflammatory events before epidermal stimulation, and the regulation of epidermal growth, may help elucidate the mechanism of psoriasis.

Treatment

Most therapies are designed to retard epidermal proliferation but have some antiinflammatory effects as well. It is not certain which of these effects produces the most successful therapeutic results.

Topical steroids improve psoriasis temporarily, with the most benefit obtained from moderate- to high-potency glucocorticosteroids. Low-potency topical steroids such as 1% hydrocortisone are ineffective in childhood psoriasis.[1] The maximal benefit is obtained with 2 to 3 weeks of daily therapy, and remissions are shorter than with phototherapy. Topical steroid therapy may be followed with phototherapy to maintain the remission.

Ultraviolet light (UVL) with artificial ultraviolet (UV) sources (phototherapy) is effective in the management of psoriasis. In general, psoriatic children have better therapeutic response to UVL if done in a structured phototherapy protocol rather than sunbathing. Lubrication of the skin surface with mineral oil or petrolatum before UVL produces uniform penetration of UVL by reducing the reflection of light from the disrupted skin surface.[16] UVL (290 to 320 nm ultraviolet B [UVB]) three times weekly for 18 to 25 treatments may be quite successful.

For the scalp, softening the scales with salicylic acid 3% in mineral oil or olive oil or use of a phenol and saline scalp solution, massaged in and left in overnight, is useful. Then the scalp can be shampooed with a tar shampoo and the scales mechanically removed with a comb and brush. This is repeated daily until the scales are gone. The tar shampoo may be drying, and a commercial shampoo followed by a conditioner may be substituted if the child's hair appears weathered.

Topical calcitriol (1,25-hydroxyvitamin D_3) may be equally effective as midpotency steroids in the management of childhood psoriasis, requiring 4 weeks to clearing.[17]

Children with guttate psoriasis and evidence of streptococcal infection should be treated with antibiotics to eliminate the infection.[5,6]

Systemic steroids are contraindicated in childhood psoriasis because psoriatic erythroderma may follow withdrawal, resulting in fever, hypoalbuminuria, and other metabolic changes associated with generalized skin involvement.[9]

Anthralin is a tricyclic hydrocarbon that is efficacious in the management of psoriasis by inhibiting epidermal proliferation through downregulation of the epidermal growth factor TGF-alpha and its receptor, the epidermal growth factor receptor.[18] The so-called "short-contact" protocols are particularly useful. Anthralin 1% ointment is applied once daily to the psoriatic lesions for 20 minutes, then neutralized with a pH 7.0 soap, such as Dove soap, thoroughly washing off all the anthralin. If not washed off, it produces considerable skin irritation. Anthralin stains the skin and clothing brown. Most patients require 3 to 8 weeks of daily anthralin therapy to clear. There is no benefit from adding topical steroids to anthralin.[18]

Photochemotherapy with methoxsalen and long-wave UVL (320 to 400 nm ultraviolet A [UVA]), so-called PUVA (psoralen ultraviolet A-range) therapy, is reserved for children who have failed on standard therapies.[19] Because of potential mutagenicity,[18] PUVA should be administered only by experienced dermatologists.

Cyclosporin has been demonstrated to be efficacious in childhood psoriasis, but renal toxicity restricts its use to only the most recalcitrant cases.[20]

Oral retinoids are efficacious in severe forms of childhood psoriasis, such as generalized pustular psoriasis and psoriatic erythroderma,[9] but their effects on growing bones prohibit their long-term use in childhood.[21] Retinoids should never be considered the drug of first choice in the management of childhood psoriasis. Antimetabolites, such as methotrexate, inhibit the formation of epidermal deoxyribonucleic acid (DNA), but are reserved for the most severe, disabling forms of psoriasis because of their significant side effects. The use of antimetabolites in children should generally be avoided, with the exception of psoriatic arthritis.[10,11]

Patient education

Children with psoriasis have a chronic disease, and education is a crucial aspect of overall care. Patients and parents should understand that the disease is the result of both a genetic susceptibility and environmental factors. Childhood-onset psoriasis tends to increase in severity in adult life.[1-4] One should emphasize that good remission and good control of psoriasis can be achieved, but that sometimes childhood psoriasis is difficult to treat. One should explain that good treatments require 4 to 6 weeks to obtain significant improvement. It should also be stated that even if psoriasis clears, there is a hereditary susceptibility for psoriasis, and it can reappear in the future. Adolescents in particular need considerable emotional support. The occurrence of exacerbations at times of emotional stress is well recognized.

Patients should understand that trauma to the skin induces psoriasis, but severe restriction of activities is unwarranted. Not scratching psoriasis lesions should be stressed. In childhood guttate psoriasis, prompt administration of antibiotics with each sore throat or respiratory illness should be stressed, and children who have multiple episodes of poststreptococcal guttate psoriasis in a year might require prophylactic antibiotics.

Staphylococcus aureus can be cultured in large numbers from the skin surface in psoriasis. Occlusive dressings should be avoided, since they enhance the overgrowth of skin bacteria. Hospitalized children with psoriasis will shed bacteria continually into the room air.

Follow-up visits

Patients should be seen every 2 weeks during therapy to evaluate their response and provide supportive care. Dermatology nurse specialists or psoriatic day-care centers are ideal for this type of specialized care. An advantage of phototherapy protocols is that emotional support for the patient can be provided with each treatment, and the parents and patient can develop a better understanding of the condition and the care required to successfully control psoriasis.

PITYRIASIS ROSEA

Clinical features

Pityriasis rosea is most commonly seen in adolescents and children,[22] but has been described at all ages including infancy.[23] It may be preceded by a prodrome of pharyngitis, lymphadenopathy, headache, and malaise, but in most children no history of constitutional symptoms is given. An annular, scaly, erythematous lesion (the herald patch) precedes the appearance of the remainder of the lesions by 1 to 30 days[22] (Fig. 9-15). The herald patch is present in 80% of children. It is usually on the trunk, but may appear on the face or extremities. The herald patch, unlike the other lesions, shows central clearing and may mimic tinea corporis.[22]

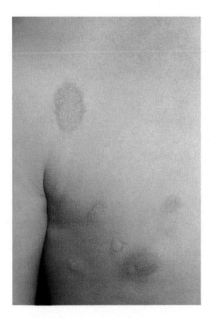

Fig. 9-15
Pityriasis rosea. Herald patch, which is larger than other papules, is seen on the child's chest.

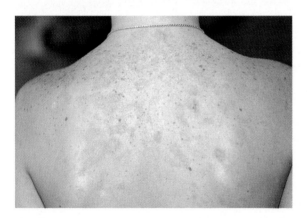

Fig. 9-16
Lesions of pityriasis rosea following a "Christmas tree" distribution.

The cutaneous lesions consist of multiple erythematous macules progressing to small, red papules and appear over the trunk (Fig. 9-16). The papules enlarge, becoming oval. The long axes of the oval lesions tend to be parallel to each other and follow the lines of skin stress (Fig. 9-17). A thin scale develops in the center of the oval lesions.[22] Individual lesions may be atypical in

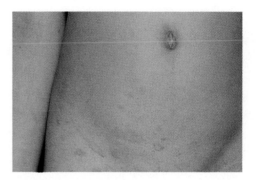

Fig. 9-17
Inverse pityriasis rosea with lesions seen in inguinal creases.

appearance, including vesicular, crusted, and purpuric types.[24] Asymptomatic oral lesions may be noted in 16%.[25] In black skin, lesions over the proximal extremities, inguinal and axillary areas, and neck often predominate, with few lesions on the trunk[22] (Fig. 9-18). Despite the different distribution, the course is similar. The lesions last 4 to 8 weeks. Mild itching is common during the first week of the generalized eruption, but the lesions are asymptomatic thereafter.

Differential diagnosis
The herald patch is often confused with tinea corporis before the appearance of the generalized eruption. If an antifungal agent is used, the generalized papular eruption may be mistaken for a drug reaction to the antifungal. The herald patch may also be confused with a lesion of nummular eczema. Nummular eczema usually is crusted in contrast to the dry, scaly herald patch. The generalized papular eruption may mimic urticaria, the viral exanthems, morbilliform drug eruptions, post–bone marrow transplantation eruption, or guttate psoriasis (see Box 9-2), but the presence of the herald patch is a useful distinguishing feature. As the lesions become more oval, secondary syphilis should be considered. Although secondary syphilis is usually characterized by lesions of the oral and genital mucosa and ham-colored macules on the palms and soles, the adolescent with "pityriasis rosea" accompanied by palmar lesions, fever, or lymphadenopathy should have a Venereal Disease Research Laboratories (VDRL) test

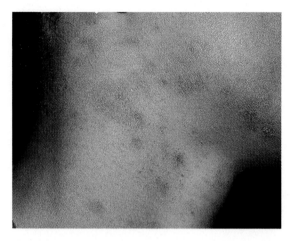

Fig. 9-18
Inverse pityriasis rosea with oval plaques with central scale on the neck of a black child.

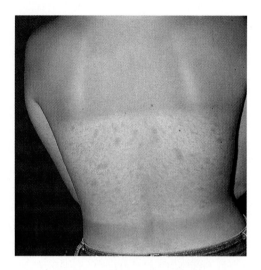

Fig. 9-19
The effect of sunlight on pityriasis rosea. Lesions present only in untanned areas of a child's back.

to exclude secondary syphilis. The oval lesions may also be confused with guttate parapsoriasis.

Pathogenesis

Since epidemics occur in a susceptible age group, pityriasis rosea has long been considered to be an infectious process. However, no viral or other microbial agent has been discovered in pityriasis rosea. Pathologic changes consist only of mild inflammation, with edema of the epidermis and dermis, and a mild perivascular accumulation of lymphocytes. Focal areas of parakeratosis are seen.

Treatment

Most children and adolescents require no therapy. A single dose of UVL, either natural sunlight exposure to redness or one minimal erythema dose of sunlamp exposure, will stop itching and hasten the disappearance of the lesions[26] (Fig. 9-19). Oral antihistamines are rarely necessary. Topical steroids do not influence the lesions.

Patient education

The long duration of the lesions should be explained, with assurance that they will disappear, leaving normal-appearing skin. A repeat episode of pityriasis rosea may cause concern, but multiple episodes occasionally occur and do not indicate need for concern.[22]

Follow-up visits

Follow-up visits are usually unnecessary except for follow-up on syphilis serology.

LUES (SECONDARY SYPHILIS)

Clinical features

Secondary syphilis is characterized by discrete pink macules or pink papules with a fine scale distributed over the trunk, associated with lymphadenopathy (see Chapter 5). Skin lesions erupt 3 to 6 weeks after the appearance of the chancre. Serologic tests for syphilis are always positive at the time of the secondary cutaneous eruption. A list of the cutaneous signs of secondary syphilis is presented in Box 9-3. The major signs include maculopapular lesions, condylomata lata, and mucous patches.

Condylomata lata are moist, warty papules seen in the perineum and other intertriginous areas, such as under the breast and in the interdigital webs and axillae. The mucous patch is a papular lesion seen

Box 9-3 Cutaneous signs of secondary syphilis

Major
- Papular lesions
- Condylomata lata
- Mucous patches

Minor
- Annular
- Nodular
- Pustular crusted lesions
- Alopecia
- Keratotic macules of palms and soles
- Usually associated with generalized lymphadenopathy

most often on the tongue as a red papule lacking tongue papillae. On the buccal mucosa, palate, tonsils, vaginal mucosa, glans penis, and coronal sulcus, it appears as a papule with a central erosion.

The maculopapular lesions, condylomata lata, and mucous patches contain hundreds of spirochetes and are infectious. Generalized lymphadenopathy accompanies these features in 85% of cases; low-grade fever, lethargy, and arthralgias accompany the eruptions in 50% of cases.

Minor variants of secondary syphilis include the following: annular lesions of the face, neck, and genitalia, most commonly seen in blacks; acral nodules that are few in number; sterile pustules and crusted lesions that mimic ecthyma; a "motheaten" alopecia of the eyebrows and scalp hair; and keratotic, ham-colored macules of the palms and soles.

Untreated secondary syphilis may progress to nephrotic syndrome, cranial nerve palsies, meningismus, osteolytic lesions, syphilitic hepatitis, or neurosyphilis.

Differential diagnosis
Syphilis is well known to mimic a wide variety of cutaneous conditions (Box 9-2), but most commonly, pityriasis rosea. The generalized eruptions may be differentiated from pityriasis rosea by the involvement of the palms and soles, lymphadenopathy, mucous patches, and a positive VDRL flocculation test.

Condylomata lata must be distinguished from venereal warts by the VDRL flocculation test or dark-field microscopic examination.

Mucous patches may be confused with geographic tongue, aphthous stomatitis, angular cheilitis, or other mucocutaneous syndromes.

For pathogenesis, treatment, patient education, follow-up visits, and References, see Chapter 5.

PARAPSORIASIS

Clinical features
Parapsoriasis, an uncommon disorder, may be seen in two distinct childhood forms: acute parapsoriasis (Mucha-Habermann disease) (pityriasis lichenoides et varioliformis acuta [PLEVA]) and guttate parapsoriasis (pityriasis lichenoides chronica).[27] Both forms may occur in the same patient, or one form may progress to the other. Thus they are considered two forms of the same disease.[27-29] The diseases usually have their onset between 5 and 15 years.[27,29] In acute parapsoriasis, the eruption consists of recurrent crops of red papules 2 to 4 mm in diameter (Fig.

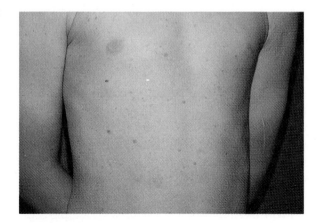

Fig. 9-20
Acute parapsoriasis. Red papules with central purpura or crusts and vesicles scattered over a 10-year-old child's trunk.

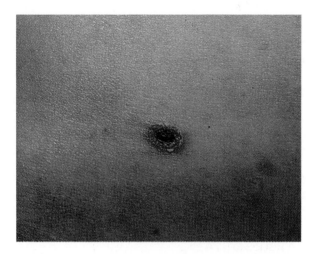

Fig. 9-21
Characteristic red papule with central crust in acute parapsoriasis.

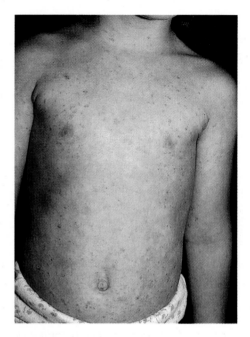

Fig. 9-22
Chronic parapsoriasis. Discrete, oval salmon-colored papules with a thin scale seen on a child's trunk.

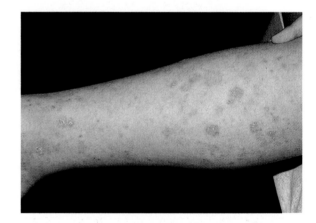

Fig. 9-23
Chronic parapsoriasis. Multiple scaly plaques on child's leg.

9-20). The papules have central petechiae and progress to crusting (Fig. 9-21). Lesions in different stages are seen, particularly on the trunk. They heal with depressed scars. The eruption lasts approximately 9 to 12 months and is occasionally associated with low-grade fever.

In guttate parapsoriasis, salmon-colored, oval papules with central thin scales are seen primarily in the perineal area, thighs, and trunk[28] (Figs. 9-22 and 9-23). They are few in number, but may persist for 2 to 3 years.[29] Both forms are seldom associated with itching.

Differential diagnosis
Acute parapsoriasis mimics varicella, and a child with "prolonged varicella" should bring acute parapsoriasis to mind. Occasionally insect bites or necrotizing vasculitis are confused with acute parapsoriasis. In acute parapsoriasis at least some lesions have a purpuric center, which is helpful to distinguish it from varicella or insect bites. The presence of lesions in many different stages is useful in separating acute parapsoriasis from vasculitis. In a few children lesions appear similar to those of acute parapsoriasis, but the infiltrating cells will demonstrate abnormal nuclear shapes and size. This condition is called *lymphomatoid papulosis*. A few children with lymphomatoid papulosis may develop a cutaneous T cell lymphoma, mycosis fungoides.[29,30] A skin biopsy will distinguish.[28,29]

The guttate form mimics pityriasis rosea, and thus "prolonged pityriasis rosea" should alert one to the diagnosis of guttate parapsoriasis. Dry skin dermatitis, nummular eczema, secondary syphilis, guttate psoriasis, and tinea corporis sometimes confuse the diagnosis (see Box 9-2). The long duration and sparse number of lesions help distinguish.

Pathogenesis

Acute parapsoriasis is a vascular injury, with extravasation of erythrocytes, a superficial perivascular lymphohistiocytic infiltrate, and necrosis of the overlying epidermis.[28] Focal parakeratosis is also seen. In contrast to necrotizing vasculitis, no fibrinoid necrosis of the vessel walls is seen, neutrophils are not present, and nuclear fragments are not found around vessels. The mechanism of the disease remains unknown.

The histologic findings in guttate parapsoriasis are similar to those of pityriasis rosea. The mechanism of the disease is unknown.

Treatment

Treatment with oral erythromycin, at 40 mg/kg/day for 1 to 2 months, may benefit some children.[31] For children who fail erythromycin therapy, a conservative approach is recommended, with therapy much like that for psoriasis; UVB phototherapy may control the disease and some authorities believe it is the treatment of choice for parapsoriasis.[32] Topical steroids do not influence the disease, and claims for efficacy from high-dose tetracycline or low-dose methotrexate cannot be substantiated.

Box 9-4   The "P's" of lichen planus

Planar (flat-topped)
Pruritic (itchy)
Purple
Polygonal (angulated borders)
Papules
Penile

Patient education

The prolonged course of these disorders should be emphasized.

Follow-up visits

A visit in 1 month is useful to reevaluate the child's disease state and determine response to therapy. In the child with persistent lesions over 2 years, reevaluation every 6 to 12 months is suggested with consideration of rebiopsy because of the possibility of development of a cutaneous T cell lymphoma.[29,30]

LICHEN PLANUS

Clinical features

Lichen planus is a chronic papular skin disorder characterized by the appearance of purple, flat-topped papules.[33,34] The list in Box 9-4 is helpful in recalling the major features. The classic polygonal purple papules occur on the wrist and extensor surfaces of the forearm (Fig. 9-24). On the knees, feet, and lower legs, thick scaling is found over thickened, purple plaques (hypertrophic lichen planus) (Fig. 9-25). Bullae or erosions may be seen on the feet or head and neck.[33] The shaft of the penis is commonly involved (Fig. 9-26). Lichen planus may be inherited

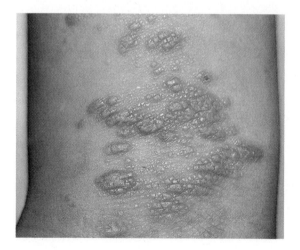

Fig. 9-24
Childhood lichen planus. Purple papules on wrist and forearm.

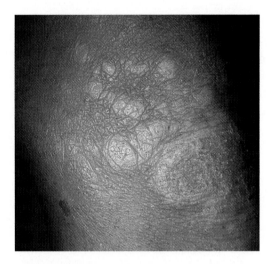

Fig. 9-25
Thick, scaly, purple plaques over the knee in a child with lichen planus.

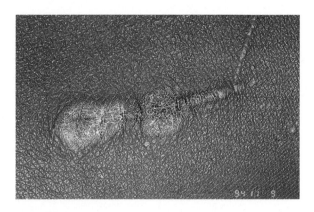

Fig. 9-27
Isomorphic phenomenon in childhood lichen planus. Linear extension of lichen planus along the line of a scratch.

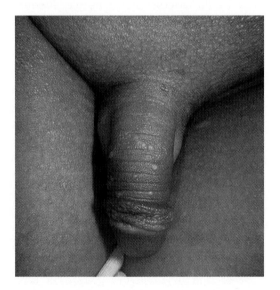

Fig. 9-26
Linear purple papules on the penis in a child with lichen planus.

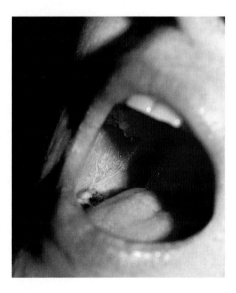

Fig. 9-28
Lacy white thickening of the buccal mucosa in an adolescent demonstrating mucosal involvement in lichen planus.

in an autosomal dominant manner.[33,34] The isomorphic phenomenon may be prominent (Fig. 9-27).

Oral lesions are seen most commonly on the buccal mucosa as white, thickened papules in a lacy pattern[35] (Fig. 9-28). Erosions or thickening of the tongue or gingivae may be seen.

In the scalp a circumscribed area of hair loss with replacement of follicles by scarring rarely occurs.[36]

The nail changes of lichen planus are rare in children, but a roughening of the nail surface (trachyonychia) may be seen.[37] Total destruction of all 20 nails with synechiae formation may precede, accompany, or

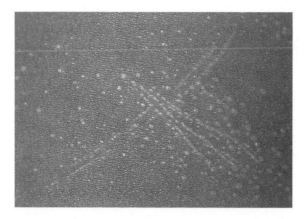

Fig. 9-29
Hundreds of discrete, pinpoint, white flat-topped papules on a child with lichen nitidus.

follow the onset of skin lesions.[38] The nail is narrowed, with an overgrowth of fibrous tissue from the proximal nail fold across the nail plate to the tip of the digit. A few children with lichen planus will present with only nail involvement, which is often labeled 20-nail dystrophy of childhood until a nail biopsy is done or other mucocutaneous lesions of lichen planus develop.[38]

Itching is severe in lichen planus, and the isomorphic phenomenon occurs commonly with the appearance of lichen planus papules along an area of skin trauma.[33] Localized forms also occur in children. The natural history of lichen planus is to resolve in 9 to 18 months, leaving hyperpigmented areas in sites where lesions occurred.

A variant of lichen planus, called lichen nitidus, has histologic features identical to those of lichen planus, yet is more focal in nature.[39] It demonstrates tiny (1 to 2 mm) hypopigmented, flat-topped papules occurring in clusters, usually over the trunk (Fig. 9-29). Lesions may demonstrate the isomorphic phenomenon.[39] They do not itch. Lesions of lichen nitidus have been found in 25% of children with lichen planus.

Differential diagnosis
The characteristic purple color, with flat-topped papules with angulated borders, distinguishes lichen planus from other papulosquamous disorders (see Box 9-2). The hypertrophic lesions on the lower legs

mimic psoriasis. Erosive lesions in the mouth mimic aphthous stomatitis and herpes simplex, and the white, lacy appearance of the buccal mucosa may be confused with premalignant leukoplakia or a white sponge nevus. A skin biopsy may be required to confirm the diagnosis of lichen planus.[33]

A variety of drugs can produce an eruption identical to lichen planus, including thiazide diuretics, atabrine, chloroquine, quinine, quinidine, and gold, but these agents are rarely used in children.

Lichen nitidus may mimic keratosis pilaris, but the inspissated, dry, scaly follicular plugs of keratosis pilaris are not seen, and lichen nitidus lesions are smooth-topped.[39]

Pathogenesis
Lichen planus results from an acute injury to the basal cells of the epidermis such that liquefaction degeneration of basal cells occurs, and the dermal-epidermal junction is obscured. In bullous lichen planus the epidermis separates from the dermis. Amorphous colloid bodies representing degenerating basal cells combined with immunoreactants such as immunoglobulin A (IgA), immunoglobulin G (IgG), immunoglobulin M (IgM), complement, and fibrin are seen in the basal layer or just beneath it. The damaged basal cells have decreased ability to divide. Thus there are features of prolonged retention of cells in the epidermis, with acanthosis, hyperkeratosis, and a thickened granular layer. The exact mechanism of the epidermal basal cell injury is unknown, but it is thought to be due to inflammatory injury by mononuclear cells that interact with the basement membrane.

In lichen nitidus the same pathologic changes occur, but they are limited to a single dermal papilla.

Treatment
Topical glucocorticosteroids are effective in controlling the itching and resolution of the lesions. They are used twice daily, and 4 to 8 weeks of therapy are often required for remission. In children with severe generalized lichen planus, prompt relief from prednisone, 1 to 2 mg/kg/day in a single morning dose, can be expected in 2 weeks, although the lichen planus may

return as the steroids are reduced. Oral lesions are usually asymptomatic, but when painful, will respond to topical steroid or topical isotretinoin gels applied to the mucosa. Lichen nitidus need not be treated.

Patient education

Patients should be informed of the prolonged nature of lichen planus and the tendency for dyspigmentation to occur on healing. It should be emphasized that topical steroids are the most effective method to relieve the itching, but that the clearing of individual lesions will be slow.

Follow-up visits

Follow-up visits every 2 to 4 weeks are needed to monitor the course of the disease and the response to therapy.

LUPUS ERYTHEMATOSUS

Clinical features

Lupus erythematosus (LE) occurs more often in females than in males.[41] The prevalence may be three times higher in black, Asian, or Hispanic children than in whites.[42] In approximately 15% of all patients with LE, the onset is between the ages of 9 and 15 years,[41] and the incidence is estimated at 0.6 per 100,000.[42]

A cutaneous eruption is present in 80% of adolescents with LE, and in 25% it is the presenting sign. The most frequent cutaneous sign is the erythematous maculopapular eruption over the cheeks and nose with a "butterfly" distribution[41] (Fig. 9-30). It is covered by a fine scale and occurs in one third to one half of the patients.[41,42] Next most common is the discoid lesion, a chronic, persistent skin change that progresses to scarring and pigmentary changes; in black patients, severe hypopigmentation may be seen[43] (Fig. 9-31). Discoid lesions are seen most frequently over the face and hands, ears, and scalp, where scarring hair loss results[41,43] (Fig. 9-32). More transient annular papulosquamous lesions limited to sun-exposed areas of skin are observed in subacute cutaneous lupus[41,42] (Fig. 9-33). Subacute cutaneous lupus is more likely to occur in early childhood and be associated with genetic complement deficiencies and the presence of anti-Ro and anti-La autoantibodies.[41,44]

Other kinds of skin involvement may occur in adolescents with LE, including telangiectatic erythema on the thenar and hypothenar eminences of the palms and

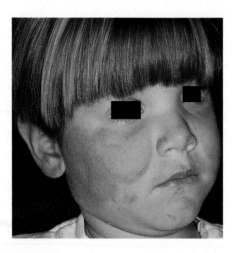

Fig. 9-30
Bright red, scaly plaques on cheeks of a girl with acute systemic lupus erythematosus.

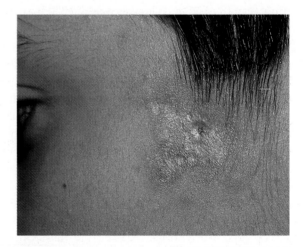

Fig. 9-31
Atrophy, erythema, and scaling of preauricular skin of a child with discoid lupus erythematosus.

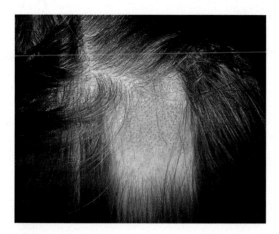

Fig. 9-32
Scarring hair loss with redness and scaling of the underlying scalp in an 8-year-old girl with discoid lupus erythematosus.

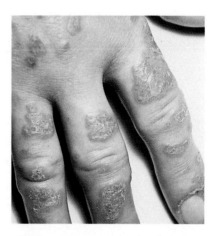

Fig. 9-34
Scaly plaques between the knuckles in systemic lupus erythematosus. Compare with Figs. 9-40 and 9-41.

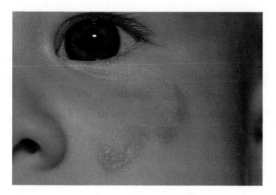

Fig. 9-33
Subacute cutaneous lupus erythematosus. Annular, scaly red plaque of a child's cheek.

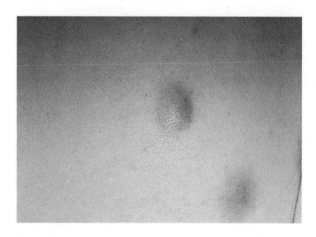

Fig. 9-35
Red-purple nodules on the upper arm of a girl with lupus profundus (panniculitis).

the pulps of the fingers and diffuse erythema and telangiectasia of the cuticle, with erythematous, scaly macules occurring over the dorsa of the fingers between the knuckles[41,42] (Fig. 9-34). Bullous lesions may occasionally occur. A mottling of the extensor surface of the extremities, the so-called livedo reticularis, occasionally occurs.[41] Features of cutaneous vasculitis, such as subcutaneous nodules, splinter nail hemorrhages, purpuric acral infarcts, palpable purpura, and distal gangrene, may be seen. Raynaud's phenomenon, a two-phase color change of the digit upon cold exposure with pallor and cyanosis, occurs in 35% of adoles-

cents. Rarely, persistent, tender, red-purple nodules on the cheeks, proximal extremities, or trunk—which represent lupus panniculitis—will be seen in children[41] (Fig. 9-35). A distinct history of sun sensitivity may not be obtained in children with lupus, and careful questioning may be required to uncover photosensitivity.

Diagnosis depends on a constellation of clinical, pathologic, and serologic findings. Use of American Rheumatism Association (ARA) criteria for LE is recommended.[41]

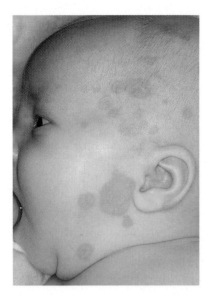

Fig. 9-36
Neonatal lupus syndrome. Four-week-old female with dozens of scaly, annular red macules on the forehead and cheeks.

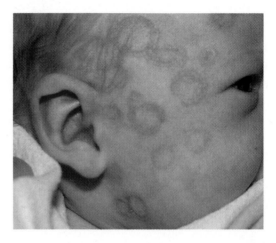

Fig. 9-37
Neonatal lupus syndrome. Five-week-old baby with annular papulosquamous lesions of the head.

The neonatal lupus syndrome is characterized by congenital heart block or annular papulosquamous skin lesions or both[45-49] (Figs. 9-36 and 9-37). Although affected infants do not meet ARA criteria for lupus, the association with maternal lupus or Sjögren's syndrome and the clinical skin lesions, skin pathology, and distinctive pattern of autoantibodies similar to those found in subacute cutaneous lupus permit the use of lupus in the diagnosis of this neonatal lupus syndrome. The skin lesions fade by 6 to 7 months of age, but the heart block will persist. Residual telangiectasia may persist for several years. Five percent of babies with neonatal lupus syndrome will have liver disease or thrombocytopenia.[47,48]

The most useful serologic test in the diagnosis of lupus is the fluorescent antinuclear antibody (ANA) test, which is positive in over 90% of children with LE. Sensitivity is improved if human, rather than rodent, tissue substrates are used.[41,50,51] Autoantibodies in LE are directed against a variety of nuclear components. The most specific is that directed against the nuclear acidic chromosomal proteins, such as the Sm antigen. It is very specific, but is found in only 30% of patients. In addition to screening with a fluorescent ANA test, in some children in whom lupus is suspected, an ANA profile in which immunodiffusion tests are done against soluble nuclear antigens may be performed. This is especially useful in detecting antibodies to Sjögren's syndrome A (SS-A) (Ro), which is a diagnostic marker for neonatal lupus syndrome and is found in 98% of reported babies.[45-51] A few babies will have autoantibodies to U1-RNP rather than anti-Ro.[47]

Depressed complement levels, especially the C4 level, are useful for detecting active vasculitis, particularly in the central nervous system and kidney. Direct immunofluorescence of skin biopsy specimens of involved skin are positive for granular deposits of IgG or C3 at the dermal-epidermal junction in 90% of patients. IgG deposits over basal keratinocytes are observed in subacute cutaneous lupus and neonatal lupus.[52]

The initial evaluation of patients with suspected LE should include the tests listed in Box 9-5.

In general, patients with discoid cutaneous lesions, subacute cutaneous lupus, or lupus panniculitis have a low incidence of disease in other organs, whereas those with the butterfly maculopapular eruption or vasculitis lesions are likely to have renal, central nervous system, or other vital organ involvement.[41]

Box 9-5   Initial laboratory evaluation of lupus

Skin biopsy, formalin fixed for routine histologic study
Skin biopsy, frozen section, for immunofluorescence
Serum for antinuclear antibody and ANA profile
Serum for total hemolytic complement and complement components
Urinalysis
Complete blood cell count with differential and platelet count

---

Box 9-6   Drugs responsible for inducing lupus-like syndromes

High risk
   Hydralazine
   Procainamide
   D-Penicillamine
   Practolol
Moderate risk
   Isoniazid
   Phenytoin
   Ethosuximide
   Propylthiouracil
   Trimethadione

Differential diagnosis

Childhood dermatomyositis and lupus may present with similar cutaneous features. The photosensitive butterfly eruption may be seen in children with dermatomyositis or drug-induced photosensitivity, such as seen with the phenothiazines, naproxen, or thiazide diuretics. A butterfly eruption may also be seen in polymorphous light eruption. Skin biopsy and immunofluorescence will be useful in distinguishing lupus erythematosus from these processes. The eruption may be scaly enough to consider psoriasis, lichen planus, or other papulosquamous disorders (see Box 9-2). Dermatophyte facial infection (tinea faciei) must be excluded by KOH examination of the scales.

Biopsy is necessary to differentiate discoid lesions of the face from psoriasis and lichen planus, and the discoid lesions of the scalp from other causes of circumscribed alopecia.

Drug-induced LE syndromes rarely cause cutaneous eruptions, but sometimes may mimic LE. The drugs likely to produce LE syndromes are listed in Box 9-6. The livedo reticularis pattern is seen in dermatomyositis, scleroderma, and other collagen vascular diseases, as is Raynaud's phenomenon, palmar erythema, and cuticular telangiectasia.

Careful examination of the dorsa of the hands may help distinguish LE from dermatomyositis. In LE, scaly erythematous macules are seen between the knuckles on the dorsum of the hand, whereas in dermatomyositis, scaly macules or papules are seen over the knuckle pads. Compare Fig. 9-34 with Fig. 9-40.

The annular papulosquamous lesions of subacute cutaneous LE may mimic tinea corporis, erythema infectiosum, or pityriasis rosea, but a skin biopsy will distinguish.

The red-purple nodules of lupus panniculitis may be confused with vascular tumors or cutaneous lymphomas or leukemias.

Pathogenesis

Lupus erythematosus is associated with circulating immune complexes, which may account for many of the vasculitis features in the joints, kidneys, and central nervous system. In the skin there is an injury to epidermal basal cells with liquefaction degeneration, which may lead to dermal-epidermal separation.[41,52] A patchy accumulation of lymphocytes around dermal blood vessels and hair follicles is seen. These findings are found in acute, subacute, chronic (discoid), and neonatal skin lesions. In addition, discoid lupus shows epidermal atrophy and follicular plugs of scale.[52] Usually no evidence of necrotizing vasculitis is found in the skin, although antigen-antibody complexes have been eluted from the skin. In lupus panniculitis, there is usually a dense lymphocytic infiltrate around subcutaneous vessels between fat lobules, without the superficial skin injury observed in other forms of cutaneous lupus.

The exact mechanism of skin injury and photosensitivity is unknown. A possible association with viruses or virus-induced tissue injury is suggested from animal models of LE-like diseases.

Treatment

It is beyond the scope of this book to discuss the treatment of systemic LE. The chronic cutaneous lesions respond to potent topical fluorinated glucocorticosteroids applied twice daily. In the discoid lupus form, response is slow, over many months. Although chloroquine has been demonstrated to be efficacious in discoid LE, particularly that associated with arthritis, it produces a cardiomyopathy in prepubertal children, and must be used with careful monitoring. In older adolescents, hydoxychloroquine, 200 mg twice daily, may be efficacious. Prior visual screening should be obtained by ophthalmologic consultation, and regular 3-month eye examinations given. In lupus panniculitis, superpotent topical steroids and hydroxychloroquine have been used successfully.[41,53]

In children and adolescents with systemic involvement, skin lesions clear with immunosuppressive agents in the doses used to treat renal disease. Sometimes skin lesions require additional topical therapy with potent or superpotent topical steroids for control.

Photoprotection should be a mainstay of therapy for cutaneous LE, even when photosensitivity is uncertain. Protective clothing and regular use of sunscreens are recommended.

Patient education

Sun sensitivity should be discussed and the use of photoprotective agents strongly emphasized. Daily use of a sunscreen of at least SPF-30 is advised. In addition, it is advisable for the patient to avoid sun exposure between the hours of 10 A.M. and 4 P.M., during which time 60% of UVL reaches the earth's surface. The patient should be advised to wear a hat to protect the face. Severe sunburn has resulted in systemic exacerbations of LE. Cosmetic coverings are helpful, both as sunscreens and for disguising unsightly skin lesions.

Follow-up visits

After the initial visit, a visit in 1 week is useful for the evaluation of laboratory evidence, which may indicate potential systemic involvement. Often adolescents presenting with acute symptoms such as fever, acute arthralgias, or renal disease must be hospitalized. It is important to remember that in 5% to 10% of those presenting with cutaneous lesions only, the disease may progress to involvement of internal organs. Thus reevaluation every 3 months is recommended.

DERMATOMYOSITIS

Clinical features

The onset of most cases of childhood dermatomyositis is between 4 and 12 years.[54] The incidence is estimated as 1 per 100,000.[54,55] Childhood dermatomyositis often presents with a photosensitive facial rash involving the malar areas and the upper eyelids.[56] Photosensitivity in juvenile dermatomyositis is more frequent than in LE[56] (Fig. 9-38). Periorbital edema and a violaceous hue to the eyelids are seen. Over the elbows and knees, erythematous plaques with a fine scale are observed (Fig. 9-39), and flat-

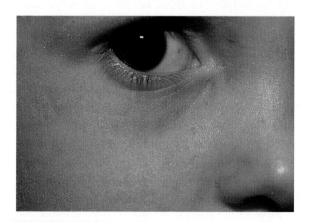

Fig. 9-38
Dermatomyositis. Purple-red discoloration of the eyelids and cheeks in a "butterfly" distribution, which mimics lupus.

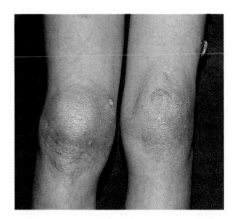

Fig. 9-39
Dermatomyositis, Scaly, rosy-colored plaques over knees, which mimic psoriasis.

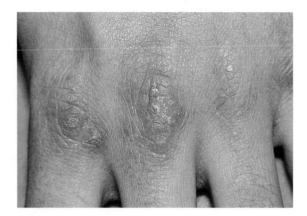

Fig. 9-41
Gottron's papules over the knuckles in juvenile dermatomyositis.

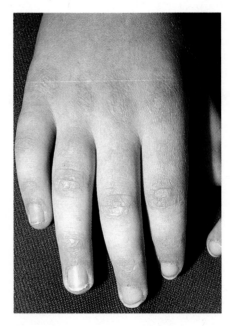

Fig. 9-40
Dermatomyositis. Scaly red papules over the knuckles (Gottron's papules) in childhood dermatomyositis. Compare with Fig. 9-34.

topped red papules over the knuckles (Gottron's papules) are found[54,55] (Figs. 9-40 and 9-41). Cuticular or eyelid margin telangiectasia is seen. A livedo reticularis pattern on the extremities may be prominent. The skin changes may precede, occur simultaneously with, or follow signs of muscle disease. Occasionally the cutaneous features are present for months before muscle symptoms are noted.[57] Children with dermatomyositis appear ill, with low-grade fever, malaise, and anorexia noted.

Weakness, with or without pain in the proximal muscles, is the most frequent symptom. Inability to run and climb stairs, easy fatiguability during play, and inability to comb hair or reach upward may be presenting symptoms.[52,58] Dysphagia is found in 10% of patients from pharyngeal muscle weakness.

As the disease slowly progresses, muscle weakness may be so profound as to make the child bedridden.[58] Calcinosis of skin and muscle eventually develops in 40% of children and becomes a major problem.[52,58] Skin calcinosis is seen as crusted papules or plaques around joints or as nonhealing sores. Muscle calcification may result in contractures or severe muscular pain.

Differential diagnosis

LE is most often confused with dermatomyositis because of the facial photosensitive eruption. Examination of the dorsa of the hands (see lupus) will help differentiate, as will muscle signs and symptoms. Muscle enzyme levels, particularly creatine phosphokinase (CPK), serum glutamate oxaloacetate transaminase (SGOT), and aldolase may be elevated.

Muscle biopsy or electromyography may assist in the diagnosis. Skin biopsy findings are not diagnostic.

The scaly plaques on elbows and knees are often confused with psoriasis. In dermatomyositis the scale is thin, not thick, and there are associated muscle findings; the child appears ill in contrast to psoriasis.

The livedo reticularis pattern may also be found in periarteritis nodosa and lupus; and the cuticular telangiectasias are found in a number of collagen vascular diseases.

Pathogenesis

The mechanism of cutaneous injury is unknown.[59] Skin biopsies show edema of the upper dermis with a sparse perivascular mononuclear cell infiltrate, and immunofluorescent studies are usually nonspecific. A skin biopsy may be most useful to detect calcification. Children with dermatomyositis may have autoantibodies to muscle proteins such as Jo-1, PM/SCL, or Mi and have positive ANAs. Of interest is the dermatomyositis syndrome produced by enteroviruses in children with congenital immunodeficiencies.[52] Whether dermatomyositis is a viral disease is as yet unproven.

Treatment

Systemic steroids and steroid-sparing drugs such as azathioprine are the primary modes of therapy in dermatomyositis.[52] Skin lesions usually are controlled by systemic therapy, but occasionally potent or superpotent topical steroids will be required in addition. Low-dose coumarin may be useful in preventing or reversing cutaneous calcification.

Patient education

It should be emphasized that a multidiscipline approach to care for children with dermatomyositis is required. Children should be treated in settings where muscle disease specialists, dermatologists, and rheumatologists can coordinate the care, and physical therapy and nutritional support are available. Parents must recognize the serious and disabling nature of the condition, be prepared for long-term therapy, and be apprised of the potential complications of the disease and the long-term immunosuppressive therapy.

Follow-up visits

If not hospitalized, the child should be seen weekly until good control of the disease is achieved.

LICHEN STRIATUS

Clinical features

Lichen striatus is a disorder peculiar to childhood, characterized by linear, shiny, hypopigmented papules limited to one extremity[60] (Fig. 9-42). It does not follow vascular or neural structures, but tends to follow the lines of Blaschko[60] (Fig. 9-43). It is most

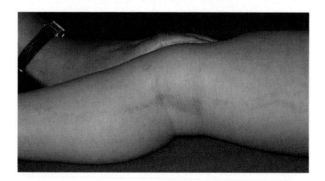

Fig. 9-42
Lichen striatus. Linear, red, scaly papules extending down flexor surface of a child.

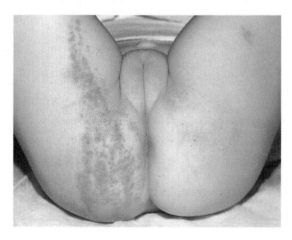

Fig. 9-43
Lichen striatus lesions, which follow the lines of Blaschko.

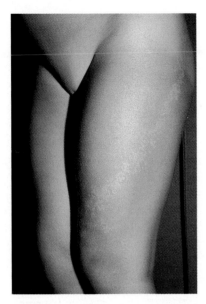

Fig. 9-44
Hypopigmented residual macules in healing lichen striatus.

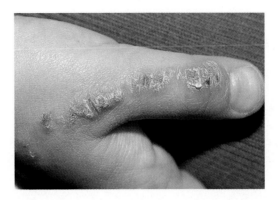

Fig. 9-45
Lichen striatus extending down the digit.

common in ages 2 to 12 years, with a mean age of 4 years.[60] Although the lesions begin as pink or dull-red papules, they quickly become hypopigmented (Fig. 9-44). Characteristically, the lesions begin on a buttock and spread down the leg, or begin on the shoulder and progress down the arm.[60,61] They may first be noticed distally, however. The lesion may extend down the digit (Fig. 9-45) and produce a linear nail dystrophy.[62] Occasionally lesions will be noted on the face. The lesions last 1 week to 3 years, with a mean of 9 months, then spontaneously disappear.[60] Hypopigmented macules occur in 50% and may persist for additional months.[60] Relapses of short duration have been noted after complete clearing.[60]

Differential diagnosis
The linear lesions are so characteristic that they are seldom confused with other lesions. The isomorphic phenomenon, seen in lichen planus, lichen nitidus, or psoriasis, may be confused with lichen striatus, but lesions will be present in other areas of the skin in these diseases. Epidermal birthmarks may be confused, but they are irregular on the surface rather than shiny and are present from birth, rather than being acquired later in life. Porokeratosis of Mibelli may be confused, but does not transcend an entire extremity nor follow the lines of Blaschko. A skin biopsy will distinguish, but is usually not required.

Pathogenesis
A chronic dermatitis is seen on histologic sections, but the mechanism of the disease is unknown. There is considerable overlap between the pathology of linear lichen planus and lichen striatus.[61]

Treatment
Treatment is unnecessary. Topical steroids are of little help.

Patient education
The benign nature and complete resolution of these lesions should be emphasized.

Follow-up visits
A follow-up visit in 4 weeks is useful to examine for skin lesions in other areas to rule out other papulosquamous conditions.

POROKERATOSIS OF MIBELLI

Clinical features
Porokeratosis of Mibelli may appear as a segmental single lesion or as a group of lesions that may mimic

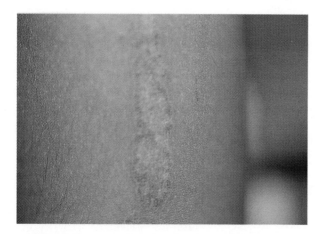

Fig. 9-46
Porokeratosis of Mibelli. Linear, scaly plaque with moatlike border in a 9-year-old child.

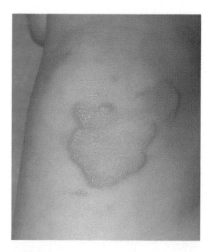

Fig. 9-47
Porokeratosis of the knee of a child.

lichen striatus or an epidermal nevus[63] (Fig. 9-46). The condition occurs more frequently in males and has a predilection for the face, neck, forearms, and hands, although the knees (Fig. 9-47), buttocks, and feet may also occasionally be involved. Individual lesions appear as craterlike areas on the skin with a scaly, irregular, oval border.[63] The crateriform area may measure from 5 to 50 mm in diameter, and several craters may be grouped together. The most important diagnostic feature of porokeratosis of Mibelli is the appearance of a scaly border in which a double row of scales surmounted by a furrow is observed. Diagnosis is by biopsy of the border of the lesion.

Differential diagnosis

Porokeratosis of Mibelli may be confused with lichen striatus or with epidermal nevi. However, in contrast to lichen striatus, lesions are often segmental and do not completely extend down an extremity. In contrast to epidermal nevi, they are never present at birth but develop later in childhood, and do not have as verrucous a surface. Biopsy is often useful in distinguishing among these possibilities.

Pathogenesis

The characteristic biopsy finding demonstrates focal areas of parakeratosis within the epidermis and, if proper sectioning of the double ridge has been obtained, a pair of focal parakeratotic columns with a normal or slightly thinned epidermis sandwiched between them.[63,64] Sparse or moderate inflammation may be seen beneath the parakeratotic columns. It is believed that this represents hyperplastic clones of sweat duct keratinocytes, perhaps transformed by a papillomavirus.[64] This would explain its generalized nature in immunosuppressed patients or in patients with chronic sun damage.[63]

Treatment

The lesions of porokeratosis may produce some concern about cosmetic appearance in the parents, but no satisfactory therapy has been developed. Progressive growth may occur over 2 to 3 years and some spontaneous resolutions have been reported. Topical keratolytic agents have not been of use in therapy, and topical 5-fluorouracil (5-FU) solution has been reported to be efficacious, although it should be used cautiously in children. Some promising results have been obtained with combinations of topical tretinoin and 5-FU.

Patient education

The parents must be told that the cause is unknown, and the likelihood of spontaneous remission within a few years is high. They must be warned against rushing into cosmetic surgery for improvement because the scarring after surgery may be worse than the lesion itself. The advantages of a conservative approach to such lesions should be emphasized. It should be stated that the malignant potential in children is unknown.

Follow-up visits

A follow-up visit in 6 to 12 months may be useful to determine the course of the lesion in the child.

PITYRIASIS RUBRA PILARIS (PRP)

Clinical features

Pityriasis rubra pilaris (PRP) has its onset between the ages of 2 and 9 years.[65-67] The first sign is commonly salmon-colored diffuse thickening of the palms and soles, with exaggerated scaling in the fissures[65] (Figs. 9-48 and 9-49). The involvement extends beyond the dorsopalmar and dorsoplantar junctions, often involving the knuckle pads (Fig. 9-50).

In 20% of children the condition will remain restricted to the palms and soles.[65] In 60% of children the disease also involves other areas of skin, such as circumscribed salmon-colored plaques of elbows and knees with a fine scale. The disease may also produce 2- to 6-mm red follicular papules, particularly over the distal extremities (Fig. 9-51). In 20% of children widespread involvement of the trunk and face may be seen, and in 4% progress to exfoliative erythroderma.[65] One feature frequently observed is the presence of an area of uninvolved skin entrapped within a large plaque of involved skin.[67] These so-called "islands of sparing" were once considered a diagnostic feature (Fig. 9-52), but most now believe this can be seen in

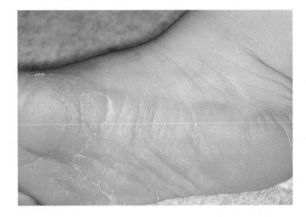

Fig. 9-49
Salmon-colored thickening of the sole in childhood pityriasis rubra pilaris.

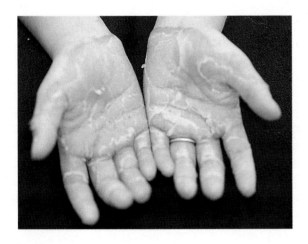

Fig. 9-48
Salmon-colored scaly palms in childhood pityriasis rubra pilaris.

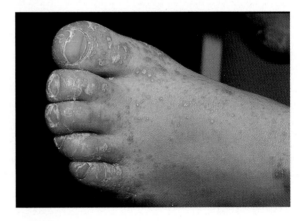

Fig. 9-50
Involvement extending to the dorsa of the foot and toes in childhood pityriasis rubra pilaris.

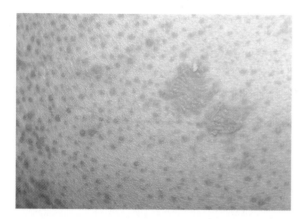

Fig. 9-51
Follicular papules in childhood pityriasis rubra pilaris.

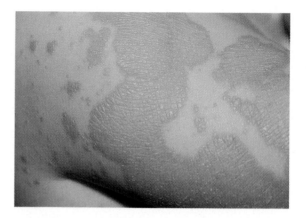

Fig. 9-52
Red plaques on the trunk with "island of sparing" in childhood pityriasis rubra pilaris.

drug eruptions, psoriasis, and other conditions.[65-67] Despite widespread involvement, the child with PRP usually has minimal to no itching. Scalp involvement has been reported, as has an asymptomatic white lacy change of the oral mucosa. Most clinicians appreciate that a wide spectrum of disease may be observed, and as the condition evolves over many weeks, different skin sites may be affected.[67] The condition tends to be persistent and last many months.

Differential Diagnosis

All the papulosquamous eruptions may be considered in the differential diagnosis at some point (see Box 9-2). Psoriasis and guttate parapsoriasis are the most likely to be confused. Drug eruptions may mimic PRP, and the involvement of the palms and soles may mimic poststreptococcal desquamation. However, the prolonged duration of PRP and the characteristic salmon-colored thickenings should lead to a suspicion of PRP. Skin biopsies are not diagnostic, but may suggest the diagnosis because of the "moundlike" parakeratosis around follicular openings accompanied by hyperkeratosis and irregular acanthosis.[65,67]

Pathogenesis

The cause of the condition is unknown. In early-onset PRP an autosomal dominant pattern of inheritance has been suggested.[65] Thickening of the epidermis,

with increased keratinocyte proliferation and differentiation, is found.

Treatment

Childhood PRP is quite difficult to treat.[67] It is unresponsive to topical steroids and phototherapy.[65] Some children may respond to topical calcipotriol.[68] Oral retinoids, such as isotretinoin, have been successful as has etretinate.[67,69] Methotrexate has had variable results, and oral vitamin A has no therapeutic index in this condition.[69] Currently a 4-month trial of isotretinoin, 1 mg/kg/day, has the highest success rate. Management should be done by an experienced dermatologist.

Patient education

Patients and parents should understand that this is a condition that can be quite persistent, and therapeutic responses are slow. One should state that the cause is unknown, and the therapy available treats the epidermal proliferation and not the triggering factors. The side effects of the systemic agent chosen should be carefully explained, and the risks and benefits of each therapy discussed.

Follow-up visits

Follow-up visits should be at two weekly intervals until the response to therapy and side effects are determined. It is usually not necessary to treat until every skin area is cleared, and if using retinoids, provide a "drug holiday" after 4 months of treatment.

References

1. Krueger GG, Duvic M: Epidemiology of psoriasis: clinical issues, *J Invest Dermatol* 102:14s, 1994.

2. Smith AE, Kassab JY, Rowland Payne CM, et al: Bimodality in age of onset of psoriasis, in both patients and their relatives, *Dermatology* 186:181, 1993.

3. Elder JT, Nair RP, Voorhees JJ: Epidemiology and genetics of psoriasis, *J Invest Dermatol* 102:24S, 1994.

4. Braathen LR, Botten G, Bjerkedal T: Psoriasis in Norway. *Acta Derm Venereol Suppl (Stockh)* 142:1, 1989.

5. Telfer NR, Chalmers RJG, Whale K, et al: The role of streptococcal infection in the initiation of guttate psoriasis. *Arch Dermatol* 128:39, 1992.

6. Patrizi A, Costa AM, Fiorillo I, et al: Perianal streptococcal dermatitis associated with guttate psoriasis and/or balanoposthitis: a study of five cases, *Pediatr Dermatol* 11:168, 1994.

7. Atherton DJ, Kahana M, Russell-Jones R: Naevoid psoriasis, *Br J Dermatol* 120:843, 1989.

8. Akinduro OM, Venning VA, Burge SM: Psoriatic nail-pitting in infancy, *Br J Dermatol* 130:800, 1994.

9. Matsuoka Y, Okada N, Yoshikawa K: Familial cases of psoriasis vulgaris and pustulosis palmaris et plantaris. *Int J Dermatol* 20:308, 1993.

10. Judge MR, McDonald A, Black MM: Pustular psoriasis in childhood, *Clin Exp Dermatol* 18:97, 1993.

11. Ivker RA, Grin-Jorgensen CM, Vega VK, et al: Infantile generalized pustular psoriasis associated with lytic lesions of bone, *Pediatr Dermatol* 10:277, 1993.

12. Biondi-Oriente C, Scarpa R, Oriente P: Prevalence and clinical features of juvenile psoriatic arthritis in 425 psoriatic patients, *Acta Derm Venereol Suppl (Stockh)* 186:109, 1994.

13. Ansell B, Beeson M, Hall P, et al: HLA and juvenile psoriatic arthritis, *Br J Rheumatol* 32:836, 1993.

14. Tomfohrde J, Silverman A, Barne R, et al: Gene for familial psoriasis susceptibility mapped to the distal end of human chromosome 17q, *Science* 264:1141, 1994.

15. Onuma S: Immunohistochemical studies of infiltrating cells in early and chronic lesions of psoriasis, *J Dermatol* 21:223, 1994.

16. Hudson-Peacock MJ, Diffey BJ, Farr PM: Photoprotective action of emollients in ultraviolet therapy of psoriasis, *Br J Dermatol* 130:361, 1994

17. Saggese G, Federico G, Battini R: Topical application of 1,25-dihydoxyvitamin D3 (calcitriol) is an effective and reliable therapy to cure skin lesions in psoriatic children, *Eur J Pediatr* 152:389, 1993.

18. Mahrle G, Bonnekoh B, Wevers A, et al: Anthralin: How does it act and are there more favourable derivatives? *Acta Derm Venereol Suppl (Stockh)* 186:83, 1994.

19. Sarda S, Karahalil B, Karakaya AE, et al: Mutagenic risk in psoriatic patients before and after 8-methoxypsoralen and long-wave ultraviolet radiation, *Mutat Res* 312:79, 1993.

20. Carcovich A, Gatti M, Olivetti G, et al: Short-term treatment with cyclosporin in severe psoriasis; four years experience, *Acta Derm Venereol Suppl (Stockh)* 186:92, 1994.

21. Rosinka D, Wolska H, Jablonska S, et al: Etretinate in severe psoriasis, *Pediatr Dermatol* 5:266, 1988.

22. Parsons JM: Pityriasis rosea update: 1986, *J Am Acad Dermatol* 15:159, 1986.

23. Hendricks AA, Lohr JA: Pityriasis rosea in infancy, *Arch Dermatol* 115:896, 1979.

24. Pierson JC, Dijkstra JW, Elston DM: Purpuric pityriasis rosea, *J Am Acad Dermatol* 28:1021, 1993.

25. Vidimos AT, Camisa C: Tongue and cheek: oral lesions in pityriasis rosea, *Cutis* 50:276, 1992.

26. Arndt KA, Paul BS, Stern RS, et al: Treatment of pityriasis rosea with ultraviolet radiation, *Arch Dermatol* 119:381, 1983.

27. Ross S, Sanchez JL: Parapsoriasis: a century later, *Int J Dermatol* 29:329, 1990.

28. Menni S, Piccinno R, Crosti L, et al: Parapsoriasis in two children: immunophenotypic and immunogenotypic study, *Pediatr Dermatol* 11:151, 1994.

29. Rogers M: Pityriasis lichenoides and lymphomatoid papulosis, *Semin Dermatol* 11:73, 1992.

30. Rogers M, De Launey J, Kemp A, et al: Lymphomatoid papulosis in an eleven-month old infant, *Pediatr Dermatol* 2:124, 1984.

31. Truhan AP, Hebert AA, Esterly NB: Pityriasis lichenoides in children: therapeutic response to erythromycin, *J Am Acad Dermatol* 15:66, 1986.

32. Honig B, Morison WL, Karp D: Photochemotherapy beyond psoriasis, *J Am Acad Dermatol* 31:775, 1994.

33. Cottoni F, Ena P, Tedde G, et al: Lichen planus in children, *Pediatr Dermatol* 10:132, 1993.

34. Kumar V, Garg BR, Baruah MC, et al: Childhood lichen planus (LP), *J Dermatol* 20:175, 1993.

35. Scully C, de Almeida OP, Welbury R: Oral lichen planus in childhood, *Br J Dermatol* 130:131, 1994.

36. Nayar M, Schomberg K, Dawber RP, et al: A clinico-pathologic study of scarring alopecia, *Br J Dermatol* 128:533, 1993.

37. Joshi RK, Abanmi A, Ohman SG, et al: Lichen planus of the nails presenting as trachyonychia, *Int J Dermatol* 32:54, 1993.

38. Peluso AM, Tosti A, Piraccini BM, et al: Lichen planus limited to the nails in childhood, *Pediatr Dermatol* 10:36, 1993.

39. Maeda M: A case of generalized lichen nitidus with Koebner's phenomenon, *J Dermatol* 21:273, 1994.

40. Voute AB, Schulten EA, Langendijk et al: Fluocinonide in an adhesive base for the treatment of oral lichen planus. A double-blind placebo-controlled study, *Oral Surg Oral Med Oral Pathol* 75:181, 1993.

41. Laman SD, Provost TT: Cutaneous manifestations of lupus erythematosus, *Rheum Dis Clin North Am* 20:195, 1994.

42. Lehman TJA: *Systemic lupus erythematosus in childhood and adolescence*. In Wallace DJ, Hahn BH, editors: *Dubois' lupus erythematosus*, Philadelphia, 1993, Lea & Febiger, p 431.

43. George PM, Tunnessen WW Jr: Childhood discoid lupus erythematosus, *Arch Dermatol* 129:613, 1993.

44. Perkins W, Stables GI, Lever RS: Protein S deficiency in lupus erythematosus secondary to hereditary angioedema, *Br J Dermatol* 130:381, 1994.

45. Topper SF, Agha A, Hashimoto K: Annular scaly plaques in an infant. Neonatal lupus erythematosus (NLE), *Arch Dermatol* 130:105, 1994.

46. Watson RM, Scheel JN, Petri M, et al: Neonatal lupus erythematosus. Report of serological and immuno-genetic studies in twins discordant for congenital heart block, *Br J Dermatol* 130:342, 1994.

47. Lee LA: Neonatal lupus erythematosus, *J Invest Dermatol* 100:9s, 1993.

48. Lee LA, Reichlin M, Ruyle SZ, et al: Neonatal lupus liver disease, *Lupus* 2:333, 1994.

49. Ishimaru S, Izaki S, Kitamura K, et al: Neonatal lupus erythematosus: dissolution of atrioventricular block after administration of corticosteroid to the pregnant mother, *Dermatology* 189 (suppl 1):92, 1994.

50. Zappi E, Sontheimer R: Clinical relevance of antibodies to Ro/SS-A and La/SS-B in subacute cutaneous lupus and related conditions, *Immunol Invest* 22:189, 1993.

51. Lee LA, Frank MB, McCubbin VR, et al: Auto-antibodies of neonatal lupus erythematosus, *J Invest Dermatol* 102:963, 1994.

52. David-Bajar KM, Bennion SD, DeSpain JD, et al: Clinical, histologic and immunofluorescent distinctions between subacute cutaneous lupus erythematosus and discoid lupus erythematosus, *J Invest Dermatol* 99:251, 1992.

53. Yell JA, Burge SM: Lupus erythematosus profundus treated with clobetasol propionate under a hydrocolloid dressing, *Br J Dermatol* 128:103, 1993.

54. Olson JC: Juvenile dermatomyositis, *Semin Dermatol* 11:57, 1992.

55. Hiketa T, Matsumoto Y, Ohashi M, et al: Juvenile dermatomyositis: a statistical study of 114 patients with dermatomyositis, *J Dermatol* 19:470, 1992.

56. Cheong W-K, Hughes GRV, Norris PG, et al: Cutaneous photosensitivity in dermatomyositis, *Br J Dermatol* 131:205, 1994.

57. Euwer RL, Sontheimer RD: Amyopathic dermato-myositis (dermatomyositis sine myositis), *J Am Acad Dermatol* 24:959, 1991.

58. Miller LC, Michael AF, Youngki K: Childhood dermatomyositis: clinical course and long term follow-up, *Clin Pediatr* 26:561, 1987.

59. Plotz PH, et al: Current concepts in the idiopathic inflammatory myopathies: polymyositis, dermato-myositis and related disorders, *Ann Int Med* 111:143, 1989.

60. Taieb A, El Youbi A, Grosshans E, et al: Lichen striatus: a Blaschko linear acquired inflammatory skin eruption, *J Am Acad Dermatol* 25:637, 1991.

61. Herd RM, McLaren KM, Aldridge RD: Linear lichen planus and lichen striatus—opposite ends of the spectrum, *Clin Exp Dermatol* 18:335, 1993.

62. Karp DL, Cohen BA: Onychodystrophy in lichen striatus, *Pediatr Dermatol* 10:359, 1993.

63. Bencini PL, et al: Porokeratosis: immunosuppression and exposure to sunlight, *Br J Dermatol* 116:113, 1987.

64. Otsuka F: Porokeratosis has neoplastic clones in the epidermis: Microfluorimetric analysis of DNA content of epidermal cell nuclei, *J Invest Dermatol* 92:231S, 1989.

65. Piamphongsant T, Akaraphant R: Pityriasis rubra pilaris: a new proposed classification, *Clin Exp Dermatol* 19:134, 1994.

66. Shahidullah H, Aldridge RD: Changing forms of juvenile pityriasis rubra pilaris, *Clin Exp Dermatol* 19:254, 1994.

67. Cohen PR, Prystowsky JH: Pityriasis rubra pilaris: a review of diagnosis and treatment, *J Am Acad Dermatol* 20:801, 1989.

68. Van de Kerkhof PC, Steijlen PM: Topical treatment of pityriasis rubra pilaris with calcipotriol, *Br J Dermatol* 130:675, 1994.

69. Dicken CH: Treatment of pityriasis rubra pilaris, *J Am Acad Dermatol* 31:997, 1994.

10
Sun Sensitivity

Sun exposure in children may result in sunburn or abnormal reactions in the skin. Abnormal reactions occur in the skin areas predominantly exposed to sunlight: the face, ears, back of the neck, "V" of the neck, and extensor surfaces of the arms and hands. Sun sensitivity is suspected when the distribution of the cutaneous eruption is limited to these areas. Three diseases account for the majority of cases of sun sensitivity in children: polymorphous light eruption, erythropoietic protoporphyria (EPP), and lupus erythematosus (LE) (see Chapter 9). These conditions should be considered in every child with sun sensitivity.

SUNBURN

The result of excessive sun exposure is sunburn. Sunburn readily occurs in fair-skinned children, who have less melanin protection than darker-skinned children. However, intense sun exposure can produce sunburn in children with dark skin as well. Any child who seeks medical assistance because of sunburn should be questioned about exposure to agents that make individuals sun sensitive.

Clinical features

Erythema and skin tenderness begin 30 minutes to 4 hours after sun exposure, depending on the intensity of the exposure and the degree of the child's natural protection against the sun; peak at 24 hours; and may last up to 72 hours[1] (see Box 10-1; Fig. 10-1). On the face, sunburn is usually most prominent on the nose and cheeks, with sun-protected areas under the nose, the chin, and upper eyelids uninvolved (Fig. 10-2). On the extremities and trunk, protective clothing may produce sharp borders between burned and nonburned areas (Figs. 10-1 and 10-3). After intense sun exposure, edema and blistering occur (Fig. 10-3). Some 2 to 7 days after intense sun exposure, 5 to 10 cell layers of epidermis are shed in one piece as a white scale (desquamation). With acute sunburn, sleep is often disturbed because of the tenderness of the skin. Extensive sunburn causes a reduction in the sweating rate and may contribute to collapse from heatstroke. Sunburn over large areas of the body in a child may result in fever, headache, and fatigue.

Differential diagnosis

It is occasionally difficult to determine in children what constitutes overexposure to sunlight (see Box

Box 10-1   Skin types and sun sensitivity

Skin Type	Description
I	Fair skin; always burns; never tans
II	Fair skin; usually burns, sometimes tans
III	Lightly pigmented; usually tans; sometimes burns
IV	Pigmented; always tans; never burns
V	Moderately pigmented; never burns
VI	Heavily pigmented (black) skin

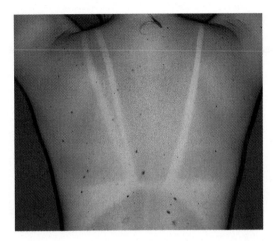

Fig. 10-1
Acute sunburn in an adolescent female. Note the sharp lines of demarcation between uninvolved skin protected by clothing and unprotected skin.

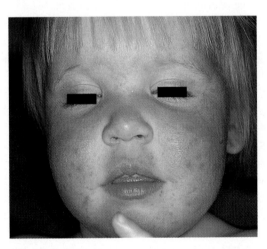

Fig. 10-2
Sunburn of an infant's face. Note protection of the upper eyelids, nasolabial folds, beneath the nose, and under the hair. Note the red papules of sweat duct obstruction.

10-2). In such a case one should consider the presence of a photosensitizing agent that would induce a sunburn reaction in an unusually short period (5 to 30 minutes of sun exposure). Agents that cause photosensitivity are listed in Chapter 18. Most have been associated with photosensitivity in adults, but they may also occur in children. Burning pain in the skin following 5 minutes of sun exposure should suggest EPP. In contrast, sunburn alone requires at least 30 minutes to produce symptoms. Rapid onset of sunburn and persistent sunburn reactions may be early clues to xeroderma pigmentosum (XP). In LE the eruption occurs 1 to 7 days after sun exposure and is characterized by scaling and erythema, which is persistent for several weeks. Many viral exanthems appear primarily or are exacerbated in sun-exposed areas (see Chapter 8). The laboratory evaluation of photosensitivity, listed in Box 10-3, should be considered when involved in the differential diagnosis of sun sensitivity.

Pathogenesis

The tanning or burning rays from the sun represent ultraviolet radiation. The exact cause of ultraviolet radiation damage to the skin is unknown, but is thought to be a combination of direct effects, generation of toxic oxygen species, and the production of inflammatory mediators.[1] The skin attempts to protect itself against ultraviolet radiation by tanning. Thus tanning is always a sign of ultraviolet injury to the skin. Ultraviolet radiation effects are cumulative as well, with many types of cutaneous cells retaining the additive effects of years of radiation exposure.[2] Long-term effects are expressed as fine and deep wrinkling; scaly, red patches (actinic keratoses); and, ultimately, skin cancer formation.[3] Basal and squamous cell carcinomas of the skin are associated with chronic expo-

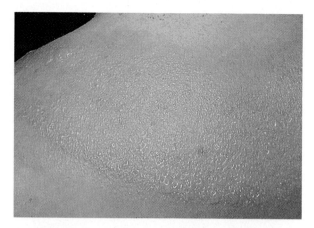

Fig. 10-3
Acute sunburn with vesiculation of the back of the neck. Note sharp demarcation of the area protected by clothing.

sure to ultraviolet radiation, whereas malignant melanoma is more commonly seen in those patients with a history of multiple severe blistering sunburns.

In acute ultraviolet injury the skin changes noted reflect immediate effects of radiation damage.[1] The first changes noted after prolonged sun exposure are vasodilatation of the dermal blood vessels. There is evidence to implicate several prostaglandins as mediators of a portion of the pain and erythema of sunburn, but total inhibition of ultraviolet radiation-induced prostaglandin formation only inhibits sunburn by 30%. Metabolic changes then occur within epidermal cells, and individual epidermal cells within the midepidermis demonstrate clumping of tonofilaments and abnormalities of cytoplasmic and nuclear shape, producing the rounded, so-called sunburn cell. Such cells lose their epidermal cell attachments; with increased sun exposure, a large number of these cells appear within the epidermis and produce an intraepidermal blister cavity.

Treatment
The pain and erythema of sunburn can be relieved by the use of wet dressings or cool compresses. Inhibitors of prostaglandin synthesis, such as aspirin or indomethacin, may modify sunburn if given within 48 hours of exposure. There is no convincing evidence that systemic or topical glucocorticosteroids are beneficial in the treatment of sunburn. Topical anesthetics, such as benzocaine, are sensitizing and transient in their relief of pain and thus not recommended. *Sunburn is 100% preventable, and prevention is by far the superior treatment.*

Patient education
Over 80% of lifetime sun exposure is received before the age of 18 years.[2] Thus it is extremely important to protect infants, children, and adolescents against sun exposure. Sun protection habits should be formed at an early age, because adolescents either do not realize or do not admit that they are sun sensitive, and they are likely to be noncompliant.[4] Also, many parents do not recognize the degree of sun sensitivity of their children. Infants younger than 6 months should not be subjected to sun exposure because of the decreased sweating rate

---

Box 10-4 Sunscreen sun protection factor

$$SPF = \frac{MED \text{ of sunscreened skin}}{MED \text{ of unprotected skin}}$$

MED, Minimal erythema dose—that is, the minimal amount of UVB energy required to produce erythema to human skin.

Box 10-5 Recommendations for sunscreen use in children

Use a broad-spectrum sunscreen with UVB SPF of
   15 or greater
Select a waterproof sunscreen preparation
Apply at least 30 minutes before sun exposure
Reapply every 1 to 2 hours

Box 10-6 Types of available sunscreens

UVB
   PABA (*p*-aminobenzoic acid)
   PABA esters
   Cinnamates
   Salicylates
   Combinations of *above* ingredients
UVA
   Dioxybenzones
UVB plus UVA
   Benzophenones
   Anthranilates
   Physical agents that block light

---

and the likelihood of heatstroke.[5] For those older than 6 months, clothing and umbrellas are good sun protection. Special sun-protective clothing such as Solumbra and Frogskin are available. Sunscreen agents with SPF (sun protection factor) of 15 or greater are recommended (see Boxes 10-4, 10-5, and 10-6). Because of the increasing evidence that ultraviolet A (UVA) radiation is also damaging to the skin, many sunscreens now contain agents that block both ultraviolet B (UVB) and UVA[6,7] (Box 10-6). It must be remembered that sunburn is a gross sign of sun damage, and that cellular damage to the skin can occur even with the use of SPF-15 sunscreens or higher. These creams and lotions should be applied to the skin 30 minutes before sun exposure. Regular daily use throughout the spring and summer months, as well as the winter in sunny climates, is the best method of protection. Physical sun blocks, such as zinc oxide pastes and titanium dioxide, have become more cosmetically acceptable and are good sun-protective agents. Although local reactions to sunscreens are common, these reactions are almost always due to the sunscreen vehicle and not to the active ingre-

dient.[8] Sun avoidance, such as planning outdoor activities before 10:00 A.M. and after 4:00 P.M., is advisable.

Follow-up visits
Follow-up visits are unnecessary.

POLYMORPHOUS LIGHT ERUPTION

Clinical features
Polymorphous light eruption comprises a group of related sun-sensitive conditions that are sometimes separated by distinct clinical patterns. Four major types are reported[9] (see Box 10-7).

Papular polymorphous light eruption is the most common type. The process begins in the spring and improves throughout the summer. In 75% of patients onset of the disease is sudden, occurs within the first 3 decades of life, and affects predominantly females (87%). New lesions appear within hours to days of sun exposure, remain 1 to 7 days, and usually heal without scarring. The clinical lesions are discrete erythematous papules and plaques (Fig. 10-4), occurring in sun-exposed areas. For unknown reasons, not all sun-exposed skin is affected. The majority of patients

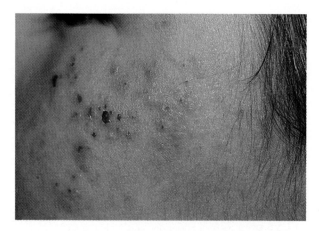

Fig. 10-4
Erythematous papules and plaques in a 9-year-old male with papular polymorphic light eruption.

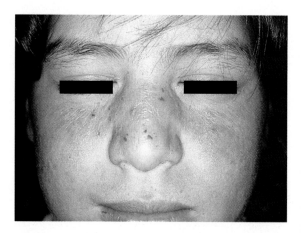

Fig. 10-6
Chronic polymorphous light eruption with lichenification by midsummer.

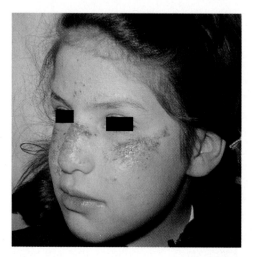

Fig. 10-5
Polymorphous light eruption. Photodermatitis of a North American Indian child, with vesicles and crusting of the face at springtime onset.

> **Box 10-7 Types of polymorphous light eruption**
>
> Papular polymorphous light eruption
> Actinic prurigo
>   Photodermatitis of North American Indians
> Juvenile spring eruption (hydroa aestivale)
> Hydroa vacciniforme

improve with age, and in some patients the disease may totally subside.

Hutchinson's summer prurigo (actinic prurigo) and photodermatitis of North American Indians have many overlapping features. They begin as a dermatitis predominantly occurring on the face and extensor surface of the forearms of school-age children. Actinic prurigo has been described in the United Kingdom and north-ern Europe, and the related form is seen in the Plains Indians of North America.[10] Both characteristically start in the early spring, when sufficient sunlight energy reaches the earth's surface. Lesions occur by age 5 years in 35% of children, and by age 10 years in 70%; the eruption develops during adolescence in the remainder. The initial eruption consists of an itchy, acute facial or forearm dermatitis with edematous papules (Fig. 10-5) and vesicles. As the spring progresses, the dermatitis becomes subacute, with crusting on the surface and epidermal thickening or lichenification (Fig. 10-6). Papular lesions may predominate on the face. In the summer the eruption may spontaneously clear, to recur again the next spring. Some very sun-sensitive children will have the eruption throughout the year. It is characteristic that several patches of

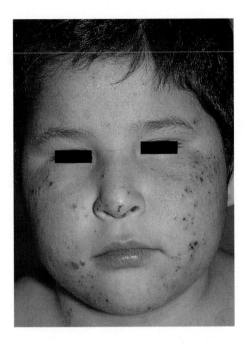

Fig. 10-7
Involvement of the lower lip with redness, edema, and fissures in polymorphous light eruption.

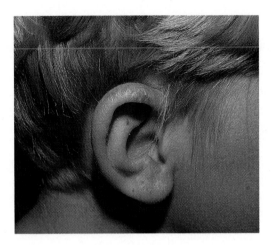

Fig. 10-8
Vesicles and crusts on the tops of the ears in a child with juvenile spring eruption.

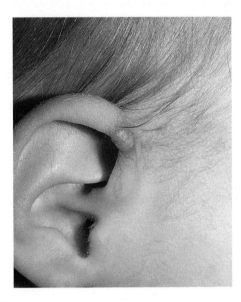

Fig. 10-9
Deep-seated vesicle on the ear of a child with hydroa vacciniforme.

skin are involved, with uninvolved areas of skin in between. In North American Indians the disease differs in two respects: (1) a chronic cheilitis of the lower lip is frequently observed (Fig. 10-7), which may be related to living in regions of intense sunlight, and (2) a family history of the disease is often obtained. Overlap with atopic dermatitis that worsens with summer heat is frequent in both actinic prurigo and photodermatitis of North American Indians.

Juvenile spring eruption (hydroa aestivale) is described in European children, mainly boys aged 5 to12 years. It characteristically begins as 2- to 3-mm discrete papules or vesicles on the ears and cheeks of fair-skinned children. The episode lasts 1 week and reappears the next spring (Fig. 10-8). A small percentage (22%) of patients with juvenile spring eruption will at other times in their lives develop lesions more typical of plaque-type polymorphous light eruption.[11]

Hydroa vacciniforme is characterized by a few discrete, deep-seated vesicles on the ears or nose that heal with scarring (Fig. 10-9). They are frequently persistent, lasting up to 4 weeks, and more episodes may occur with further sun exposure. The eye may be affected with keratitis, and uveitis is observed. This is the rarest of all forms of polymorphous light eruption.

It is unclear how these clinical patterns are inter-related, but, until pathologic or biochemical tests can distinguish, they are catalogued under the broad term *polymorphous light eruption*. Biopsy of early lesions shows an acute dermatitis, whereas biopsy of papular, crusted, and lichenified forms shows a chronic dermatitis.

In American Plains Indians and Spanish-Americans living in western North America, polymorphous light eruption occurs as an autosomal dominant condition. Females predominate 2:1. Non-Indian children may also have polymorphous light eruption, but the hereditary pattern is not defined. As in any dermatitis, itching may be severe, and scratching, resulting in secondary bacterial infection, may occur.

Differential diagnosis

Atopic dermatitis, in addition to other photosensitive states, may mimic polymorphous light eruption (see Box 10-2). During hot weather, sweating in children with atopic dermatitis may induce itching and dermatitis on the face and sun-exposed areas. A family history of atopic dermatitis, and the finding of flexural dermatitis in addition to photodermatitis, are useful differentiating features. Acute sensitivity to airborne substances may also lead to the appearance of a contact dermatitis predominantly on sun-exposed areas. In airborne contact dermatitis, the upper eyelids are usually involved, in contrast to polymorphous light eruption. LE, EPP, dermatophyte infections of the face, and sunburn are likely to be confused. Laboratory tests listed in Box 10-3 should be considered. Photodermatitis due to drugs characteristically produces a diffuse involvement of sun-exposed areas, rather than the patchy areas of dermatitis seen with polymorphous light eruption.

EPP and XP have an onset in early infancy rather than childhood, and they may have symptoms out of proportion to skin changes. They usually do not develop dermatitis-like changes.

Pathogenesis

The mechanism of any form of polymorphous light eruption is unknown. Patients with polymorphous light eruption are generally more likely to be sensitive to UVA than UVB, or both UVA and UVB.[9,10] The biochemical change responsible for initiating the dermatitis following sun exposure is unknown.

Treatment

Treatment of polymorphous light eruption involves the use of topical glucocorticosteroids in an ointment base applied twice daily for the dermatitis. In addition, wet dressings in the form of a face mask made of a damp washcloth, with eye, nose, and mouth holes, will serve to enhance the steroid effect on the face. This may be used for 2 to 3 days. Secondary bacterial infection is best treated with systemic antibiotics.

Sun avoidance is crucial is such patients and should be the mainstay of any treatment program. The child should restrict outdoor activities to the hours before 10 A.M. and after 4 P.M. Further photoprotection with a wide-brimmed hat, long-sleeved shirts, and sunscreens of UVB SPF greater than 30, as well UVA protection may be necessary (see Box 10-6).

Children with polymorphous light eruption who are sensitive to the UVA spectrum of light and remain symptomatic despite adequate sun avoidance and UVA sunscreen may be treated with beta carotene capsules, 40 to 120 mg/day to achieve a serum carotene level of 600 to 800 μg/ml. Approximately 20% of all children with polymorphous light eruption will respond to beta carotene.

In cases of severe polymorphous light eruption, treatment with a psoralen and UVA may be considered. Although it appears contradictory to treat a photosensitive disorder with a photosensitizing agent, low-dose oral psoralen and UVA will induce melanin pigmentation and epidermal thickening, increasing the natural protection to sunlight.

Patient education

The concept of sun sensitivity must be understood by patients and their parents. Sun protection methods should be carefully explained and reexplained at each visit. Because of the delayed nature of the eruption, the relationship of the disease to sun exposure is difficult to comprehend. Many parents are reluctant to accept sun avoidance or to restrict their children's activities at school or play.

Follow-up visits

A visit 1 week after initial therapy is useful to assess the therapeutic response. Visits at 4-week intervals thereafter are advised until the condition has cleared.

ERYTHROPOIETIC PROTOPORPHYRIA

Clinical features

EPP is an inherited disorder of porphyrin metabolism. In many children EPP shows an autosomal dominant pattern of inheritance, but other modes of inheritance have been described.[12] The preschool child experiences burning, stinging, or itching sensations in the skin. Often this occurs after a sun exposure of only 1 to 10 minutes. Despite the severe discomfort the child suffers, no skin lesions may be found. The child soon learns to stay indoors. Intense sun exposure may result in facial edema, erythema, or urticaria, followed by petechiae primarily on the face. Less often, vesiculation and crusting of the face appear (Figs. 10-10 and 10-11).

More commonly, however, acute skin changes do not occur, and chronic changes are apparent. Chronic changes usually do not appear until late childhood.

Slightly thickened skin-colored papules appear over the dorsa of the hands (Fig. 10-12), nose, and cheeks. Pitted scars on the face (Figs. 10-10 and 10-11) and perioral linear skin-colored papules may result from previous vesicular injury.

Skin biopsy specimens from sun-exposed skin show thickening of the small blood vessels of the papillary dermis, with a perivascular deposit of periodic acid-Schiff (PAS)–positive material. Direct immunofluorescence of such lesions demonstrates deposits of immunoglobulins, mostly immunoglobulin G (IgG),

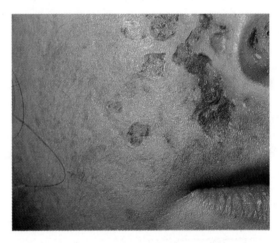

Fig. 10-11
Crusting of the cheek and atrophic scarring in severe erythropoietic protoporphyria.

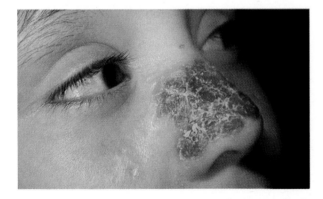

Fig. 10-10
Crusting of the nose after acute sun exposure in erythropoietic protoporphyria. Note depressed scars on the cheek from a prior episode.

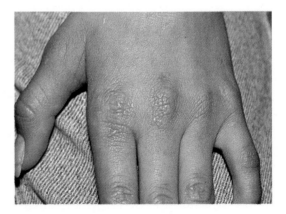

Fig. 10-12
Thickened papules over the dorsa of the left hand of a 12-year-old female with erythropoietic protoporphyria.

around superficial dermal blood vessels. Of children with EPP, 5% may suffer cholelithiasis with porphyrin stones in the gallbladder and varying degrees of liver injury. Nine deaths from hepatic failure and EPP have been reported in children and adolescents. Mild anemia may also occur.

The diagnosis can be confirmed by laboratory tests. Heparinized blood diluted 1:10 in unpreserved saline solution can be examined with a fluorescence microscope for coral-red fluorescence of red blood cells. It is important that the blood be withdrawn in a light-protected tube, since exposure may allow protoporphyrin to be converted to a nonfluorescent metabolite. In normal children less than 1% of red blood cells fluoresce, whereas in those with EPP, from 5% to 30% of the total erythrocytes fluoresce. Quantitative red blood cell protoporphyrins are also useful.

Differential diagnosis

Most other photosensitive states (see Box 10-2), such as polymorphous light eruption, LE, sunburn, and drug photosensitivity, can be excluded by the striking history of cutaneous burning seen in children with EPP, by a positive family history, and by laboratory studies. Occasionally the family is unable to relate the symptoms to exposure to sunlight, and airborne allergens are suspected. This is particularly true if facial edema or urticaria is a major feature. A careful history, however, will reveal the role of sun exposure.

Pathogenesis

Abnormally elevated tissue levels of protoporphyrin IX, a normal precursor of heme, are found in EPP. The increased levels of protoporphyrin IX are due to a defect in the enzyme ferrochelatase. Excessive protoporphyrin IX has been found in the circulating erythrocytes, plasma, liver, and bone marrow. Protoporphyrin IX absorbs light at 409 nm and becomes a molecule with an altered energy state. The molecule then transfers energy to molecular oxygen; toxic oxygen products are thought to be responsible for the injury to vascular membranes, and perhaps to lysosomal membranes, with subsequent inflammation.

Light-producing 409-nm wavelengths are found in sunlight, reflected sunlight, sunlight traveling through window glass, and fluorescent lighting. Thus a child could develop symptoms indoors or through window glass.

Treatment

Oral administration of beta carotene is the treatment of choice. In children, a dosage of 40 to 120 mg/day will raise serum carotene levels to 600 to 800 µg/100 ml, the desired therapeutic range. The child becomes carotenemic, but sun tolerance is greatly increased. Children who previously refused to go outdoors may play for 3 to 4 hours outside without symptoms.

Conventional sun protection methods have been uniformly unsuccessful because of the poor ability of sunscreen to protect in the 409-nm range and the small amount of light necessary to induce symptoms.

Pyridoxine has been used successfully to treat the photosensitivity of EPP in some patients unresponsive to beta carotene. Pyridoxine treatment does not alter protoporphyrin IX levels, and its mechanism of action is unknown.[13]

Patient education

The hereditary nature of the disease should be discussed with the patient and the parents, and all family members should be screened by protoporphyrin level determinations. Liver function tests may be performed on family members as well. It must be emphasized that photosensitivity can occur with fluorescent lamps, such as those in overhead lighting in school.

Follow-up visits

During the initiation of therapy a visit every 2 to 3 weeks is useful to ascertain the response and to adjust the therapeutic dosage of beta carotene. After 4 weeks the serum carotene levels may be used to monitor for the correct dosage. After an effective therapeutic response is achieved, visits every 6 months to examine the patient for possible liver involvement are valuable.

PHYTOPHOTODERMATITIS

Clinical features

Redness and blisters that occur in bizarre shapes, such as linear streaks, and that leave intense hyperpigmentation are characteristic of phytophotodermatitis (Figs. 10-13 and 10-14). Exposure to plants in the spring and summer months from outdoor activities is the usual history. Some children present with only the hyperpigmented streaks, without a distinct history of erythema or blistering. Exposure to limes or certain perfumes may also produce the syndrome.

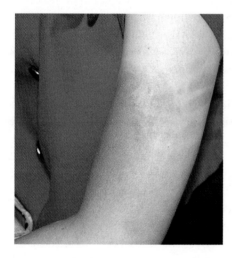

Fig. 10-13
Irregular erythema and hyperpigmentation secondary to contact with riverside grasses followed by sun exposure.

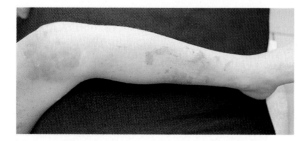

Fig. 10-14
Phytophotodermatitis. Linear and bizarre shapes of hyperpigmentation in an 8-year-old boy from a fight with his brother; they were hitting each other with plants found along a lakeshore.

Differential diagnosis

The linear streaks of blisters may be confused with acute allergic contact dermatitis from plants such as poison ivy, whereas the hyperpigmented macules can be confused with incontinentia pigmenti because of the linear arrangement or irregular café-au-lait spots. The bizarre shapes and simultaneous, sudden onset of phytophotodermatitis lesions help differentiate from contact dermatitis.

Pathogenesis

Plants that contain the furocoumarin psoralen are responsible. This includes the celery (Fig. 10-15) family and certain grasses and limes. The plants produce the psoralen transiently, usually after a rainy week. The child gets the psoralen onto the skin from the plant touching the skin (the epicutaneous application of a photosensitizer). The psoralen, when exposed to sunlight, produces a photodermatitis with blister formation, followed by intense stimulation of melanin production. The resultant hyperpigmentation may last for months.

Treatment

The acute dermatitis phase is treated as an acute allergic contact dermatitis with moderate-potency topical steroid ointments twice daily for 2 weeks.

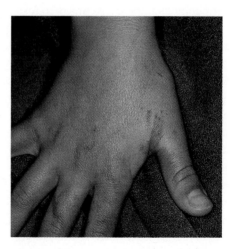

Fig. 10-15
Hyperpigmentation from exposure to celery and sunlight.

The hyperpigmentation phase usually is not treated, but bleaching creams may be used if cosmetically important areas are involved.

Patient education

Patients and parents should be advised that once hyperpigmentation occurs, it may persist for 6 to 12 months. They should be told of the nature of the photosensitizing chemical from plants and should avoid play in the area where the plants were contacted.

Follow-up visits

A follow-up visit in 4 weeks to evaluate the progress of the condition is recommended.

XERODERMA PIGMENTOSUM

Clinical features

XP is an autosomal recessive disorder of sun sensitivity in which eight different forms have been recognized. Onset of skin lesions by 18 months of age is characteristic, with early sunburn reactions from minimal sun exposure and numerous freckles as the predominant findings. An important clue is that the sunburn may persist for several weeks rather resolve within a week. Telangiectasia of the sun-exposed areas and cutaneous atrophy develop within a few years of the other cutanous findings. Actinic keratoses, which appear as persistent red, scaly, rough macules in sun-exposed skin are found next, and the child's skin appears prematurely aged. In dark-skinned children these findings may be difficult to appreciate. Skin cancers may develop by the age of 6 to 8 years, with basal cell carcinomas, squamous cell carcinomas, and malignant melanomas reported before puberty. Skin-colored or pigmented papules should be regarded as suspicious for skin cancers, and biopsy should be done promptly. The majority of precancerous and cancerous skin lesions occur on the head and neck. Early death from metastatic skin cancers is reported, with 10% of the patients dead before puberty. Up to 20% of affected patients have ocular or neurologic disease, or both. Photophobia may be a prominent symptom, and decreased vision is observed. Mild to severe mental retardation is found, as well as hearing loss and areflexia. Most cases of mental retardation are found in children with the De Sanctis-Cacchione type of XP. Diagnosis and classification of suspected XP are accomplished by examination of abnormal deoxyribonucleic acid (DNA) repair by the patient's cells following ultraviolet light exposure.

Differential diagnosis

The early freckling should be differentiated from lentigines observed in multiple lentigines syndromes and the LEOPARD (lengitines, EKG abnormalities, ocular hypertelorism, pulmonary stenosis, abnormalities of genitalia, retardation of growth, and deafness) and NAME (nevi, atrial myxoma, myxoid neurofibroma, ephelides) syndromes. Freckling is earlier in onset, macular, and tan, whereas lentigines are slightly raised and brown. Ordinary freckles usually begin between the ages of 3 and 5 years, rather than before 2 years, in children with XP and are not accompanied by skin changes that make the child appear old. Actinic keratoses and skin cancers in prepubertal children may be seen in the basal cell nevus syndrome or in Bazex's syndrome, but not at an age as young as in children who have XP, nor do these children develop the other skin changes associated with XP.[14] Diagnosis is confirmed by skin biopsy showing severe actinic skin damage at an early age. Confirmation is made by culture of skin cells with evaluation of DNA repair.

Pathogenesis

Enzymes involved in several steps of DNA repair may be abnormal.[15] Thus far at least eight different defects in DNA repair can be found by the fusion of cultured cells from different patient groups with each other to determine if normal DNA repair is restored. Molecular biology techniques will eventually precisely define the specific defects in DNA repair. Failure to repair ultraviolet light damage results in carcinogenesis, and XP patients are an important model in the ultimate understanding of sun-induced cancers.

Treatment

Sun avoidance is essential to minimize skin damage and skin cancer formation. Children with XP should avoid sunlight, wear protective clothing, and use sunscreens with maximal SPF each day. Biopsy of any suspect skin lesion is necessary. Referral to a center with experience in management of this condition is recommended. Dermatologic, ophthalmologic, and neurologic consultations should be obtained.

Patient education

The autosomal recessive inheritance of this disease should be emphasized. Twenty percent of reported patients have parents who are cousins. A great deal of effort stressing the critical role of sunlight in producing skin cancers is required. The need for frequent evaluations must be emphasized because many skin cancers are preventable or cured if detected early and removed.

Follow-up visits

A cutaneous examination every 3 months is necessary, preferably at a center with experience in XP. At the follow-up visit, careful examination for skin cancers should be done, with biopsy of any suspect lesions. An evaluation of the child's sun protection program should be performed at each visit.

References

1. Soter NA: Acute effects of ultraviolet radiation on the skin, *Semin Dermatol* 9:11, 1990.
2. Truhan AP: Sun protection in childhood, *Clin Pediatr* 12:676, 1991.
3. Browder JF, Beers B: Photoaging. Cosmetic effects of the sun, *Postgrad Med* 8:74, 1993.
4. Grob JJ, Guglielmina C, Gouvernet J, et al: Study of the sunbathing habits in children and adolescents: application to the prevention of melanoma, *Dermatology* 186:94, 1993.
5. Morelli JG, Weston WL: What sunscreen should I use for my 3 month old baby? *Pediatrics* 6:882, 1993.
6. Stiller MJ, Davis IC, Shupack JL: A concise guide to topical sunscreens: state of the art, *Int J Dermatol* 8:544, 1992.
7. Menter JM: Recent developments in UVA protection, *Int J Dermatol* 6:389, 1990.
8. Foley P, Nixon R, Marks R, et al: The frequency of reactions to sunscreens: result of a longitudinal population-based study on the regular use of sunscreens in Australia, *Br J Dermatol* 5:512, 1993.
9. Norris PG, Hawk JLM: Polymorphic light eruption, *Photodermatol Photoimmunol Photomed* 7:186, 1990.
10. Lane PR, Hogan DJ, Martel MJ, et al: Actinic prurigo: clinical features and prognosis, *J Am Acad Dermatol* 26:683, 1992.
11. Berth-Jones J, Norris PG, Graham-Brown RAC, et al: Juvenile spring eruption of the ears: a probable variant of polymorphic light eruption, *Br J Dermatol* 124:375, 1991.
12. Norris PG, Nunn AV, Hawk JLM, et al: Genetic heterogeneity in erythropoietic protoporphyria: a study of the enzymatic defect in nine affected families, *J Invest Dermatol* 95:260, 1990.
13. Ross JB, Moss MA: Relief of the photosensitivity of erythropoietic protoporphyria by pyridoxine, *J Am Acad Dermatol* 22:340, 1990.
14. Shumrick KA, Coldiron B: Genetic syndromes associated with skin cancer, *Otolaryngol Clin North Am* 26:117, 1993.
15. Downes CS, Ryan AJ, Johnson RT: Fine tuning of DNA repair in transcribed genes: mechanisms, prevalence and consequences, *Bioessays* 15:209, 1993.

11

Bullous Diseases and Mucocutaneous Syndromes

Blister formation in the skin of children usually brings to mind an acute dermatitis, viral infection, or bullous impetigo. However, a large variety of noninfectious blistering skin diseases may be seen. These may be spontaneously occurring blisters, such as seen in the immunobullous disorders, or trauma-produced blisters (mechanobullous disorders). A history of trauma-induced blisters is important in distinguishing mechanobullous disorders from immunobullous disorders. Blisters on the palms and soles often have a thick roof of stratum corneum and appear deceptively deep in tissue when they are within the epidermis or at the dermal-epidermal junction. In contrast, blisters on mucous membranes shed their roofs quickly, so that only blister bases (erosions) are seen. Infectious blisters are discussed in detail in Chapters 5 and 8, and mechanobullous diseases are discussed in Chapter 18.

SPONTANEOUS VESICULOBULLOUS ERUPTIONS

Viral blisters (see Chapter 8), bullous impetigo (see Chapter 5), chemical or thermal burns, papular

urticaria, and acute dermatitis (see Chapter 4) are the most common forms of blisters that appear spontaneously. The injury in thermal burns is similar to that in sunburn. Erythema multiforme (EM) is a recurrent blistering disease of the skin. Stevens-Johnson syndrome (SJS) and toxic epidermal necrolysis (TEN) are uncommon but serious blistering mucocutaneous syndromes in children. Miliaria, aphthous ulcers, and geographic tongue are common, more benign, forms of spontaneous vesiculobullous diseases, whereas the immunobullous diseases are quite uncommon to rare. Bullous mastocytosis, an uncommon blistering condition, is discussed in Chapter 14. Kawasaki disease is included in this chapter, although not truly a bullous disease,[2] because it mimics the major mucocutaneous syndromes.

ERYTHEMA MULTIFORME

Clinical features

EM is a syndrome characterized by the acute onset of oval or round, fixed, erythematous skin lesions appearing symmetrically on the skin.[1,2] Each lesion

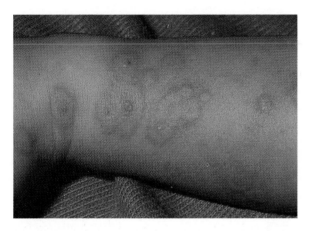

Fig. 11-1
Early fixed papules with a central dusky zone on the dorsum of the hand of a child with erythema multiforme due to herpes simplex virus.

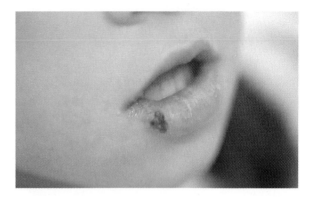

Fig. 11-3
Herpes labialis crusted lesion present on child's lip at the onset of erythema multiforme.

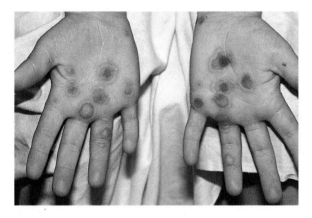

Fig. 11-2
"Target" or "iris" lesions with characteristic central dusky zone on palms of a child with erythema multiforme due to herpes simplex virus.

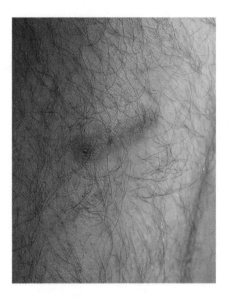

Fig. 11-4
Isomorphic (Koebner) phenomenon in adolescent with EM.

remains at the same site at least 7 days, and often for 2 or 3 weeks[1,2] (Fig. 11-1). The lesions progress over several days to form concentric zones of color change where the central zone becomes dusky. These colored lesions are called target or iris lesions[2] (Fig. 11-2). Occasionally, the central dusky zone will develop a blister. Prodromal symptoms in EM are conspicuously absent.[2] EM lesions are frequently recurrent and preceded by a lesion of herpes labialis[1-3] (Fig. 11-3). Skin lesions initially involve the dorsal surface of the hands and the extensor aspects of the extremities.[1,2] The palms and soles are frequently involved, the flexor aspects of the extremities less frequently. The isomorphic (or Koebner) phenomenon has been reported in EM[1,2] (Fig. 11-4). Systemic symptoms and signs are absent in EM. Usually there are no mucosal lesions, but when present, only the oral mucosa is involved and lesions are few (5 to 10) in contrast to

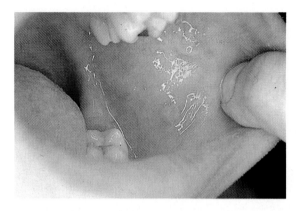

Fig. 11-5
Oral involvement in erythema multiforme.

hundreds on the skin[1,2] (Fig. 11-5). EM lasts an average of 3 weeks. It is most common in adolescents but may occur at all ages.[3] Recurrences may occur yearly but may occasionally recur every 1 or 2 months, particularly if the child has been treated with systemic steroids.[1-3] There is no evidence that EM progresses to SJS or TEN.[1,2]

Differential diagnosis

Acute urticaria is most often confused with EM.[4] This confusion results from the fact that urticaria may frequently have lesions with concentric color changes, with a pale edematous center and an erythematous border. In particular, giant urticaria, with large polycyclic lesions, which is often accompanied by angioedema of the hands and feet, may be confused.[4] However, urticarial lesions are transient, usually lasting 24 hours or less, whereas EM lesions are fixed and stay at the same site for at least 7 days. Further, the first concentric zone of color change seen in EM minor is not pale in the center, as seen in urticaria, but rather a dusky-blue color. Urticarial lesions will clear with subcutaneous epinephrine, and EM minor will not.[4] Skin biopsy will also distinguish EM from urticaria.[2]

Oral mucous lesions that are confused with EM include aphthous ulcers, bullous pemphigoid, pemphigus, and epidermolysis bullosa. Exfoliative cytologic study of the blister base will demonstrate epidermal giant cells of herpes simplex.

Pathogenesis

EM is thought to be due to a herpes simplex virus (HSV) specific host response to HSV antigens expressed on keratinocytes within the target lesion.[1-3] There is compelling evidence to show that HSV antigens and deoxyribonucleic acid (DNA) are present within the skin lesions even when a distinctive preceding HSV episode is not observed.[3] Children with recurrent lesions may have recurrent HSV preceding most, but not all, EM episodes. HSV may reside within keratinocytes of previously involved skin and may reactivate at the same sites.[5] The central necrotic zone of a target lesion shows individual keratinocyte necrosis and inflammatory cells around superficial dermal blood vessels and up into the epidermis.[6] The outer red zone shows dilation of vessels and minimal inflammation. Sheets of necrotic epithelium, as observed in SJS or TEN, are conspicuously absent. In a few children, HSV may not be the precipitating agent. Epstein-Barr virus (EBV) and other human herpesviruses have been implicated.

Treatment

For EM, symptomatic relief may be obtained from wet compresses or oral antihistamines. There is no evidence to support the use of systemic steroids in EM.[2,7] In patients with recurrent episodes of EM, prophylaxis with oral acyclovir may be considered.[7]

Patient education

Patients should be informed of the role of HSV in EM, and children with recurrent episodes should attempt to reduce sun exposure or other factors that might precipitate the antecedent HSV infection.

Follow-up visits

A visit in 24 to 48 hours is wise early in the disease to determine the progress of EM.

STEVENS-JOHNSON SYNDROME AND TOXIC EPIDERMAL NECROLYSIS

Clinical features

Because cutaneous features and etiologies of SJS and TEN may be indistinguishable, they will be consid-

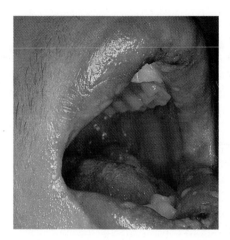

Fig. 11-6
Early oral involvement in Stevens-Johnson syndrome.

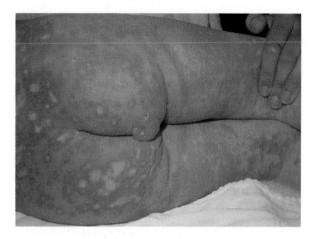

Fig. 11-8
Bullous macules with islands of uninvolved skin in Stevens-Johnson syndrome/toxic epidermal necrolysis.

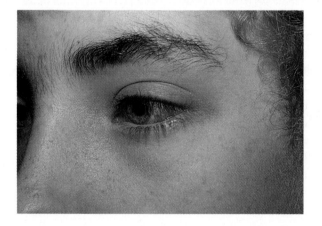

Fig. 11-7
Early eye involvement in Stevens-Johnson syndrome.

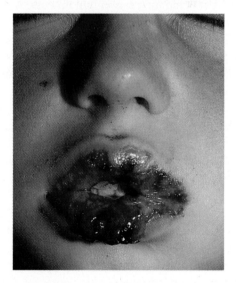

Fig. 11-9
Hemorrhagic crusts on the lips of a child with Stevens-Johnson syndrome.

ered together.[8,9] Both are serious, potentially life-threatening conditions, characterized by large areas of epithelial necrosis.[8,9] SJS in contrast to EM has a distinct prodrome lasting 1 to 14 days and is characterized by fever, headache, sore throat, malaise, and, sometimes, cough, vomiting, and diarrhea. Mucosal involvement is severe, with extensive mucosal necrosis, and it always involves at least two mucosal surfaces[8,9] (Figs. 11-6 and 11-7). The oral mucosa (Fig. 11-6) and eyes (Fig. 11-7) are the most frequently involved, but vaginal and urethral necrosis and widespread gastrointestinal or lower respiratory tract necrosis may develop.[8-10] The initial cutaneous

lesions mimic those found in EM, but progress rapidly within hours from central blisters to severe epidermal necrosis with loss of the epidermis leaving a denuded skin. Large sheets of epidermis or mucosa may be lost[8-10] (Fig. 11-8). The mouth is affected in every case of SJS.[8-10] Hemorrhagic crusts often appear on the lips (Fig. 11-9). Mucous membrane involvement often precipitates hospitalization in children because of severe limitation of the ability to eat.

Redness, swelling, bullae, or denuded erosions may be seen on the conjunctivae with pain and photophobia. Conjunctival scarring may be severe.

TEN has similar cutaneous findings that may occur in the absence of mucosal involvement. Although lesions first begin on the extremities in a pattern similar to that noted in EM, extensive truncal and facial involvement soon follows.[8,9] A large percentage of the skin may be lost, leading to complications similiar to a thermal burn.[8,9] Healing with scarring and contractures may occur, and loss of hair and nails may ensue. Permanent areas of depigmentation may develop.

There may be considerable overlap in the clinical conditions of SJS and TEN. SJS may be mucosal only, but more likely will have mucosal and necrotic skin lesions together. TEN may only involve skin but also may exhibit severe necrosis of oral mucosa. Attempts at classification of these two entities have been of help in clarifying the conditions, but the clinician should appreciate that there are overlapping clinical features and that early on it may be difficult to predict areas of involvement. Most authorities now accept four major types of SJS/TEN. The typical SJS usually has only a few red macules with blisters, which accompany the mucous membrane involvement, and less than 10% of the body surface is involved.[8,9] The "overlap" SJS/TEN has 10% to 30% of body surface involved. Two types of TEN are recognized: one in which large confluent areas of skin are involved on the face and trunk, and more than 30% of the body surface is involved; and one with "spots," in which many red macules with blisters are seen involving more than 10% of the body surface.[8,9] The course of SJS and TEN disease is more prolonged and accompanied by systemic symptoms of fever, dehydration, cough, and lymphadenopathy. The child is often sick 3 or 4 weeks. SJS and TEN are more likely to occur in children aged 2 to 10 years, younger than those with EM. Complications tend to be severe, with pseudomembrane formation of mucosa leading to mucosal scarring and loss of function in SJS.[8,9,11] As in a severe burn, fluid and electrolyte imbalance, renal and respiratory complications, and secondary bacterial infections complicate TEN.[8-11]

Differential diagnosis

SJS and TEN must be distinguished from the staphylococcal scalded skin syndrome and acute graft-versus-host disease by skin biopsy. SJS and TEN show full-thickness epidermal necrosis and subepidermal rather than intraepidermal blister formation[8,9] (Fig. 11-10). In graft-versus-host disease there is satellite cell necrosis in the epidermis and severe injury to cutaneous vessels not seen in SJS. Early in the course of disease, SJS may be confused with Kawasaki disease. In SJS there is necrosis of mucous membranes; whereas in Kawasaki disease there is redness and edema, but necrotic crusts and severe erosions are not seen. SJS may also be confused with the mucositis produced by chemotherapeutic agents in the child with cancer or with severe herpes stomatitis.[12] Medication history and culture or rapid diagnostic test for herpes will distinguish.

Pathogenesis

In SJS and TEN there is increasing evidence that the toxic injury to keratinocytes and mucosal epithelial cells may be the result of genetic susceptibility to injury.[9,11] Most SJS and TEN is related to drug ingestion, with nonsteroidal antiinflammatory agents, sulfonamides, and anticonvulsants the most often incriminated.[8-10] Since the skin is a large organ involved in drug detoxification, toxicity is thought to be related to the accumulation of arene oxides in ker-

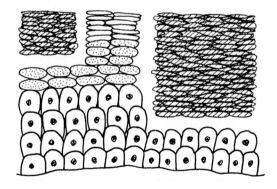

Fig. 11-10
Pathologic differentiation of scaled skin syndrome (*left*) and toxic epidermal necrolysis (*right*). Dark areas represent necrosis.

atinocytes as the result of cytochrome P-450 action on the parent drug. The detoxification of arene oxides, which bind to keratinocyte ribonucleic acids (RNAs), depends on epoxide hydrolases, which may be genetically decreased in children susceptible to SJS or TEN.[8-10] In a few cases infections with *Mycoplasma pneumoniae* or HSV have been associated with SJS. The mechanism of epithelial damage with those infectious agents is not known.

Treatment

Patients with EM major or TEN require treatment as burn patients, preferably in a burn unit.[2,7,13-15] The offending drug must be discontinued. Careful attention to fluid and electrolyte balance, respiratory toilet, fever control, and prevention of secondary bacterial infection of the denuded skin is required.[2,7,11,13-15] Most affected children cannot eat or drink, and parenteral nutrition must be supplied. Ophthalmologic consultation should be obtained, and efforts to prevent conjunctival scarring initiated. There is no evidence that systemic steroids are of benefit.[8,9,11-15]

Patient education

With SJS and TEN, the drugs thought to be associated should be avoided and patients informed that they may be genetically susceptible to develop the condition. Each complication should be discussed with the patient and parents, making them aware of potential sequelae.

Follow-up visits

For hospitalized patients, follow-up should be directed by their complications. Long-term follow-up will be required for those children who develop sequelae of mucosal or skin scarring.

KAWASAKI DISEASE (MUCOCUTANEOUS LYMPH NODE SYNDROME)

Clinical features

The child presents with a high fever of abrupt onset that lasts longer than 5 days and is accompanied by conjunctival injection[16-18] (Fig. 11-11). One of three oral changes occurs: (1) erythema, fissures,

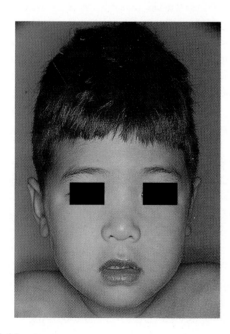

Fig. 11-11
Red, swollen lips and injected conjunctivae in a child with Kawasaki disease.

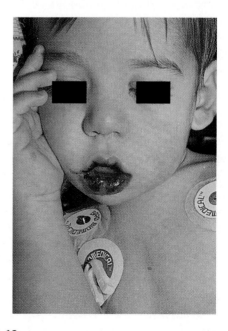

Fig. 11-12
Red, swollen, and slightly crusted lips in a child with Kawasaki disease.

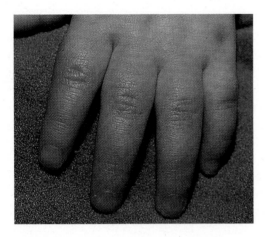

Fig. 11-13
Red, swollen fingers in an infant with Kawasaki disease.

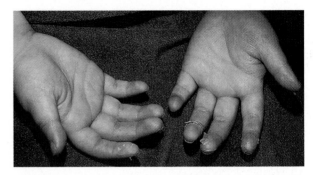

Fig. 11-14
Peeling of fingertips from distal to proximal in Kawasaki disease.

redness, and crusting of the lips (Fig. 11-12); (2) diffuse erythema of the oropharynx; or (3) strawberry tongue.[16-18] One of four changes is seen in the extremities: (1) prominent edema and induration of the hands and feet (Fig. 11-13), (2) erythema of the palms and soles, (3) desquamation beginning at the tips of the digits and spreading proximally in transverse nail grooves (Fig. 11-14), or (4) an erythematous eruption that is polymorphous in character at one point in time but mostly scarlatiniform and generalized.[16-18] Lymph node masses greater than 1.5 cm, particularly in the cervical lymph nodes, may be noted.[16-18] Kawasaki disease is often a diagnosis of exclusion, so that other forms of acute febrile syndromes must be considered first. Laboratory tests in Kawasaki syndrome disease are nonspecific, including an increased sedimentation rate of red cells, elevated nonspecific acute-phase reactants, mild anemia, and thrombocytosis that can be quite striking.[16-18]

Aneurysms of the coronary artery occur in 10% to 20% of patients with Kawasaki disease, and 2% of all patients will die from thrombosis of the aneurysms of coronary vessels.[16-18] Echocardiography may detect coronary aneurysms when present, but coronary angiography may be required.[16-18] Although there is some evidence that coronary aneurysms may heal spontaneously, careful cardiac monitoring and involvement of a pediatric cardiologist are recommended. Other complications of vasculitis may occur, including gangrene of digits.[16]

Kawasaki disease was originally described in Japan, but cases have been reported from virtually all areas of the world.[16] It is recurrent in 4% of children.[16]

Differential diagnosis

Many diseases with fever and mucocutaneous symptoms can be confused. The most common conditions that mimic Kawasaki disease are SJS, measles, toxic shock syndrome, staphylococcal scarlet fever, and acute infections such as leptospirosis. By rigidly adhering to the United States Communicable Disease Center criteria for Kawasaki disease, one may be able to distinguish one condition from another.[16-18] Cultures can be very helpful in differentiating toxic shock syndrome and staphylococcal scarlet fever from Kawasaki disease.

Pathogenesis

Kawasaki disease is a segmental vasculitis with major involvement of coronary vessels that mimics infantile periarteritis nodosa.[16] The pathogenesis is unknown, although the clustering of cases in winter and spring and close grouping have implicated an infectious agent. Although a number of infectious agents have been implicated, the most compelling evidence supports an association with parvovirus B19 infection, particularly in view of the association of the virus with periarteritis nodosa.[19] More than one infectious agent may be responsible for the syndrome. Coronary artery aneurysms develop during or following the acute inflammation.

Treatment

Intravenous gamma globulin, if given within 10 days of the onset of fever along with low-dose salicylate therapy, has been recommended to prevent aneurysms.[16,18,20,21] Intravenous gamma globulin is usually given as 2 g/kg in a single dose, although 400 mg/day for 4 days is also efficacious.[16] Retreatment may be required in patients with persistent fever.[20] High-dose steroids are contraindicated and may increase the prevalence of heart disease in this syndrome. Careful cardiac monitoring for arrhythmias is required. Involvement of a pediatric cardiologist is recommended.

Patient education

Patients should be informed that Kawasaki disease is likely the result of a yet unknown infectious agent. They should be further advised of the seriousness of the heart disease, which may eventually prompt the need for careful monitoring of cardiac signs and symptoms. It should be encouraged that any restrictions of activities or long-term diagnostic tests be obtained under the care of a pediatric cardiologist.[16,21]

Follow-up visits

Frequently the child is hospitalized, and regular hospital follow-ups are performed. Management as an outpatient should be done only when good cardiac consultation and follow-up care are available. Long-term follow-up should follow the American Heart Association guidelines.[21]

APHTHOUS ULCERS

Clinical features

Recurrent, shallow erosions of the gums, tongue, palate, lips, and buccal mucosa are seen in aphthous ulcers[12,22] (Fig. 11-15). The erosions are 1 to 10 mm in diameter and have a gray-yellow base (Fig. 11-16). Burning and tenderness may occur.[22] Healing occurs in 7 to 10 days, without scarring.[22] Recurrences are usually irregular, several months apart, and consist of two to four lesions.[12,22] In a more severe form, recurrences with numerous large (under 10 mm) lesions are frequent, so that the child is seldom free from discomfort. Aphthae are limited to the mouth, but associated ulcers on genitalia are seen in complex aphthosis, and oral and genital aphthae may be observed in association with iritis or uveitis, erythema nodosum, and central nervous system disease in the rare Behçet's syndrome. Minor aphthae may be associated with inflammatory bowel disease or an upper respiratory tract illness.[22]

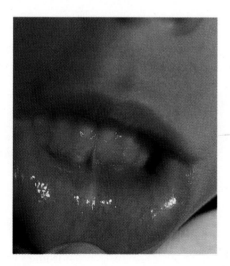

Fig. 11-15
Minor aphthous ulcer with red border in a child's mouth.

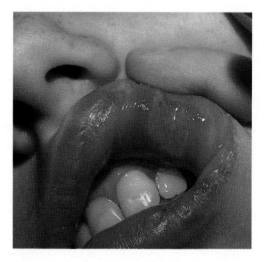

Fig. 11-16
Large aphthous ulcer with gray center.

Differential diagnosis

Aphthous ulcers must be distinguished from herpes simplex and other viral oral ulcerations, from autoimmune blistering diseases such as pemphigus, and from EM. Exfoliative cytologic study of the erosion will identify the epidermal giant cells of herpes simplex, and viral culture will distinguish the disorder from herpes simplex, coxsackieviruses A5, A10, and A16, and other enteroviruses. EM may present with oral erosions, but the symmetric target skin lesions will suggest the disorder. Erosions of the autoimmune blistering diseases will persist for many months, in contrast to days with aphthous ulcers.

Pathogenesis

The mechanism of aphthous ulcers is unknown. Several studies have demonstrated lymphocytotoxic activity against oral epithelium, suggesting an autoimmune phenomenon.[2] Biopsy shows ulceration of the epidermis and a mixed inflammatory infiltrate. Recent studies suggest that herpes simplex viral antigens may be present in oral epithelial cells within aphthous ulcer lesions, even though virus cannot be cultured. Other human herpesviruses have also been implicated.[22] The cytotoxic response that produces the injury to oral epithelium may therefore be virus specific.

Treatment

Treatment is symptomatic. Mild attacks may respond to liquid antacids[12,22] or oral cyanoacrylate dental adhesives.[23] Many mild episodes require no treatment.[12,22] Severe lesions may require topical steroids, such as triamcinolone acetonide in a base that adheres to mucous surfaces.[22] Oral prednisone, 1 to 2 mg/kg/day for 3 to 5 days, may be necessary for severe involvement that impairs eating.[12,22] Sucralfate suspension has been useful in some.[24] Antiviral agents against human herpesviruses may prove useful in future therapy of this disease.

Patient education

The recurrent nature of this disorder should be discussed and the lack of effective therapy emphasized. It should be clearly stated that the cause is unknown, and therefore therapy is nonspecific and aimed at symptomatic relief.

Follow-up visits

Follow-up visits are necessary only when attacks occur.

GEOGRAPHIC TONGUE

Clinical features

Children under 4 years of age are most commonly affected by geographic tongue, a benign inflammatory disorder. Multiple annular, smooth patches that mimic blister bases on the tongue have a gray, slightly elevated border (Fig. 11-17). There are usually no symptoms, but occasionally a child will complain of tenderness. The pattern of involvement changes from day to day and spontaneous remissions occur.

Differential diagnosis

Diagnosis is usually easy, since the migratory pattern occurs exclusively in geographic tongue. A dry tongue usually has fissures and is not migratory. Malnutrition usually produces diffuse redness and swelling of the entire tongue. Aphthous ulcers, EM, and viral ulcers do not migrate from day to day, and once established remain fixed for at least 3 to 5 days.

Pathogenesis

Pathologic changes in the annular border of the lesion of the tongue are surprisingly similar to those in pso-

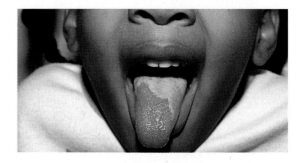

Fig. 11-17
Geographic tongue.

riasis. There are microabscesses in the epithelium and epithelial thickening, but the pathogenesis is unknown. Although the smooth area looks like an erosion clinically, the epithelium is intact and there is no blister formation.

Treatment

Treatment is usually unnecessary because the lesions are asymptomatic. Oral liquid antacids taken before meals may help if pain occurs upon eating.

Patient education

The benign nature of this condition should be emphasized.

Follow-up visits

Follow-up visits are unnecessary.

MILIARIA (HEAT RASH)

Clinical features

There are two forms of miliaria: miliaria crystallina and miliaria rubra. Miliaria crystallina occurs in newborn infants or in areas of sunburn. Miliaria rubra (heat rash) occurs primarily in infants who have induced sweating or heat retention. Airtight occlusion predisposes to miliaria.

Miliaria crystallina is characterized by clear thin-walled vesicles that are 1 to 2 mm in diameter, without erythema. The vesicles rupture within 24 to 48 hours and leave a white scale. They are seen on the head and neck and upper trunk in newborn infants and within areas of sunburn in other children.

The characteristic finding in miliaria rubra consists of 2- to 4-mm papules or papulovesicles surrounded by erythema (Fig. 11-18). Lesions are seen in flexural areas, such as the neck, axilla, and groin, following excessive sweating. The face and upper chest may be involved. Miliaria rubra may occur in a localized skin area where airtight occlusion has occurred—for example, in an immobilized or comatose child lying on a plastic bed cover.

Both forms of miliaria may be secondarily infected by *Staphylococcus aureus,* producing pustules in the sweat pores (miliaria pustulosa), which is particularly troublesome in tropical or subtropical areas. If continued sweating occurs, repeated daily episodes of miliaria result. Allowing the skin to cool and dry produces mild desquamation and healing in a few days.

Differential diagnosis

Box 11-1 presents the conditions to be considered in the differential diagnosis of miliaria crystallina and miliaria rubra. Miliaria crystallina can be distinguished from viral infections of skin or from acute dermatitis by the lack of erythema and the negative exfoliative cytologic findings. On smear of miliaria crystallina lesions, neither giant cells nor inflammatory cells are seen.

Miliaria rubra may be confused with neonatal acne, viral exanthems, candidiasis, or drug eruptions, but it is so characteristic that it is seldom misdiagnosed. The febrile child who receives an antibiotic may be mistakenly called drug allergic when the eruption with fever was miliaria.

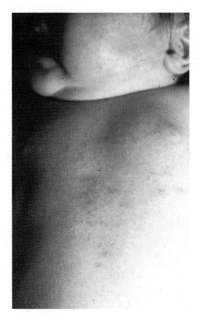

Fig. 11-18
Red pinpoint papules on chest of infant with miliaria rubra.

Box 11-1   Differential diagnosis of spontaneous vesiculobullous diseases

Commonly seen
Acute dermatitis
Bullous impetigo
Viral vesicles (HSV, varicella-zoster virus [VZV])
Thermal or chemical burns
Friction blisters
Miliaria

Uncommon disorders
Erythema multiforme
Stevens-Johnson syndrome
Toxic epidermal necrolysis
Autoimmune blistering disorders
Dermatitis herpetiformis, linear IgA
dermatosis, pemphigus, pemphigoid
epidermolysis bullosa acquisita
Mechanobullous diseases
Epidermolysis bullosa types,
especially simplex
Mastocytosis
Bullous insect bite reactions
Lupus erythematosus
Lichen planus
Polymorphous light eruption
Incontinentia pigmenti
Bullous ichthyosis

Pathogenesis

Occlusion of sweat ducts following sweating, with rupture of the sweat duct as it spirals through the epidermis, is seen in miliaria (Fig. 11-19). In miliaria crystallina the duct rupture is within the stratum corneum, whereas in miliaria rubra it occurs in the lower epidermis. Induction of sweating, overheating of the skin, and mechanical occlusion of the sweat pores are essential to the production of miliaria. The baby who is overclothed is particularly susceptible to miliaria.

Treatment

The treatment of choice consists of avoidance of further sweating and allowing the skin surface to dry and cool. If pustule formation occurs and secondary staphylococcal infection appears, systemic anti-staphylococcal antibiotics should be administered. Cooling lotions and other agents used for miliaria are not effective unless sweating is reduced. Avoidance of overclothing the baby will be preventive.

Patient education

The role of overheating the skin and the ease of sweat duct obstruction should be emphasized. The parent or care giver who overdresses the infant or child should be duly informed. Avoidance of all airtight dressings such as plastic occlusion and the need for cooling the skin must be emphasized.

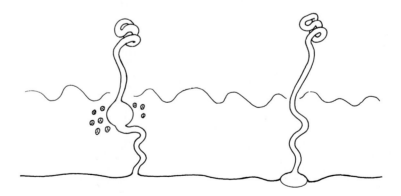

Fig. 11-19
Superficial sweat duct obstruction in miliaria crystallina (*left*) does not result in inflammation, in contrast to midepidermal sweat duct obstruction in miliaria rubra (*right*).

Follow-up visits

Follow-up visits are unnecessary.

THE IMMUNOBULLOUS DISEASES

One should suspect an immunobullous disease in the circumstance of a persistent blistering condition, particularly if present for over a month. Immunobullous diseases may present with intraepidermal blister formation, which results in a flaccid, easily eroded blister or a subepidermal blister that is tense. All are chronic diseases and as a group are quite uncommon to rare. All are characterized by the presence of autoantibodies; the immunobullous diseases are also called the autoimmune blistering diseases. In most diseases the autoantibodies are thought to play a role in the pathogenesis of the blister formation. The most common of this group of diseases is dermatitis herpetiformis, characterized by severely pruritic vesicles (Figs. 11-20 and 11-21), which

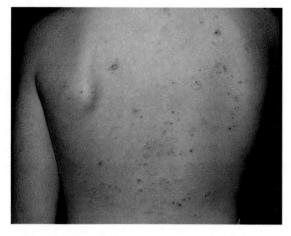

Fig. 11-20
Blisters and excoriated papules on the back of an adolescent with dermatitis herpetiformis.

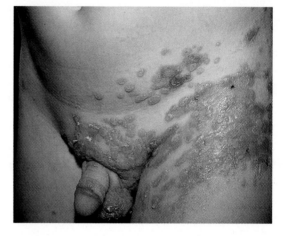

Fig. 11-22
Numerous sausage-shaped tense bullae and crusted lesions in the pelvic area of a toddler with linear IgA dermatosis.

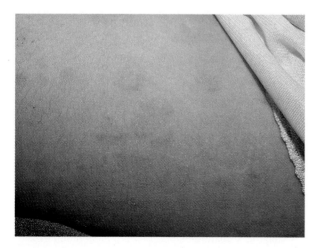

Fig. 11-21
Urticarial papules preceding blister formation on the thigh of an adolescent with dermatitis herpetiformis.

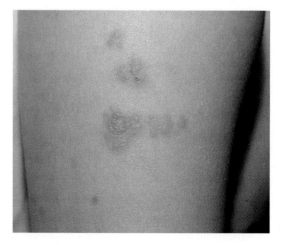

Fig. 11-23
Rosette of blisters on the leg of a child with linear IgA dermatosis.

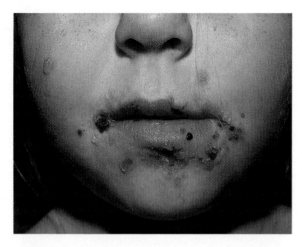

Fig. 11-24
Moist crusts and blisters in perioral distribution in a child with linear IgA dermatosis.

Box 11-2   Differential diagnosis of mechanobullous disease

Friction blisters
Recurrent bullous eruption of hands and feet (Weber-Cockayne disease)
Epidermolysis bullosa simplex (generalized and superficialis types)
Epidermolysis bullosa dystrophica, recessive and dominant types
Epidermolysis bullosa letalis (fatal and nonfatal types)
Porphyria cutanea tarda

---

usually has its onset in adolescence. The second most common is linear immunoglobulin A (IgA) dermatosis (chronic bullous disease of childhood), which has its onset in infants or toddlers (Figs. 11-22, 11-23, and 11-24). All the remaining immunobullous diseases are rare.

There are frequent errors made in the diagnosis of this group of diseases, particularly if one relies on clinical features alone. It should be emphasized that the diagnosis of immunobullous diseases is based on a combination of clinical, histologic, and immunofluorescent findings. Immunofluorescence of a skin biop-sy is frequently the diagnostic test for these diseases, and one must select noninvolved skin adjacent to a blister for biopsy. One should never biopsy an old blister or a crusted lesion. Obtaining a serum for the examination of circulating autoantibodies is most useful. These diseases are presented in Box 11-2 in order from most common to least common.

References

1. Huff JC, Weston WL: Recurrent erythema multiforme, *Medicine* 168:133, 1989.
2. Brice SL, Huff JC, Weston WL: Erythema multiforme minor in children, *Pediatrician* 18:188, 1991.
3. Weston WL, Stockert SS, Jester JD, et al: Herpes simplex virus in childhood erythema multiforme, *Pediatrics* 89:32, 1992.
4. Weston JA, Weston WL: The overdiagnosis of erythema multiforme, *Pediatrics* 89:802, 1992.
5. Zaim MT, Giorno RC, Golitz LE, et al: An immunopathological study of herpes-associated erythema multiforme, *J Cutan Pathol* 14:257, 1987.
6. Brice SL, Leahy MA, Ong L, et al: Examination of non-involved skin, previously involved skin and peripheral blood for herpes simplex virus DNA in patients with recurrent herpes-associated erythema multiforme. *J Cutan Pathol* 21:406, 1994.
7. Barton P, Flowers F: Controversies in the management of erythema multiforme and toxic epidermal necrolysis, *Curr Opin Dermatol* 2:27, 1995.
8. Bastuji-Garin S, Rzany B, Stern RS, et al: Clinical classification of cases of toxic epidermal necrolysis, Stevens-Johnson syndrome and erythema multiforme, *Arch Dermatol* 129:92, 1993.
9. Roujeau J-C: The spectrum of Stevens-Johnson syndrome and toxic epidermal necrolysis: A clinical classification, *J Invest Dermatol* 102:28s, 1994.
10. Kaufman DW: Epidemiologic approaches to the study of toxic epidermal necrolysis, *J Invest Dermatol* 102:31s, 1994.
11. Stewart MG, Duncan NO III, Franklin DJ, et al: Head and neck manifestations of erythema multiforme in children, *Otolaryngol Head Neck Surg* 111:236, 1994.
12. Hebert AA, Berg JH: Oral mucous membrane diseases

of childhood: I. Mucositis and Xerostomia. II. Recurrent aphthous stomatitis. III. Herpetic stomatitis, *Semin Dermatol* 11:80, 1992.

13. Parsons JM: Toxic epidermal necrolysis, *Int J Dermatol* 31:749, 1992.

14. Green D, Law E, Still JM: An approach to the management of toxic epidermal necrolysis in a burn centre, *Burns* 19:411, 1993.

15. Barone CM, Bianchi MA, Lee B, et al: Treatment of toxic epidermal necrolysis and Stevens-Johnson syndrome in children, *J Oral Maxillofac Surg* 51:264, 1993.

16. Beitz LO, Barron KS: Kawasaki syndrome, *Curr Opin Dermatol* 2:114, 1995.

17. Yamamoto LG, Martin JE: Kawasaki syndrome in the ED, *Am J Emer Med* 12:178, 1994.

18. Dajani A, Taubert K, Gerber M, et al: Diagnosis and therapy of Kawasaki disease in children, *Circulation* 87:1776, 1993.

19. Nigro G, Zerbini M, Kryzszrofiak A, et al: Active or recent parvovirus B19 infection in children with Kawasaki disease, *Lancet* 343:1260, 1994.

20. Sundel R, Burns J, Baler A, et al: Gamma globulin retreatment in Kawasaki disease, *J Pediatr* 123:657, 1993.

21. Dajani A, Tauber K, Takahashi M, et al: Guidelines for long-term management of patients with Kawasaki disease, *Circulation* 89:916, 1994.

22. Brice SL: Aphthous stomatitis, *Curr Probl Dermatol* 3:107, 1991.

23. Jasmin JR, Muller-Giamarchi M, et al: Local treatment of minor aphthous ulceration in children, *AJDC J Dent Child* 60:26, 1993.

24. Rattan J, Schneider M, Arber N, et al: Sucralfate suspension as a treatment of recurrent aphthous stomatitis, *J Intern Med* 236:341, 1994.

25. Dawson TA Jr: Microscopic appearance of geographic tongue, *Br J Dermatol* 81:827, 1969.

26. O'Brien JP: The pathogenesis of miliaria, *Arch Dermatol* 86:267, 1962.

27. Kirtschig H, Wojnarowska F: Autoimmune blistering diseases: an update of diagnostic methods and investigations, *Clin Exp Dermatol* 19:97, 1994.

28. Kirtschig G, Wojnarowska P, Marsden RA, et al: Acquired bullous diseases of childhood: reevaluation of diagnosis by indirect immunofluorescence examination of 1 m NaCl split skin and immunoblotting, *Br J Dermatol* 130:610, 1994.

29. Grunwald MH, Zamora E, Avinoach I, et al: Pemphigus neonatorum, *Pediatr Dermatol* 10:169, 1993.

30. Tope WD, Kamino H, Briggaman RA, et al: Neonatal pemphigus vulgaris in a child born to a woman in remission, *J Am Acad Dermatol* 29:480, 1993.

31. Leibowitz MR, Voss SP: Juvenile pemphigus foliaceous: response to dapsone, *Arch Dermatol* 129:910, 1993.

32. Oranje AP, van Joost T: Pemphigoid in children, *Pediatr Dermatol* 6:267, 1989.

33. Levine V, Sanchez M, Nestor M: Localized vulvar pemphigoid in a child misdiagnosed as sexual abuse, *Arch Dermatol* 128:804, 1992.

34. Saad RW, Domloge-Hultach N, Yancey KB, et al: Childhood localized vulvar pemphigoid is a true variant of bullous pemphigoid, *Arch Dermatol* 128:807, 1992.

35. McCuaig CC, Chan LS, Woodley DT, et al: Epidermolysis bullosa acquisita in childhood, *Arch Dermatol* 125:944, 1989.

36. Nagano T, Tani M, Adachi A, et al: Childhood bullous pemphigoid: Immunofluorescent, immunoelectron microscopic and western blot analysis, *J Am Acad Dermatol* 30:884, 1994.

37. Ruiz E, Deng J-S, Abell EA: Eosinophilic spongiosis: clinical, histologic and immunopathologic study, *J Am Acad Dermatol* 30:973, 1994.

38. Gawkroger DA, Vestey JP, Mahony SO, et al: Dermatitis herpetiformis and established coeliac disease, *Br J Dermatol* 129:694, 1993.

39. Zone JJ: *Dermatitis herpetiformis.* In Provost TT, Weston WL, editors: *Bullous diseases,* St. Louis, 1993, Mosby–Year Book, p 157.

40. Rico MJ: Management of autoimmune blistering diseases, *Curr Opin Dermatol* 2:22, 1995.

12

Skin Cysts and Nodules

Persistent masses in the skin often result in a child's being brought in for medical examination. Often parents are concerned that the skin lesion is cancer. Biopsy may be necessary to provide an accurate diagnosis in these conditions. They are rarely symptomatic except in weight-bearing areas. A large number of skin problems can produce skin nodules. When one observes a skin-colored nodule in an infant or child, an orderly list of possibilities does not easily come to mind. One should first remember that the most common palpable superficial nodule in infants and children is the lymph node. Occipital and cervical nodes are superficial and easily palpated, and sometimes may be mistaken for skin tumors or nodules.

The most common types of superficial skin nodules in infants and children that require skin biopsy are listed in Table 12-1.[1] An estimation of the approximate frequency of each skin nodule in infants and children is provided. Epithelial cysts and pilomatricomas together account for over two thirds of such superficial nodules, and one should particularly remember these two major causes of skin nodules when making a diagnosis.[1] Overall, only 1% of such skin nodules turn out to be malignant growths. The main factors in suspecting whether one of these nodules is malignant are listed in Box 12-1. The most important factor is rapid, progressive growth. Hemangiomas can show rapid growth in infancy (see Chapter 13) and have a benign course. If you are certain that a lesion is not a hemangioma, and you identify a skin nodule with rapid, progressive growth, you should suspect malignancy and obtain a tissue sample for diagnosis.

SKIN CYSTS

Skin cysts are often solitary in children and produce skin-colored nodules that distort skin contours. They are the most common skin nodule, found predominantly on the lateral border of the eyebrow or under the scalp, in both infants and children (Fig. 12-1).

Clinical features
Epithelial, dermoid, and branchial cleft cysts and milia
Epithelial cysts are slow-growing, firm, round nodules that reach a maximum size of 1 to 15 cm (Fig. 12-2).

Table 12-1

Skin Nodules and Cysts in Infants and Children

Type	Approximate percentage of all nodules
Epithelial cysts	59
Pilomatricomas	10
Fibromas	4
Neurofibromas	3
Lipomas	3
Lymphangiomas	3
Granuloma annulare	3
Juvenile xanthogranulomas	3
Mastocytomas	2
Miscellaneous lesions	9
Malignant tumors (usually sarcomas)	1

Box 12-1   Factors associated with likelihood of malignancy in superficial skin tumors in children*

Rapid, progressive growth
Ulceration
Fixed to deep fascia
Greater than 3 cm and firm
Occurs in first 30 days of life

*Listed in order of importance.

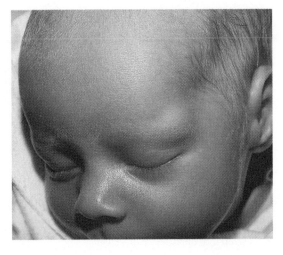

Fig. 12-1
Dermoid cyst. Cystic nodule on the lateral aspect of the left eyebrow of a newborn infant.

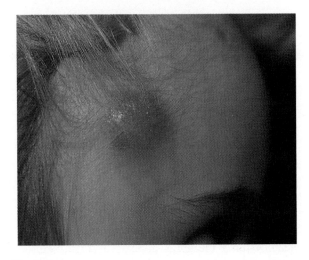

Fig. 12-2
Inflamed epithelial cyst. This lesion may be inflamed secondary to infection or spontaneous rupture and foreign body reaction.

Epidermal cysts in the newborn period are found predominantly in the lateral border of the eyebrow or in the scalp.[1] They may also be seen on the palms and soles of newborns. They may not be recognized until childhood, when the lesions grow larger. Whether these cysts contain follicular or other adnexal structures and are designated dermoid cysts does not vary their location or clinical features. Presence of midline pits or cysts on the nose poses a special problem related to possible intracranial connection.[2] Papules, cysts, or draining sinus tracts on the lateral aspect of the neck may be associated with branchial cleft cysts or sinus tracts[3] (Fig. 12-3).

In adolescence, solitary cysts appear on the scalp, face, neck, and trunk in the region where acne vulgaris is seen. Multiple cysts in children or adolescents should suggest Gardner's syndrome. Milia are tiny, superficial cysts seen on the faces of newborns and within the scar in scarring conditions such as epidermolysis bullosa (Fig. 12-4).

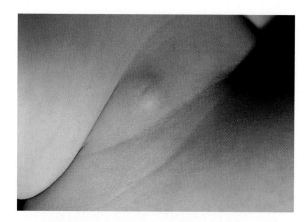

Fig. 12-3
Branchial cleft cyst on the neck of a child.

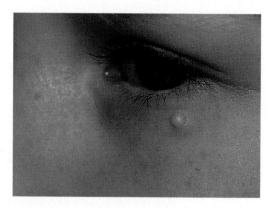

Fig. 12-4
Milia on the cheek of a child.

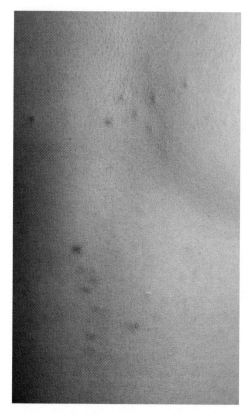

Fig. 12-5
Eruptive vellus hair cyst. Superficial cystic lesions on the mid-portion of the chest and upper aspect of the abdomen.

Steatocystoma multiplex

Steatocystoma multiplex appears as firm, skin-colored or yellowish nodules 1 to 3 cm in diameter in the axillae and on the chest and arms. The condition is inherited as autosomal dominant, begins in adolescence, and is uncommon.

Eruptive vellus hair cysts

Eruptive vellus hair cysts commonly begin between the ages of 5 and 10 years as small, skin-colored papules appearing on the lower chest and upper abdomen—areas not usually involved with epithelial or dermoid cysts[4] (Fig. 12-5). Usually five or more lesions are present.

Differential diagnosis

For a list of skin nodules and cysts that should be included in the differential diagnosis, see Table 12-1. Epithelial and dermoid cysts are difficult to distinguish from one another without a biopsy. However, since both conditions are benign, a biopsy is usually not necessary. Midline nasal dermoid lesions are the exception. These appear as a midline pit, fistula, or swelling anywhere from the glabella to the nasal tip. These lesions may have intracranial extensions. Steatocystoma multiplex similarly has a different distribution, with locations around the axilla, neck, and onto the arms. Gardner's syndrome should be considered when multiple epithelial cysts are seen. Branchial cleft cysts are usually on the lateral aspect of the neck and may show inflammation.

Pathogenesis

Epithelial cysts and milia

Although epithelial cysts are commonly called *sebaceous cysts*, they contain neither sebum nor sebaceous glands. Epithelial cysts and milia are filled with keratin in laminated layers and lined by epithelium. When they are ruptured, foreign body reactions occur around the ruptured cyst wall.

Steatocystoma multiplex

Steatocystoma multiplex consists of intricately folded cyst walls of epithelial cells, with flattened sebaceous gland lobules within or close to the cyst wall.

Dermoid cysts

Dermoid cysts represent sequestration of skin along lines of embryonic closure and contain an epithelial lining plus either mature sebaceous glands, eccrine sweat glands, or mature hair.

Branchial cleft cysts

These are defects of embryonic closure. They may drain into the pharynx or onto the skin.

Eruptive vellus hair cysts

Most authorities consider eruptive vellus hair cysts a developmental anomaly of body hair follicles. Obstruction at the neck of the follicular channel results in cystic dilation of the follicle, retention of vellus hairs, and atrophy of the hair bulbs.

Treatment

Most cysts require no treatment and may be best left alone. If cosmetic improvement can be obtained, surgical excision is the treatment of choice. Midline nasal dermoid cysts require meticulous surgical excision in an effort to prevent intracranial extension and complications. Before surgery, neuroimaging studies may help to predict intracranial involvement.[2] Branchial cleft cysts and sinus tracts require complete surgical excision to avoid recurrence. No effective therapy for vellus hair cysts is available.

Patient education

Patients should be aware of the benign nature of these growths, despite their prominent size. In children with multiple epithelial cysts, bowel examination for signs of Gardner's syndrome is indicated.

Follow-up visits

A visit 1 week after surgery to explain the pathologic findings is beneficial.

ADNEXAL TUMORS

A variety of benign growths arise from epithelial adnexal structures (sebaceous glands, hair follicles, sweat glands) and produce skin nodules or tumors. Some, such as the sebaceous nevus and epidermal nevus, appear at birth and are discussed in the section on birthmarks in Chapter 21. Most adnexal tumors do not appear until adult life, but four types—pilomatricomas, syringomas, trichoepitheliomas, and basal cell carcinoma—may be seen in childhood or adolescence.

Clinical features

Pilomatricoma

Pilomatricomas (calcifying epitheliomas) appear as solitary, hard, 2- to 5-mm papules covered by normal skin on the face or extremities[5] (Figs. 12- 6 and 12-

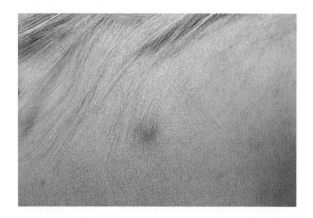

Fig. 12-6
Pilomatricoma. Firm blue papule on the face of a child.

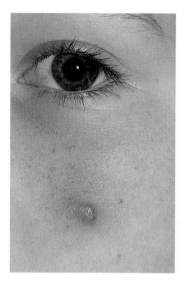

Fig. 12-7
Pilomatricoma. Firm blue papule on the face surrounded by an inflammatory reaction secondary to trauma, foreign body reaction, or infection.

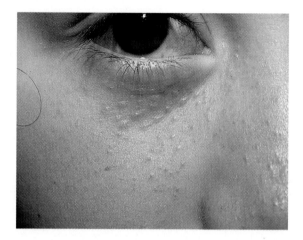

Fig. 12-8
Syringomas. Multiple skin-colored papules on the face and lower eyelid.

7). They may be blue . They often begin in infancy or during early school years, but are not hereditary. Pilomatricomas account for up to 10% of all skin nodules and tumors in children.[1] They may be present in the newborn period.

Syringoma

Syringomas appear at puberty as small (1 to 2 mm), skin-colored to yellowish soft nodules (Fig. 12-8). They occur on the eyelids, cheeks, axillae, abdomen, and vulva. They are more common in girls than in boys. Most often lesions are limited to the eyelids.[6]

Trichoepithelioma

Trichoepitheliomas appear as numerous, round, skin-colored nodules primarily on the midface (Fig. 12-9) area of children and adolescents. The nodules are 2 to 8 mm in diameter and may be seen on the upper trunk, neck, and scalp. A few fine telangiectasias may be observed over the lesions. Multiple lesions are inherited as autosomal dominant, whereas solitary lesions may appear spontaneously without a family history.

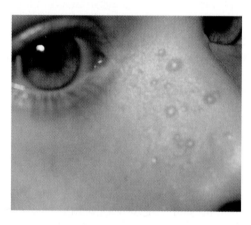

Fig. 12-9
Multiple trichoepitheliomas on the nose of a child.

Basal cell carcinoma

Basal cell carcinomas are uncommon in school-age children and adolescents.[7] They appear on the face or upper trunk as a solitary nodule with overlying telangiectasia. They may be seen in otherwise unaffected children, but their presence should suggest three syndromes: basal cell nevus syndrome,[8,9] xeroderma pigmentosum, and Bazex's syndrome (Table 12-2). Basal cell carcinoma may progress to ulceration and local invasion of the dermis and deeper tissues. They do not metastasize.

Table 12-2

Syndromes Associated with Basal Cell Carcinoma in Children

Clinical feature	Basal cell nevus syndrome	Bazex's syndrome	Xeroderma pigmentosum
Inheritance	Autosomal dominant	Autosomal dominant	Autosomal recessive
Palmar pits	Present	Present	Absent
Multiple freckles	Absent	Absent	Present
Prominent dilated pores on arms and dorsa of hands	Absent	Present	Absent
Jaw cysts	Present	Absent	Absent
Defective teeth	Present	Absent	Present

Differential diagnosis

Pilomatricomas and basal cell carcinomas are characteristically solitary and firm, in contrast to syringomas and trichoepitheliomas. Trichoepitheliomas and syringomas may be confused with acne vulgaris or the multiple angiofibromas of tuberous sclerosis, since they occur on the face. The latter are red rather than skin-colored, however. A skin biopsy will distinguish between the lesions of tuberous sclerosis, trichoepithelioma, or syringoma. Confirmatory diagnosis of all four adnexal tumors is made by skin biopsy.[10,11]

Pathogenesis

Pilomatricoma

Pilomatricoma is considered a benign hyperplasia of the cells of the hair matrix. It is a tumor located in the deep dermis, and is composed of islands of basophilic cells and anuclear "shadow" cells. Calcium deposits appear throughout the tumor.

Syringoma

Syringoma is a benign hyperplasia of the cells of the eccrine sweat ducts. Numerous small ducts are located in the middermis to upper dermis with "tennis racquet" shapes and surrounding fibrosis.

Trichoepithelioma

Trichoepitheliomas consist of multiple horn cysts and basophilic tumor islands in the middermis. They are believed to be derived from the cells of the hair follicle.

Basal cell carcinoma

Basal cell carcinomas are composed of solid masses of cells that contain a large nucleus and little cytoplasm and extend down from the epidermis. Separation from the surrounding fibrous tissue by a clear space is commonly observed. In xeroderma pigmentosum, ultraviolet light-induced deoxyribonucleic acid (DNA) damage cannot be repaired because of autosomal recessive inheritance of various enzyme deficiencies.[12] The pathogenesis of basal cell carcinomas in basal cell nevus syndrome and Bazex's syndrome is unknown.

Treatment

Excision is the treatment of choice for pilomatricomas and basal cell carcinomas. Multiple syringomas and trichoepitheliomas are difficult to treat, and treatment of multiple lesions often has poor cosmetic results.

Patient education

The benign nature and origin of pilomatricoma, syringoma, and trichoepithelioma should be discussed. Basal cell carcinomas should be considered slowly progressing malignant tumors. In the hereditary syndromes, careful evaluation of family members is necessary.

Follow-up visits

Children with basal cell carcinoma should be examined every 6 months for the appearance of further skin tumors. The importance of avoidance of exposure to the sun and the use of sunscreens should be emphasized at each visit.

SKIN NODULES

Fibroma
Clinical features

Dermatofibroma   The presenting symptom of a dermatofibroma is a small, firm, well-defined, often pigmented nodule on the leg or trunk of children, adolescents, or adults (Fig. 12-10). Dermatofibromas may follow minor skin trauma or may appear to occur spontaneously. Multiple lesions can also occur. Lateral pressure on the lesion will pro-

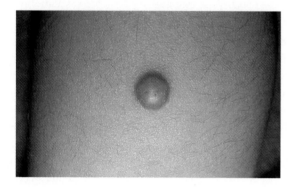

Fig. 12-10
Dermatofibroma. Firm, well-defined, pigmented nodule on the leg of an adolescent.

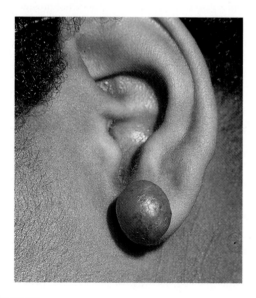

Fig. 12-11
Nodule on the ear after ear piercing.

duce dimpling of its surface. The lesions may become as large as 1 to 2 cm in diameter, and they persist indefinitely.

Hypertrophic scars   A hypertrophic scar is an overgrowth of fibrous tissue that remains at the site of the original injury (Fig. 12-11).

Keloid   Keloids are firm, progressively enlarging nodules with a shiny, hairless surface. They may be painful or may itch. They may occur on the extremities, but are predominantly located on the earlobes (Fig. 12-11), presternal area, neck (Fig. 12-12), and face following skin trauma. They often have stellate shapes. The tendency to form keloids may be inherited. They may progressively enlarge for 20 to 40 years and form lobulated or pedunculated masses.

Digital fibrous tumor of childhood   Digital fibrous tumor of childhood is a firm nodule occurring around the fingernail or toenail.[13,14] The lesion may be present at birth or will usually arise before 1 year of age. Because excision often results in rapid recurrence, the lesion is also called recurrent digital fibrous tumor. The lesion may initially grow rapidly and require a skin biopsy to confirm that it is not a sarcoma. It will usually spontaneously involute within several years.

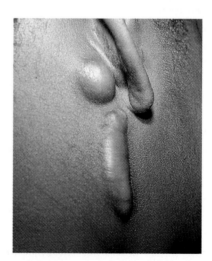

Fig. 12-12
Keloid and epithelial cyst. Superior lesion is an epithelial cyst, and the lower lesion is a keloid that formed in an excision scar of a previously excised epithelial cyst.

Differential diagnosis

Dermatofibroma Dermatofibromas may be pigmented and mimic melanoma. They are more likely to be confused with other skin nodules, however (Table 12-1).

Keloid and hypertrophic scar Although seldom misdiagnosed, early keloids mimic ordinary scars. Keloids extend beyond the bounds of the original injury, whereas hypertrophic scars remain within the area of injury.

Digital fibrous tumor of childhood Digital fibrous tumors may mimic the fibrous thickening overlying a subungual exostosis, callus, or corn. A radiograph of the digit should be obtained before biopsy.

Pathogenesis

Dermatofibroma Dermatofibromas contain numerous fibroblasts with excessive deposition of collagen and proliferation of the overlying epidermis. They are believed to be a reactive proliferation of fibroblasts in response to trauma.

Keloid and hypertrophic scar Keloids produce nodular patterns of collagen fibers associated with the new blood vessel formation, as expected in healing. However, as the vessels regress, collagen deposition continues and fails to thin as expected. Hypertrophic scars may be a similar process to a lesser degree.

Digital fibrous tumor of childhood Digital fibrous tumors show proliferating fibroblasts that contain eosinophilic cytoplasmic inclusions thought to represent myofilament.

Treatment

Dermatofibromas, if symptomatic or worrisome, may be excised. Keloids can be treated by injections of intralesional glucocorticosteroids, which results in softening and flattening. Often triamcinolone acetonide, 5 to 10 mg/ml in saline solution, is injected. Surgery alone will result in rapid reappearance of the keloid, but surgery followed by frequent intralesional injections of glucocorticosteroids may be effective therapy for large keloids. Steroid injections may result in hypopigmentation surrounding the lesion. Applications of silicone occlusive sheeting may also benefit keloids or scars.[15] Months of application may be required. Recurring digital fibrous tumors should be allowed to involute spontaneously, if possible, as surgical excision may be followed by recurrence.[13,14]

Patient education

The benign nature of these disorders should be emphasized.

Follow-up visits

Keloids may be injected at 4- to 6-week intervals.

Neurofibroma
Clinical features

Neurofibromas may be present at birth or develop later in life. The neurofibroma is a soft, skin-colored papule that may occur anywhere on the skin (Fig. 12-14). Neurofibromas may occur as solitary lesions or may be associated with neurofibromatosis.

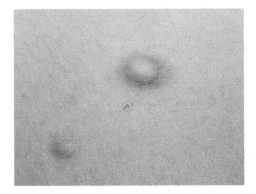

Fig. 12-13
Hypertrophic scar. Site of previous chicken pox lesions.

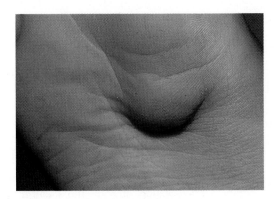

Fig. 12-14
Neurofibroma. Soft, skin-colored papule.

Box 12-2 Differential diagnosis of neurofibromas

Angiolipoma
Hemangioma
Lipoma
Lymphangioma
Mucous cyst
Melanocytic nevus

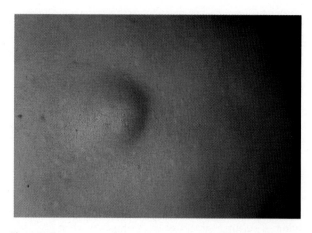

Fig. 12-15
Lipoma. Soft, subcutaneous nodule unattached to overlying skin.

Neurofibromatosis is discussed in Chapter 17. Solitary lesions may precede the other features of neurofibromatosis.

Differential diagnosis

The differential diagnosis of neurofibromas is listed in Box 12-2. A biopsy may be necessary to confirm the diagnosis.

Pathogenesis

Neurofibromas are benign tumors of nerve sheath cells.

Patient education

The nature of neurofibromas, and their association with multiple neurofibromatosis, should be carefully explained to the family, and a complete family history and evaluation of family members should be done.

Follow-up visits

Children with a solitary neurofibroma should be followed every 6 to 12 months and examined for the appearance of café-au-lait spots or other signs and symptoms of neurofibromatosis.

Lipoma
Clinical features

Lipomas are soft, subcutaneous nodules unattached to overlying skin (Fig. 12-15). They are usually solitary, begin in adolescence, and are most commonly found on the neck, upper aspect of the chest, and

arms. Angiolipomas, variants of lipomas, may present as painful subcutaneous nodules.

Differential diagnosis

Epithelial cysts, neurofibromas, and other skin nodules may mimic lipomas, but the ability to easily slide the overlying skin over the lesion helps to confirm the deep subcutaneous location of lipomas.

Pathogenesis

A lipoma is composed of nodules of normal-appearing fat cells, although unresponsiveness of fat cells to the lipolytic effects of norepinephrine occurs in multiple symmetric lipomatosis. Capillary proliferation is seen in angiolipoma in addition to an excess of normal fat cells.

Treatment

Lipomas are usually asymptomatic. Angiolipomas may be painful and may require excision for pain relief.

Patient education

The benign nature of these nodules should be emphasized.

Follow-up visits

Follow-up visits are unnecessary.

Lymphangioma

Lymphangiomas are often present at birth and are discussed in detail in the section on vascular malformations in Chapter 13. They may, however, be overlooked until later in infancy and childhood, and their presenting symptom is solitary, soft swellings of the face, neck, trunk, or extremities, showing progressive growth.

Granuloma annulare

Clinical features   Small, firm papules or nodules that form a circle or semicircle are characteristic of granuloma annulare.[16] They may be skin-colored, but more often a dusky, violaceous hue is seen. Stretching the skin reveals the ring of papules or nodules. The lesions occur predominantly in acral areas (Figs. 12-16, 12-17, and 12-18), on the digits, ankles, and wrists; 50% of affected children have a single ring of lesions. Occasionally, large firm subcutaneous nodules may be seen, or multiple small papules are found. Lesions are usually asymptomatic.

Differential diagnosis   Small, annular lesions are often mistaken for dermatophyte infections. The lack of epidermal change or scaling, and the deep palpable portion, help distinguish granuloma annulare

from tinea corporis. Large nodules of granuloma annulare may mimic rheumatoid nodules, and subcutaneous granuloma annulare may be histologically and clinically indistinguishable from rheumatoid nodules. In granuloma annulare no systemic symptoms are noted. Occasionally other annulare lesions (e.g., lichen planus, sarcoidosis, syphilis, necrobiosis

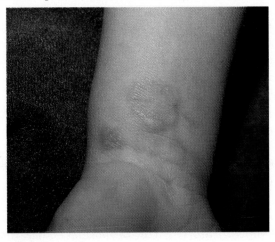

Fig. 12-17
Granuloma annulare. Large and small annular plaques on the ventral surface of the arm. Central resolution can be seen in larger lesions.

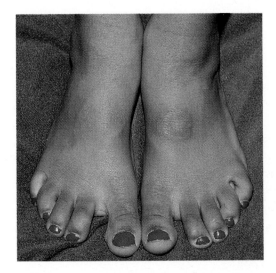

Fig. 12-16
Granuloma annulare. Unilateral oval lesion on the dorsum of the foot.

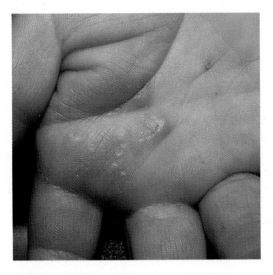

Fig. 12-18
Granuloma annulare. Grouping of firm papules on the palm of the hand.

lipoidica diabeticorum) are confused with granuloma annulare. A biopsy may be necessary to confirm the diagnosis.

Pathogenesis Focal areas of collagen degeneration surrounded by lymphocytes and epithelioid cells are seen in the middermis and reticular dermis in granuloma annulare. The mechanism of the disease is unknown.

Treatment Since lesions are asymptomatic, only reassurance is necessary. Although it is tempting to treat such conditions, spontaneous remission in several years is the rule. No effective therapy is available.

Patient education The benign nature of this disorder, and its natural history, should be stressed. Its distinct separation from rheumatoid disease states should be explained.

Follow-up visits Follow-up visits are unnecessary.

Rheumatoid nodules

Clinical features True rheumatoid nodules are uncommon in children with rheumatic disease. They are seen in rheumatoid arthritis, rheumatic fever, and systemic lupus erythematosus as 1- to 4-cm subcutaneous nodules not attached to overlying skin. They develop over bony structures, such as a joint, and are usually associated with severe rheumatoid disease with positive rheumatoid factor. The overlying skin has a normal color.

Differential diagnosis Rheumatoid nodules are most often confused with granuloma annulare (Table 12-1). However, epithelial cysts, adnexal tumors, lipomas, and other skin nodules may also be confused with rheumatoid nodules.

Pathogenesis Foci of collagen degeneration surrounded by macrophages are seen in the deep dermis and subcutaneous fat. The mechanism of production of rheumatoid nodules is unknown, but most investigators regard this condition as a form of immune complex disease.

Treatment If the nodules are symptomatic, excision is the treatment of choice. Therapy used to control other rheumatic symptoms rarely influences rheumatoid nodules.

Patient education Information about the nature of the associated disease should be given.

Follow-up visits The timing of follow-up visits should be based on the severity of the associated systemic illness.

Necrobiosis lipoidica diabeticorum

The lesions of necrobiosis lipoidica diabeticorum are irregularly shaped yellow-red plaques on the lower leg (Fig. 12-19). The lesions may show central atrophy or sclerosis. Often the lesions are bilateral and symmetric. A skin biopsy specimen of a lesion may have the histologic appearance of granuloma annulare. Children with necrobiosis lipoidica diabeticorum may have associated diabetes mellitus, and they should be evaluated with a fasting serum glucose test.

Juvenile xanthogranuloma

Clinical features In juvenile xanthogranuloma orange to yellow-brown soft nodules appear on the skin of infants and children (Figs. 12-20 and 12-21). The nodules are often multiple, numbering 5 to 10 (Figs. 12-22 and 12-23). They may be present at birth and often involute spontaneously over several years.[17,18] Lesions are seen in the iris and may be mis-

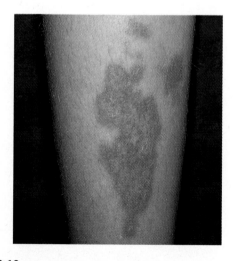

Fig. 12-19
Necrobiosis lipoidica diabeticorum. Large plaque on the lower leg of a female adolescent. Note the elevated border and yellow-red coloration.

taken for retinoblastoma, or they may cause glaucoma.[19] Although involvement is primarily in the skin, nodules have been described in the testes, lung, liver, spleen, and pericardium.

Differential diagnosis   Xanthomas, spindle and epithelioid melanocytic nevi, histiocytosis, and mastocytomas all may appear as orange or yellow-brown nodules at first presentation (see Box 12-3). Skin biopsy is necessary to distinguish juvenile xanthogranuloma from these conditions. Stroking the

skin surface covering a mastocytoma will produce urticaria within the nodule (Darier's sign).

Pathogenesis   Within the dermis, large accumulations of macrophages appear. Their cytoplasm gradually fills with lipid, creating a particular type of giant cell called the Touton giant cell. Regressing lesions show fibroblastic proliferation. There is no apparent relationship between juvenile xanthogranuloma and either abnormalities of lipid metabolism or malignant histiocytosis.

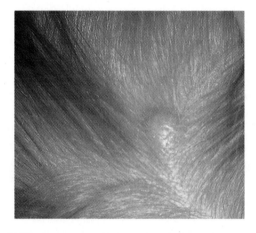

Fig. 12-20
Juvenile xanthogranuloma. Yellow-orange lesion on the scalp.

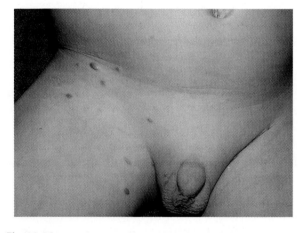

Fig. 12-22
Juvenile xanthogranuloma. Grouping of lesions on the lower aspect of the trunk and on the thigh.

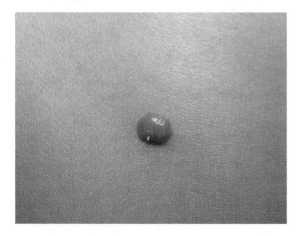

Fig. 12-21
Juvenile xanthogranuloma. Lesion on the abdomen has more of a brown-orange color.

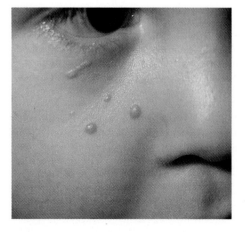

Fig. 12-23
Juvenile xanthogranuloma. Orange-brown coloration is seen on close inspection.

Box 12-3 Differential diagnosis of orange or yellow-brown nodules

Benign cephalic histiocytosis
Langerhans cell histiocytosis
Juvenile xanthogranuloma
Mastocytoma
Spindle and epithelioid cell melanocytic nevus
Xanthoma

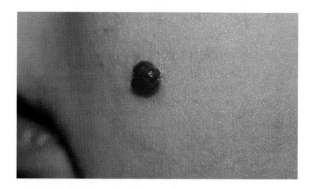

Fig. 12-24
Pyogenic granuloma. Smooth, glistening surface of an erythematous papule.

Treatment Treatment of the individual lesions is usually not necessary. Examination by an ophthalmologist may be necessary to evaluate and possibly treat eye lesions if they occur. Patients with juvenile xanthogranulomas and multiple café-au-lait spots may have an increased risk of granulocytic leukemia.[20]

Patient education The natural history of this lesion and the need for careful observation for eye involvement should be emphasized.

Follow-up visits Ophthalmologic evaluations are usually repeated semiannually or more frequently if eye lesions are present. Examination and quantitation of skin lesions can be completed during routine examinations.

Mastocytoma

Mastocytomas are usually present at birth and are discussed in detail in Chapter 14. They may not become apparent until 1 to 2 months of age as macular red or red-brown lesions usually appearing on the trunk.[21]

Pyogenic granuloma

Clinical features Pyogenic granulomas are most common in acral areas, such as the hands and fingers, and on the face (Fig. 12-24). They appear as solitary, dull-red, firm nodules that are 5 to 6 mm in diameter. The surface may be smooth and glistening, but often it is ulcerated and crusted. The lesion bleeds easily when traumatized. Removal has resulted in the appearance of multiple satellite lesions in a few instances. Pyogenic granuloma may occur at any age, but in childhood it is most common in the first 5 years

of life. The majority of patients have no history of a predisposing factor.[22]

Differential diagnosis Pyogenic granuloma is often misdiagnosed as a hemangioma, glomus tumor, melanocytic nevus, wart, molluscum contagiosum, or malignant melanoma.[23] All these lesions can ulcerate and crust if traumatized. Pathologic study distinguishes pyogenic granuloma from the other lesions.

Pathogenesis Proliferation of capillaries within a circumscribed area with flattened or ulcerated epidermis on top and epidermal proliferation at the sides, producing a "collarette" of epidermis, is seen. Pyogenic granuloma is believed to be due to an abnormal healing response.[23]

Treatment Excision is the treatment of choice. Pulse-dye laser treatment is effective for smaller lesions.

Patient education It should be explained that this growth is not malignant, but will not disappear without treatment, and represents an abnormal healing response.

Follow-up visits A visit 1 week after removal of the lesion is useful to inform the patient of the pathologic diagnosis and evaluate healing.

Smooth muscle hamartoma

Smooth muscle hamartomas are present a birth, but they may not be noted until later in infancy or childhood. The lesions may appear to have excess hair and may be hyperpigmented when compared with the normal skin. On palpation, the lesional hairs may become erect as a result of the excess smooth muscle within the lesion. Biopsy of the lesion will show abundant smooth muscle bundles within the dermis.[24]

Calcified nodules

Cutaneous calcinosis results from precipitation of insoluble calcium salts within cutaneous tissues. This can occur in congenital or acquired lesions. Solitary or multiple lesions can be present that are firm or rock hard. They are usually asymptomatic but can be painful and discharge chalky material through the skin. Underlying metabolic disease, connective tissue disease, or malignancy may be associated, or the lesion can be idiopathic. In newborn infants a solitary calcified nodule of the ear may form (Fig. 12-25), whereas in children with dermatomyositis or other collagen vascular diseases, multiple nodules may form on the extensor surfaces of hands and elbows. Biopsy confirmation is necessary before a comprehensive systemic evaluation is begun.[25]

Piezogenic pedal papules

Piezogenic pedal papules are common, sometimes painful papules that may occur on the feet (Fig. 12-26) and wrist.[26] The lesions represent herniations of fatty subcutaneous tissue into connective tissue. The herniations are seen when pressure is applied to the heel or wrist. Painful lesions can be excised or treated with orthopedic padding.[27]

Knuckle pads

Knuckle pads are thickening of the skin overlying digital joints (Fig. 12-27). The lesions grow slowly and are asymptomatic,[28] sporadic, and idiopathic. They rarely are associated with trauma. The lesions can persist indefinitely. Treatment is usually unsuccessful and unnecessary.

Panniculitis

Inflammation in the subcutaneous fat may be first seen as painful lesions that feel as if they are deep beneath the skin. Biopsy will identify the inflamma-

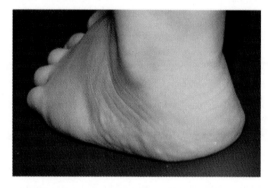

Fig. 12-26
Piezogenic pedal papules. Lesions on the foot are seen as multiple soft, compressible papules that appear when pressure is placed on the heel.

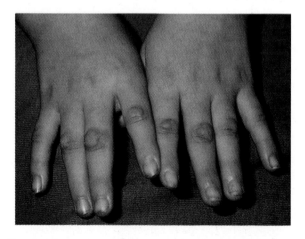

Fig. 12-27
Knuckle pads over the proximal interphalangeal joints of both hands.

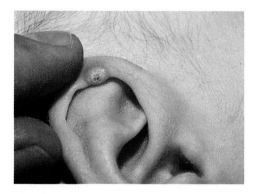

Fig. 12-25
Calcified nodule. Lesion on the ear of an infant.

tion within the fat. The cause of the panniculitis may not be found, or it can be associated with infection, trauma, or metabolic or systemic disease.[29] Biopsy confirmation may be necessary before a comprehensive systemic evaluation is begun. One type of panniculitis, subcutaneous fat necrosis of the newborn infant, is described in Chapter 21.

Sarcoidosis

Sarcoidosis a systemic disease associated with granulomas. Skin lesions can occur with or without systemic symptoms. The skin lesions may appear as indurated papules or plaques. Skin biopsy showing the granulomas of sarcoid should prompt a systemic evaluation for sarcoidosis.[30]

Corns and calluses

Clinical features   Corns and calluses are areas of thickened skin that appear on sites of prolonged pressure or friction. Patients who have these lesions often believe they are warts. Corns are more circumscribed (2 to 5 mm) and better demarcated than calluses (Fig. 12-28). Paring the surface off the lesions will reveal a central core in a corn. They are found primarily on the feet and are the result of poorly fitting shoes. Calluses are diffuse areas of thickened skin, 5 to 20 mm in diameter, on the palmar surfaces of

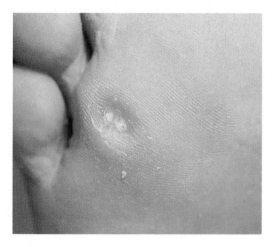

Fig. 12-28
Corn. Circumscribed epidermal thickening with central core.

hands or fingers or on the weight-bearing areas of the feet. Paring the surface of those lesions will reveal normal skin grooves.

Differential diagnosis   Plantar warts are most often confused with corns and calluses. Shaving off the skin surface with a razor blade will reveal interrupted skin ridges with a central area containing black dots in a wart, interrupted skin ridges with a central core of keratin in a corn, and normal skin ridges in a callus. Patients with unexplained focal or diffuse thickening of the palms or soles may have a variety of palmoplantar keratoderma. These conditions may be associated with metabolic or structural abnormalities and may require intensive investigation.

Pathogenesis   Prolonged pressure or friction from ill-fitting shoes produces corns and calluses on the feet. Playing a musical instrument, using playground equipment, or working with tools produces corns and calluses on the hands. The thickening is due to epidermal proliferation and an increase in the number of cells in the stratum corneum.

Treatment   Reducing the lesion with a razor blade by shaving off the excess stratum corneum, followed by covering with salicylic acid 40% plaster, left on for 1 to 7 days, will relieve the discomfort of corns and calluses.

Patient education   The patient should be told that the lesion is not a wart, and that prolonged pressure and friction are responsible for the genesis of the lesion.

Follow-up visits   Follow-up visits are unnecessary.

Histiocytosis

Clinical features   The histiocytoses include a group of benign and fatal disorders.[31-34] Lesions may be present at birth or appear during infancy or childhood (Figs. 12-29, 12-30, and 12-31). The cutaneous lesions of Langerhans cell histiocytosis (LCH) may consist of discrete red, orange, and/or yellow-brown papules or nodules. The presenting symptom may be crusted, scaling dermatitis of the scalp, postauricular, perineal, and axillary areas. Presence of red-brown purpuric papules and nodules within or peripheral to

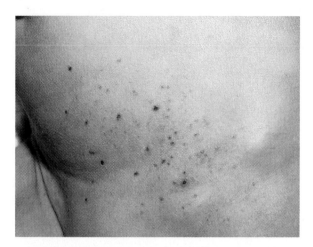

Fig. 12-29
Langerhans cell histiocytosis. Crusted purpuric papules on the lower abdomen with underlying lymphadenopathy.

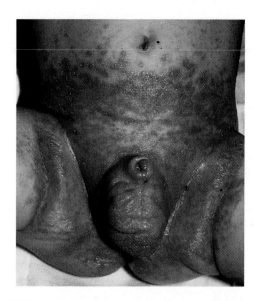

Fig. 12-31
Langerhans cell histiocytosis. More severe dermatitis in diaper area is unresponsive to conventional therapy.

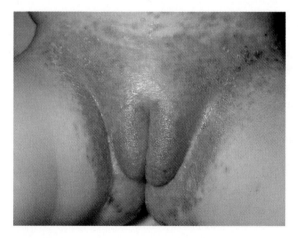

Fig. 12-30
Langerhans cell histiocytosis. Diaper dermatitis is similar to Fig. 4-12.

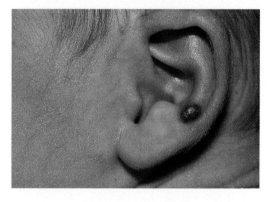

Fig. 12-32
Congenital self-healing reticulohistiocytosis. At birth, this lesion looks similar to a pyogenic granuloma.

areas of dermatitis should alert the physician to a diagnosis of LCH.

Congenital self-healing reticulohistiocytosis consists of papules and nodular lesions present at birth that can look like the lesions of LCH or a pyogenic granuloma[35.37] (Fig. 12-32). Larger lesions can demonstrate a crateriform central erosion (Fig. 12-33).

Benign cephalic histiocytosis consists of 2- to 5-mm yellow-red to tan papules that develop on the face and upper part of the body[38,39] (Figs. 12-34 and 12-35). The lesions usually begin between 6 and 12 months of age. They consist of non-Langerhans cell histiocytes.

Differential diagnosis Histiocytosis lesions include the differential diagnosis of juvenile xanthogranulomas as well as eczema, seborrheic dermatitis, diaper dermatitis, and scabies.[40] Presence of

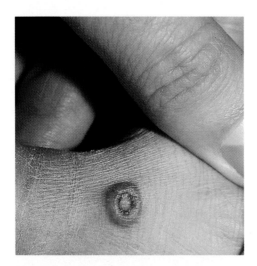

Fig. 12-33
Congenital self-healing reticulohistiocytosis. Nodule present at birth with crateriform central erosion.

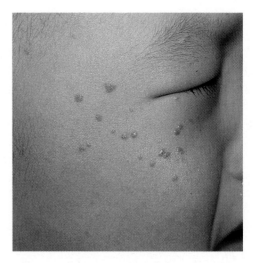

Fig. 12-35
Benign cephalic histiocytosis. Multiple red-tan papules on the face.

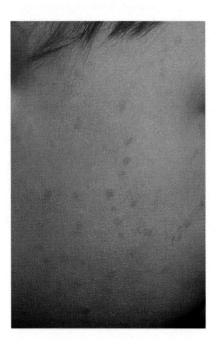

Fig. 12-34
Benign cephalic histiocytosis. Multiple tan papules on the face.

petechiae or purpura within or peripheral to areas of dermatitis suggests LCH.

Pathogenesis   The Langerhans cell is a specific monocyte-macrophage that expresses CD1a glyco-protein and contains Birbeck granules.[32] Langerhans cells are found within the epidermis of skin and within regional lymph nodes, thymic epithelium, and bronchial mucosa. The histiocyte is a monocyte-macrophage. The associated histiocytic syndromes represent infiltrations with histiocytic cells that may or may not be Langerhans cells.

The term *LCH* includes the diseases previously called histiocytosis X. The diagnostic feature of LCH is the presence of lesional histiocytes, at least some of which are phenotypically like normal Langerhans cells.[41] The lesions may contain varying proportions of LCH cells, macrophages, lymphocytes, eosinophils, neutrophils, and plasma cells. Skin, bone, spleen, liver, lungs, and lymph nodes may be affected. Great clinical heterogeneity of LCH exists despite more uniform pathologic features. LCH may be localized to bone or skin, may be associated with diabetes insipidus or exophthalmos, or may have lethal multiorgan involvement. Recent studies have suggested a relationship of human herpesvirus 6 and LCH.[42,43]

Benign cephalic histiocytosis lesions consist of non-Langerhans cell histiocytes.

Treatment   Treatment of these disorders depends on the specific diagnosis and extent of disease. A biopsy is usually necessary to confirm the diagnosis. Additional biopsies may be needed for electron microscopic examination and immunohistochemistry to confirm the specific type of histiocytosis.

Benign cephalic histiocytosis requires no therapy and should resolve during childhood. Congenital self-healing reticulohistiocytosis requires close clinical observation to confirm a benign course. LCH survival and therapy are dependent on the number of organs involved and the severity of the involvement.[44,45] Therapy for LCH may involve surgical removal of lesions, chemotherapy, or observation. Chemotherapy may include corticosteroids, alkylating agents, cytokines, or immunoglobulin. Before therapy a systemic evaluation is required to identify the extent and severity of disease.

Patient education A thorough evaluation is necessary to identify the type and extent of histiocytic syndromes. Parents should be informed of the unusual nature of LCH and should be given information on the benign or malignant course that their child can expect.

Follow-up visits Diagnosis and treatment of these conditions require coordination with a pathologist, radiologist, pediatric oncologist, and primary care physician. Follow-up visits should be arranged to inform the patient and the patient's family of the severity and extent of disease and possible therapies directed by the pediatric oncologist.

Rhabdomyosarcomas

Clinical features Rhabdomyosarcomas are the most common malignant soft-tissue tumors in childhood. They are far more common than melanomas in prepubertal children. The head (Fig. 12-36) and neck and urogenital tract are the usual sites of involvement. Two peaks of age in childhood have a higher incidence of rhabdomyosarcoma: ages 1 to 5 years and during adolescence. The tumor usually appears as a mass lesion of the neck, face, or extremity, or is seen as a subcutaneous or intradermal nodule that has normal-appearing skin. Occasionally the surface of the skin covering the tumor becomes reddened. The lesion may produce local signs of destruction,

depending on the location. For example, in the orbit, it may produce exophthalmos or ptosis; in the ear canal, a bloody discharge with a polypoid ear mass; and in the nasal passages, obstruction of one of the airways and bleeding. In the genitourinary tract, it may appear as urinary obstruction. Grapelike masses of tumor protruding from the vagina are another presentation of rhabdomyosarcoma.

Rhabdomyosarcomas may spread either by local extension or by hematogenous or lymphatic metastases. Seventy-five percent of the metastases will become apparent within 6 months of the appearance of the original lesion. The most frequent sites involved with metastases are the regional lymph nodes, lungs, liver, bone marrow, bone, and brain. Head and neck tumors have been reported to extend directly into the brain, and may occur as frequently as in one third of all cases.

Differential diagnosis The feature of rapid, progressive growth will help distinguish rhabdomyosarcoma from the other skin nodules and cysts of infants and children listed in Table 12-1. Ulceration is not an early sign of rhabdomyosarcoma, but the tumor is fixed to deep fascia, is often greater than 3 cm, and is firm in consistency.

Pathogenesis Rhabdomyosarcoma is a malignant tumor of striated muscles. There is no hereditary pattern, and there are no known precipitating factors.[46,47]

Treatment Therapy has included radiation and combination chemotherapy in the initial stages of dis-

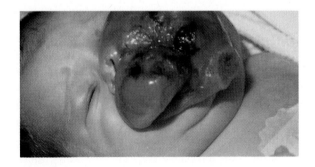

Fig. 12-36
Embryonal rhabdomyosarcoma on the face of an infant.

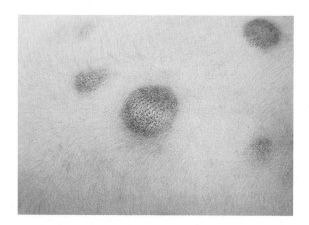

Fig. 12-37
Leukemia cutis in a child.

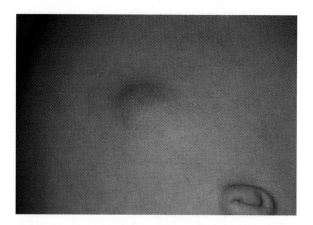

Fig. 12-38
Cutaneous neuroblastoma was the first sign of this infant's disease.

ease, following wide surgical excision. Debulking the tumor with wide surgical excision is the first treatment of choice. New therapeutic protocols are currently being evaluated.[48,49]

Patient education Prognosis should be discussed with the family, keeping in mind that a number of factors are important in the survival rate. The location of the original lesion is an important factor, with the best prognosis occurring in orbital lesions, the next best with bladder, and the worst with lesions beginning on the head and neck. Referral to a pediatric oncology facility as soon as the diagnosis is suspected is indicated.

Follow-up visits Follow-up visits should be arranged for family support, but a pediatric oncologist should be involved in determining frequency of visits.

Neuroblastoma, leukemia, and lymphoma

Lymphoma, leukemia (Fig. 12-37), and neuroblastoma (Fig. 12-38) can present as cutaneous papules or nodules.[50-52] The lesions may appear as the primary manifestation of disease or as metastases of known disease. Unknown nodules or lesions that demonstrate rapid progressive growth (*see* Box 12-1) should be biopsied for specific diagnosis. Therapy will need to be directed by a pediatric oncologist.

References

1. Knight PJ, Reiner CB: Superficial lumps in children: what, when and why? *Pediatrics* 72:147, 1983.
2. Paller AS, Pensler JM, Tomimta T: Nasal midline masses in infants and children, *Arch Dermatol* 127:362, 1991.
3. Todd NW: Common congenital anomalies of the neck. Embryology and surgical anatomy, *Surg Clin North Am* 73:599, 1993.
4. Grimalt R, Gelmetti C: Eruptive vellus hair cysts: case report and review of the literature, *Pediatr Dermatol* 9:98, 1992.
5. Taaffe A, Wyatt EH, Bury L: Pilomatricoma (Malherbe). A clinical and histopathologic survey of 78 cases, *Int J Dermatol* 7:477, 1988.
6. Pruzan DL, Esterly NB, Prose NS: Eruptive syringoma, *Arch Dermatol* 125:1119, 1989.
7. Price MA, Goldberg LH, Levy ML: Juvenile basal cell carcinoma, *Pediatr Dermatol* 11:176, 1994.
8. Howell JB: Nevoid basal cell carcinoma syndrome, *J Am Acad Dermatol* 11:98, 1984.
9. Shanley S, Ratcliffe J, Hockey A, et al: Nevoid basal cell carcinoma syndrome: review of 118 affected individuals, *Am J Med Genet* 50:282, 1994.
10. Kirchmann TT, Prieto VG, Smoller BR: CD34 staining pattern distinguishes basal cell carcinoma from trichoepithelioma, *Arch Dermatol* 130:589, 1994.

11. Marrogi AJ, Wick MR, Dehner LP: Benign cutaneous adnexal tumors in childhood and young adults, excluding pilomatrixoma: review of 28 cases and literature, *J Cutan Pathol* 18:20, 1991.

12. Kraemer KH, Levy DD, Parris CN, et al: Xeroderma pigmentosum and related disorders: examining the linkage between defective DNA repair and cancer, *J Invest Dermatol* 103:96, 1994.

13. Lauri G, Santucci M, Ceruso M, Innocenti M: Recurrent digital fibromatosis of childhood, *J Hand Surg* 15A:106, 1990.

14. Ishii N, Matsui K, Ichiyama S, et al: A case of infantile digital fibromatosis showing spontaneous regression, *Br J Dermatol* 121:129, 1989.

15. Hirshowitz B, Ullmann Y, Har-Shai Y, et al: Silicone occlusive sheeting (SOS) in the management of hypertrophic and keloid scarring, including the possible mode of action of silicone, by static electricity, *Eur J Plast Surg* 16:5, 1993.

16. Lucky AW, Prose NS, Bove K, et al: Papular umbilicated granuloma annulare, *Arch Dermatol* 128:1375, 1992.

17. Török E, Daróczy J: Juvenile xanthogranuloma: An analysis of 45 cases by clinical follow-up, light-and-electron microscopy, *Acta Derm Venereol (Stockh)* 65:167, 1985.

18. Fonseca E, Contreras F, Cuevas J: Papular xanthoma in children: report and immunohistochemical study, *Pediatr Dermatol* 10:139, 1993.

19. Collum LM, Power WJ, Mullaney J, et al: Limbal xanthogranuloma, *J Pediatr Ophthalmol Strabismus* 28:157, 1991.

20. Moier P, Mérot Y, Paccaud D, et al: Juvenile chronic granulocytic leukemia, juvenile xanthogranulomas, and neurofibromatosis, *J Am Acad Dermatol* 22:962, 1990.

21. Azaña JM, Torrelo A, Mediero IG, Zambrano A: Urticaria pigmentosa: a review of 67 pediatric cases, *Pediatr Dermatol* 11:102, 1994.

22. Patrice SJ, Wiss K, Mulliken JB: Pyogenic granuloma (lobular capillary hemangioma): a clinicopathologic study of 178 cases, *Pediatr Dermatol* 8:267, 1991.

23. Frieden IJ, Esterly NB: Pyogenic granulomas of infancy masquerading as strawberry hemangiomas, *Pediatrics* 90:989, 1992.

24. Gagné EJ, Su WPD: Congenital smooth muscle hamartoma of the skin, *Pediatr Dermatol* 10:142, 1993.

25. Foster CM, Levin S, Levine M, et al: Limited dermal ossification: clinical features and natural history, *J Pediatr* 109:71, 1986.

26. Laing VB, Fleischer AB: Peizogenic wrist papules: a common and asymptomatic finding, *J Am Acad Dermatol* 24:415, 1991.

27. Pontious J, Lasday S, Mele R: Piezogenic pedal papules extending into the arch. Case reports and discussion, *J Am Podiatr Med Assoc* 80:444, 1990.

28. Paller AS, Hebert AA: Knuckle pads in children, *Am J Dis Child* 140:915, 1986.

29. Schuval SJ, Frances A, Valderrama E, et al: Panniculitis and fever in children, *J Pediatr* 122:372, 1993.

30. Pattishall EN, Strope GL, Spinola SM, Denny FW: Childhood sarcoidosis, *J Pediatr* 108:169, 1986.

31. Ha SY, Helms P, Fletcher M, et al: Lung involvement in Langerhans' cell histiocytosis: prevalence, clinical features, and outcome, *Pediatrics* 89:466, 1992.

32. Chu T, Jaffe R: The normal Langerhans cell and LCH cell, *Br J Cancer* 70:4S, 1994.

33. Willman CL, Busque L, Griffith BB, et al: Langerhans'-cell histiocytosis (histiocytosis X)—a clonal proliferative disease, *N Engl J Med* 331:154, 1994.

34. Beverly PCL, Abbas AK: The scientific challenge of Langerhans cell histiocytosis, *Br J Cancer* 70:61S, 1994.

35. Berger TG, Lane AT, Headington JT, et al: A solitary variant of congenital self-healing reticulohistiocytosis: solitary Hashimoto-Pritzker disease, *Pediatr Dermatol* 3:230, 1986.

36. Herman LE, Rothman KF, Harawi S, et al: Congenital self-healing reticulohistiocytosis, *Arch Dermatol* 126:210, 1990.

37. Hashimoto K, Kagetsu N, Taniguchi Y, et al: Immunohistochemistry and electron microscopy in Langerhans cell histiocytosis confined to the skin, *J Am Acad Dermatol* 25:1044, 1991.

38. Barsky BL, Lao I, Barsky S, Rhee HL: Benign cephalic histiocytosis, *Arch Dermatol* 120:650, 1984.

39. Peña-Penabad C, Unamuno P, Garcia-Silva J, et al: Benign cephalic histiocytosis: case report and literature review, *Pediatr Dermatol* 11:164, 1994.

40. Talanin NY, Smith SS, Shelley D, Moores WB: Cutaneous histiocytosis with Langerhans cell features induced by scabies: a case report, *Pediatr Dermatol* 11:327, 1994.

41. Favara BE, Jaffe R: The histopathology of Langerhans cell histiocytosis, *Br J Cancer* 70:41S, 1994.

42. Leahy MA, Krejci SM, Friednash M, et al: Human herpesvirus 6 is present in lesions of Langerhans cell histiocytosis, *J Invest Dermatol* 101:643, 1993.

43. McClain K, Weiss RA: Viruses and Langerhans cell histiocytosis: Is there a link? *Br J Cancer* 70:34S, 1994

44. Ladisch S, Gardner H: Treatment of Langerhans cell histiocytosis—evolution and current approaches, *Br J Cancer* 70:41S, 1994.

45. Arceci RJ: Treatment options—commentary, *Br J Cancer* 70:58S, 1994.

46. Parham DM: The molecular biology of childhood rhabdomyosarcoma, *Semin Diagn Path* 11:39, 1994.

47. Tsokos M: The diagnosis and classification of childhood rhabdomyosarcoma, *Semin Diagn Pathol* 11:26, 1994.

48. Lukens JN: Progress resulting from clinical trials. Solid tumors in childhood cancer, *Cancer* 74:2710, 1994.

49. Wiener ES: Rhabdomyosarcoma: new dimensions in management, *Semin Pediatr Surg* 2:47, 1993.

50. Zaatari GS, Chan WC, Kim TH, et al: Malignant lymphoma of the skin in children, *Cancer* 59:1040, 1987.

51. Grosfeld JL, Rescorla FJ, West KW, Goldman J: Neuroblastoma in the first year of life: clinical and biological factors influencing outcome, *Semin Pediatr Surg* 2:37, 1993.

52. Orozco-Covarrubias MDLL, Tamayo-Sanchez L, Duran-McKinster C, et al: Malignant cutaneous tumors in children, *J Am Acad Dermatol* 30:243, 1994.

13

Hemangiomas and Vascular Malformations

Vascular birthmarks are one of the most common forms of birth defects. The classification of vascular birthmarks has in the past been confusing. We prefer the classification of Mulliken and Glowacki[1] (Table 13-1), which divides vascular birthmarks into hemangiomas and vascular malformations.[2] Although they may occasionally appear similar at birth, the natural history of these lesions is quite distinct, and within a few months of age they can usually be differentiated (Table 13-2).

HEMANGIOMAS

Clinical features

Although generally classified as vascular birthmarks, only 20% of hemangiomas are present at birth.[3] Approximately 1% to 3% of newborns will have a hemangioma noted at birth. The other 80% arise between 2 and 4 weeks of age. By 1 year of age, 10% to 12% of children will have a hemangioma. There are three major types of presentations (see Box 13-1). The most common presentation is a pale white to gray-blue macule (Fig. 13-1). The other types are the telangiectatic (Fig. 13-2) and the papular (Fig. 13-3) forms. At the time of presentation it is impossible to predict what form the hemangioma will eventually take or its final size. Because all hemangiomas are derived from the same cell type, and all have the same natural history, the terms strawberry and cavernous should not be used to describe hemangiomas.[3] These terms should be replaced by describing the location of the hemangioma within the skin (Table 13-1). Bright-red papular hemangiomas should be referred to as superficial hemangiomas (Fig. 13-4), whereas blue nodular hemangiomas should be referred to as deep hemangiomas (Fig. 13-5). The majority of hemangiomas contain both a superficial and a deep component (Fig. 13-6) and should be labeled as mixed hemangiomas (Table 13-1). At 4 to 8 weeks of age, hemangiomas undergo a rapid growth phase that continues until the infant is 6 to 9 months of age. During this time the rate of growth of the hemangioma is much greater than the growth rate of the infant. This rapid growth phase is a characteristic feature of hemangiomas.[3] Following the rapid growth phase, the hemangioma growth slows and approximates the growth rate of

Table 13-1

Classification of Hemangiomas and Vascular Malformations

Hemangiomas	Vascular malformations
Superficial	Capillary (port-wine stain)
Mixed	Telangiectatic
Deep	Hypertrophic capillary (angiokeratoma)
	Venous
	Arteriovenous
	Lymphatic
	Cutis marmorata telangiectatica congenita
	Mixed

Table 13-2

Differential Diagnosis of Hemangiomas and Vascular Malformations

Hemangiomas	Vascular malformations
Tumor of endothelial cells	Developmental abnormality
Only 20% present at birth	Always present at birth
Undergo rapid growth	Stable growth
Always undergo regression	Never regress

Box 13-1   Clinical presentation of hemangiomas

Clinical presentation of hemangiomas
Blue-gray macule
Telangiectatic
Papular

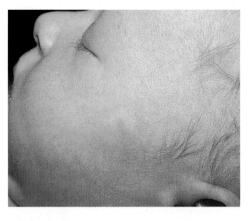

Fig. 13-1
Macular pale white presentation of a hemangioma.

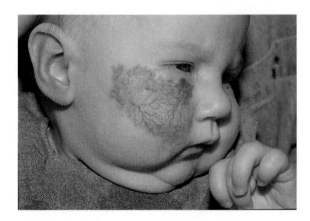

Fig. 13-2
Telangiectatic presentation of a hemangioma.

the infant. As they grow, most hemangiomas will feel soft and be easily compressible. The growth phase is eventually followed by regression of the hemangioma. This begins sometime in the second year of life. The regression phase begins with paling of the hemangioma (Fig. 13-7), followed by flattening of the tumor. This phase slowly continues, and by 5 years of age 50% of hemangiomas have reached maximal regression. By 9 years of age 90% of hemangiomas will have reached maximal regression.

Maximal regression of the hemangioma does not define a return to normal skin. Residual posthemangioma regression includes hypopigmentation, telangiectasia (Fig. 13-8), fibrofatty deposits, and scarring if the hemangioma has previously ulcerated.

Although hemangiomas are usually benign lesions, they can be associated with certain local and systemic complications[3] (Table 13-3). These include obstruction of a vital function (vision [Fig. 13-9], breathing [Fig. 13-6], eating, urination, or defecation), platelet trapping with consumption coagulopathy (Kasabach-Merritt syndrome) (Fig. 13-10), high-output cardiac failure, ulceration (Fig. 13-11), and infection. Infants with periorbital hemangiomas should always be

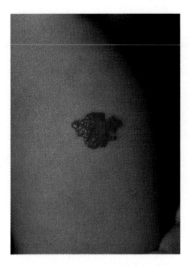

Fig. 13-3
Papular presentation of a hemangioma.

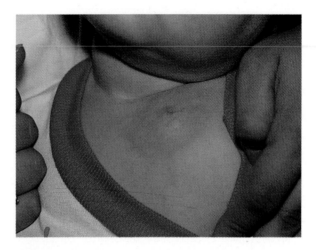

Fig. 13-5
Deep hemangioma.

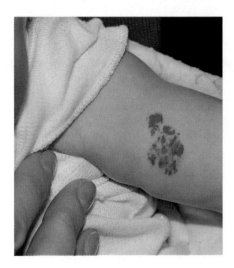

Fig. 13-4
Superficial hemangioma.

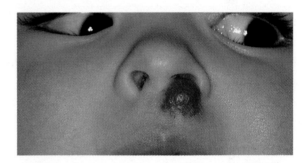

Fig. 13-6
Mixed superficial and deep hemangioma that obstructed breathing.

Table 13-3
Complications of Hemangiomas

Local	Systemic
Obstruction of vital function	Kasabach-Merritt syndrome
Ulceration	High-output cardiac failure
Infection	

referred for ophthalmologic evaluation for amblyopia and/or astigmatism.

Ulceration and subsequent infection are the most common form of complications of hemangiomas. Ulcerations occur during the rapid growth phase of hemangiomas primarily located in the diaper area.[4] Platelet trapping with consumption coagulopathy also occurs during the rapid growth phase, usually within the first 3 months of life. A large, rapidly growing,

soft, compressible hemangioma is noted to suddenly become firm and to become dark purple. Laboratory evaluation will show a decreased platelet count and abnormal blood clotting consistent with a consumption coagulopathy. Although quite rare, it is a medical emergency. A solitary cutaneous hemangioma caus-

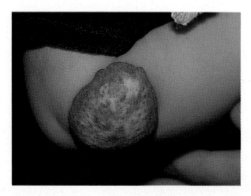

Fig. 13-7
Paling of a mixed superficial and deep hemangioma in an 18-month-old female. This is often the initial sign of regression of the hemangioma.

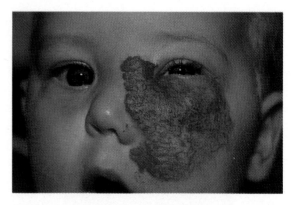

Fig. 13-9
Mixed superficial and deep hemangioma in a 4-month old male, leading to partial visual obstruction.

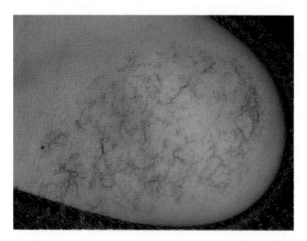

Fig. 13-8
Residual hypopigmentation and telangiectasia post-regression of a hemangioma in a 17-year-old female.

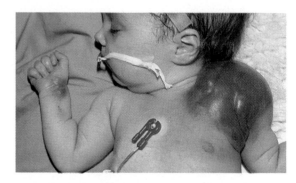

Fig. 13-10
Sudden change of a large superficial and deep hemangioma to deep purple as part of the Kasabach-Merritt syndrome.

ing high-output cardiac failure is also an exceedingly rare event.

Differential diagnosis

The differential diagnosis of a hemangioma depends on the time of presentation to the physician. A mature hemangioma that has undergone a rapid growth phase followed by the initiation of regression is difficult to confuse with anything else. The greatest difficulty in the differential diagnosis of hemangiomas occurs with those present at birth. The telangiectatic presentation of hemangiomas can easily be confused with a telangiectatic vascular malformation.[5] Only observation over time will differentiate between these two types of birthmarks. Deep hemangiomas can be mistaken for lymphatic malformations, and again time will simplify the differential. Subcutaneous sarcomas are rare but should be considered when an infant presents with a firm, rather than rubbery-feeling, rapidly growing mass. Imaging and biopsy may be required to obtain the correct diagnosis.

Pathogenesis

Hemangiomas are benign tumors of capillary endothelium.[6] Proliferating hemangiomas are associated with an overabundance of mast cells, and as the tumor regresses, the mast cell number also decreas-

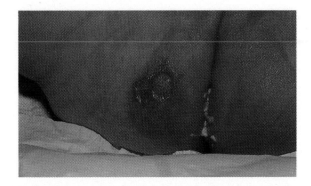

Fig. 13-11
Ulceration of a hemangioma on the buttock of a 3-month-old infant.

Box 13-2 Indications for treatment of hemangiomas

Kasabach-Merritt syndrome
High-output cardiac failure
Obstruction of vital function
Ulceration
Infection
Facial location
Diaper area location

Box 13-3 Treatment options for hemangiomas

Oral glucocorticosteroids
Interferon-α2a
Vascular-specific pulsed dye laser

es.[6] It is not unusual for mast cells to be associated with blood vessel growth, and it is unknown whether this is a primary or secondary event. Endothelial cell proliferation is enhanced by certain angiogenic factors, such as acidic and basic fibroblast growth factor, transforming growth factor α and β, and angiogenin. Regression in hemangiomas is asynchronous, with parts of the tumor regressing while other portions continue to grow. As with the beginning of growth of the tumor, the mechanism of initiation of regression remains unknown.[6]

Treatment

The first question that arises regarding treatment of hemangiomas is which ones should be treated (see Box 13-2). Certainly, all hemangiomas with the potential to interfere with a vital function should be treated. Periorbital hemangiomas may cause pressure on the eye, leading to astigmatism, or they may partially or totally obstruct vision, causing amblyopia. The Kasabach-Merritt syndrome and high-output cardiac failure, although rare, are medical emergencies and require immediate attention. Hemangiomas in the diaper area frequently ulcerate,[4] and early treatment may minimize the risk of ulceration as well as decrease the likelihood of anal or urethral obstruction. Ulcerated hemangiomas are severely painful and at risk for superinfection. Recognition of the complications associated with hemangiomas in the diaper area and early treatment of these lesions can minimize

complications and prevent the need for a diverting colostomy. Facial hemangiomas can be disfiguring, and early treatment minimizes the extent of hemangioma growth and the eventual residua. Other hemangiomas should be observed and treated only if complications arise.

For years the mainstay of treatment for hemangiomas has been oral glucocorticosteroids (see Box 13-3). Thirty to sixty percent of hemangiomas are reported to be responsive to glucocorticosteroid therapy.[7] Treatment should be started at 2 mg/kg and adjusted depending on the response of the tumor. Responsive hemangiomas will demonstrate an effect from treatment with 7 to 10 days, manifested as softening of the tumor, lightening in color, or a noticeable decrease in growth rate. Systemic glucocorticosteroids should be used as the first line of treatment for the Kasabach-Merritt syndrome, high-output cardiac failure, and those rapidly growing hemangiomas that threaten to interfere with a vital function. Heparin and fresh-frozen plasma may also be needed to control bleeding in the Kasabach-Merritt syndrome. Systemic glucocorticosteroid therapy is not

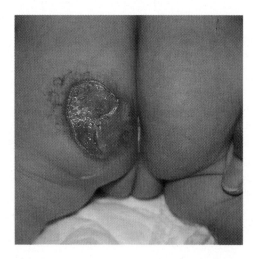

Fig. 13-12
Ulceration of a hemangioma on the buttock of a 5-month-old infant.

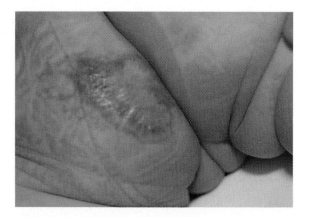

Fig. 13-13
Same hemangioma 4 weeks later following one pulsed dye laser treatment.

without side effects, and treatment should be maintained for as short a time as possible. The use of intralesional steroids has also been advocated for the treatment of hemangiomas, but we feel that this procedure should be done only by those with experience.

Recently, interferon-α2a has been demonstrated to be effective for hemangiomas that are unresponsive to glucocorticosteroids.[8] Treatment is initiated daily by subcutaneous injection at a dose of 3 million U/m^2 and continued until the hemangioma is fully in a regressive state. On the average, treatments have been continued for 8 months. Fever is the most common side effect, and long-term toxicity has not yet been identified. Despite its apparent efficacy, experience with the use of interferon-α2a is limited, and it should be reserved for hemangiomas unresponsive to glucocorticosteroids.

The vascular-specific pulsed dye laser has added another option for the treatment of hemangiomas. This form of therapy is excellent for the treatment of ulcerated hemangiomas, leading to a rapid decrease in the pain associated with the ulceration, and complete healing of 75% of the ulcerations within 2 weeks[4] (Figs. 13-12 and 13-13). Superficial papular hemangiomas prior to or early in the rapid growth phase also respond well to treatment.[9] The treatment is simple

and fast and side effects are nearly nonexistent. Vascular-specific pulsed dye laser therapy should be considered for facial and diaper area hemangiomas because it minimizes the eventual residua and decreases the risk for ulceration in at-risk tumors. It also has a role as an adjunct to steroid therapy in rapidly growing hemangiomas. Nonspecific laser therapy, such as the carbon dioxide or the neodymium:YAG (yttrium, aluminum, garnet) laser, although effective in destroying hemangiomas, often leads to scarring and a worse outcome than natural regression.

Patient education

The natural history and potential complications of hemangiomas should be discussed with the families. They should be aware of the difficulty of predicting the eventual size and type of the hemangioma, the final outcome, and the need for treatment. The need for frequent follow-up visits, until the hemangioma growth and complication pattern is evident, should be emphasized.

Follow-up visits

Hemangiomas need to be followed closely during the rapid growth phase. Initially visits should be every 2 weeks, and if no complications occur and the hemangioma growth has stabilized the time between visits can be lengthened. Children with periorbital hemangiomas should be referred for ophthalmologic evaluation and management. Measurement of the size of the lesions allows a more accurate measure of actual growth than observation alone. Once regression has begun and no complications have been noted follow-up should be on a yearly basis.

VASCULAR MALFORMATIONS

Clinical features

Vascular malformations are developmental errors of blood and/or lymphatic vessel formation. By definition, vascular malformations are always present at birth.[10] They do not undergo a rapid growth phase, but rather grow proportionally with the child. Vascular malformations should be classified according to the predominant vessel type within the birthmark[10] (Table 13-1).

Capillary malformations (port-wine stains) are the most common type of vascular malformation. They occur in 3 per 1000 births. The name *port-wine stain* derives from the dark red color that is common in mature capillary malformations (Fig. 13-14). However, most port-wine stains present as light pink macules (Fig. 13-15). The dark red color (port-wine) slowly develops as the patient ages. Along with the darkening in color, maturing port-wine stains develop progressive nodularity and blebbing, and may lead to overgrowth of the underlying soft tissue and bone. The rate of progression of any individual port-wine stain cannot be predicted, but approximately 67% of patients with facial port-wine stains will develop these changes by the fifth decade.[11] In patients with facial port-wine stains, the possibility of the Sturge-Weber syndrome should be considered. The Sturge-Weber syndrome is the association of a facial port-wine stain with central nervous system (seizures, mental retardation, hemiplegia) and ophthalmologic (glaucoma) abnormalities. The overall risk of a facial port-wine stain having the associated abnormalities of the Sturge-Weber syndrome is 8%, but the chances are increased with increasing size of the facial port-wine stain (Fig. 13-16). Infants with bilateral facial port-wine stains are at the highest risk (33%).[12] Patients with a port-wine stain or any other type of vascular malformation covering an extremity are at risk for the development of overgrowth of that extremity (Klippel-Trenaunay-Weber syndrome) (Fig. 13-17). As the child gets older the overgrowth can become enormous and can be associated with severe varicosities, venous stasis, ulceration, and recurrent infection, leading to a state of chronic lymphedema. Occasionally port-wine stains are extensive and cover large areas of skin.

Telangiectatic vascular malformations are capillary malformations in which individual rather than conflu-

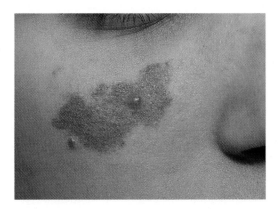

Fig. 13-14
Dark red port-wine stain with central blebbing in a 14-year-old female.

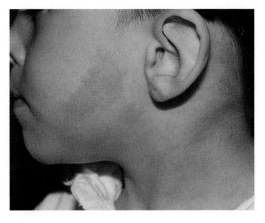

Fig. 13-15
Typical light pink port-wine stain in a 3-year-old male.

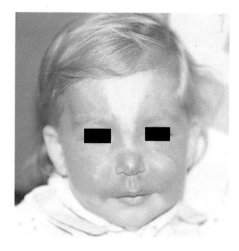

Fig. 13-16
Bilateral port-wine stain in a 2-year-old female with the Sturge-Weber syndrome.

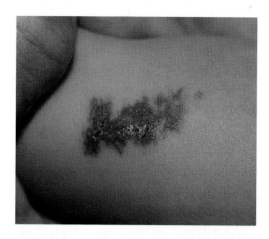

Fig. 13-18
Angiokeratoma circumscriptum in a 6-month-old female demonstrating thickened epidermis overlying a capillary malformation.

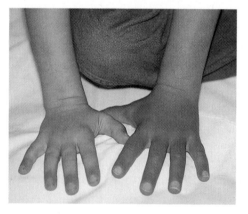

Fig. 13-17
Hypertrophy of the left arm and hand in a 6-year-old male with the Klippel-Trenaunay-Weber syndrome.

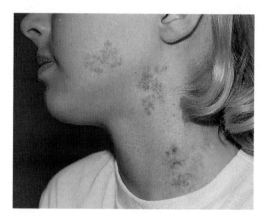

Fig. 13-19
Distinct blue venous pattern of a venous malformation in an 11-year-old female.

ent telangiectasias are the presenting feature.[5] They should be considered a variant of port-wine stains. The risk of development of the Sturge-Weber and Klippel-Trenaunay-Weber syndromes in association with telangiectatic malformations is unknown.

Hyperkeratotic capillary malformations (angiokeratomas) are distinguished by their acanthotic, hyperkeratotic epidermis overlying a capillary malformation. Five separate conditions are classified as angiokeratomas, but only angiokeratoma circumscriptum is congenital. They should be considered a mixed developmental abnormality of vessels and epidermis. They are most commonly seen on an extremity as unilateral bands or as palm-sized plaques composed of blue-black papules or nodules with a warty, hyperkeratotic surface (Fig. 13-18).

Venous malformations are developmental errors in vein formation. Their distinct venous pattern is obvious at presentation (Fig. 13-19). Occasionally, large nodules will develop within these lesions (Fig. 13-20).

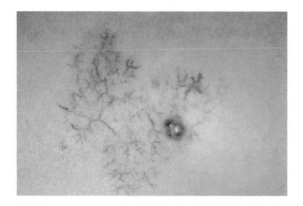

Fig. 13-20
Venous malformation with a large nodule in a 9-year-old male.

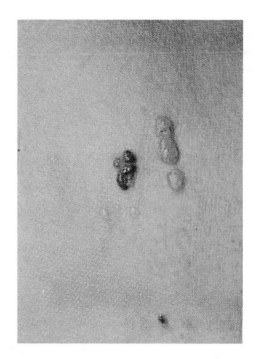

Fig. 13-22
Lymphangioma circumscriptum. After minor trauma lesions may darken, resulting from bleeding into the lesion.

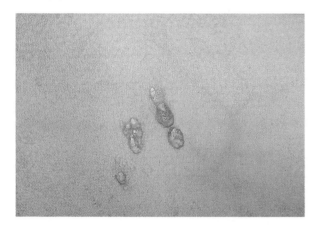

Fig. 13-21
Lymphangioma circumscriptum. Grouping of gelatinous skin-colored papules on the abdomen.

Arteriovenous malformations (fistulae) are direct connections between an artery and the venous system, bypassing the capillary bed. They are often initially trivial-appearing lesions but with time may expand rapidly. They are high-flow lesions and may have a notable pulsation and/or thrills and bruits. Localized pain, hyperhidrosis, hypertrichosis, and hyperthermia of a relatively banal-looking vascular lesion should raise the suspicion of an arteriovenous malformation.[10] Arteriovenous malformations are the rarest type of vascular malformation.

Lymphatic malformations are in general referred to as lymphangiomas—a misnomer because the lesions are developmental errors in the formation of lymphatic vessels and not tumors as the suffix *oma* designates. There are three clinical types of lymphatic malformations: solitary simple, circumscriptum, and cavernous. Solitary simple lymphatic malformations present as dermal or subcutaneous squishy nodules. Lymphangioma circumscriptum consists of multiple clusters of small vesicles covering limited skin areas, usually less than 10 cm in diameter (Figs. 13-21 and 13-22). Cavernous lymphatic malformations (cystic hygromas) present as large, ill-defined, grotesque, rubbery, skin-colored, subcutaneous nodules that may underlie areas of more superficial lymphatic malformations. They are usually solitary and involve the face, trunk, and extremities.

In cutis marmorata telangiectatica congenita, two clinical presentations may be seen. The first is a mottled pattern of blue or dusky-red erythema present at birth (Fig. 13-23). In the second form there is atrophy of the skin and larger depressed blue venous

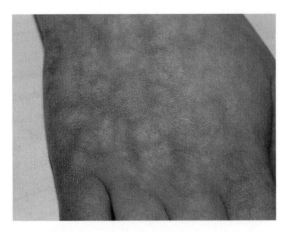

Fig. 13-23
Permanent mottled appearance of cutis marmorata telangiectatica congenita.

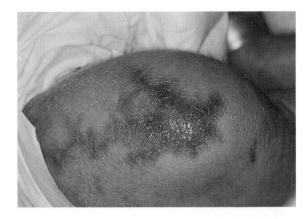

Fig. 13-24
Venous pattern of cutis marmorata telangiectatica congenita (congenital phlebectasia).

malformations (Fig. 13-24) (congenital phlebectasia). Both types may be seen in the same patient. Often a single extremity is involved, but the lesions may occur bilaterally on the extremities or on the trunk. A gradual increase in the size of the lesions is expected during the first years of life, but the lesions may become less noticeable by adult life. Rigorous natural history studies of cutis marmorata telangiectatica congenita are not available. Associations with musculoskeletal or other vascular malformations may occur.

Occasionally, vascular malformations will contain a mixture of many different types of vascular components. They present as a composite of the presentation of each individual component.

Differential diagnosis

In older children, port-wine stains and telangiectatic malformations are rather characteristic and seldom confused with other lesions. At birth, port-wine stains and telangiectatic vascular malformations must be differentiated from the macular and telangiectatic presentations of hemangiomas.[5] These lesions will eventually be distinguished by the presence or absence of a rapid growth phase.

Congenital solitary angiokeratomas and angiokeratoma circumscriptum must be differentiated his-

torically from the acquired forms of angiokeratoma. Although quite rare the development of numerous angiokeratomas at a young age should alert one to the possibility of either Fabry's disease or α-fucosidosis.

As with the capillary malformations, venous and arteriovenous malformations are usually quite characteristic. Rarely, these lesions are disfiguring and can be mistaken for vascular malignancies such as Kaposi's sarcoma and angiosarcomas.[13]

Lymphangioma circumscriptum may be mistaken for a disorder with grouped vesicles, such as herpes simplex, herpes zoster, or dermatitis herpetiformis. There is no erythematous base in circumscribed lymphangioma, however, and the lesions appear gelatinous, not fluid-filled. As noted, hemorrhage into such lesions results in darkening, which may be confused with melanoma.

Cavernous lymphatic malformations may be confused with lipomas, plexiform neurofibromas, and other soft subcutaneous masses.

In contrast to cutis marmorata telangiectatica congenita, mottling of newborn skin is a transient vasodilatation and is relieved by rewarming the skin. The livedo reticularis pattern of collagen vascular disease is flat, is not depressed over the discolored areas, is always bilateral, and is associated with systemic signs and symptoms.

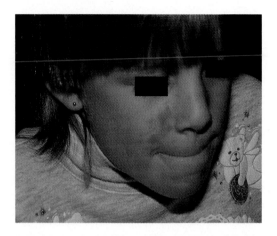

Fig. 13-25
Prelaser treatment port-wine stain in an 8-year-old female.

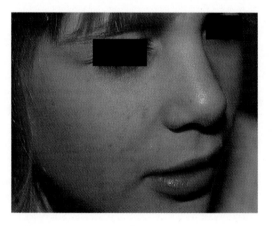

Fig. 13-26
Same patient shown in Fig. 13-25, 2 years later, after 10 laser treatments.

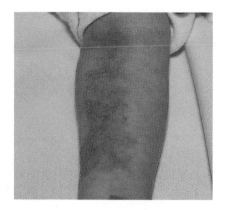

Fig. 13-27
Telangiectatic malformation in a 4-month-old female.

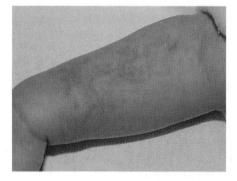

Fig. 13-28
Same patient shown in Fig. 13-27, 2 months following initial laser treatment.

Pathogenesis

All vascular malformations should be considered developmental errors in vessel formation.[14] There is no evidence at this time for a specific genetic abnormality leading to the development of any of these birthmarks.

Treatment

The vascular-specific (585 nm) pulsed (450 μsec) dye laser is recognized as the treatment of choice for capillary and telangiectatic vascular malformations.[15] Response of these lesions to treatment depends on the age of the patients at the beginning of treatment and the size of the lesion.[15-17] The younger the child at the beginning of treatment and the smaller the lesion, the increased likelihood of complete removal (Figs. 13-25 and 13-26) (personal observation). Treatments can safely be started as early as 2 weeks of age.[18] Large lesions are improved by treatment, but total removal is less likely. Response to treatment is slow, and even small lesions in very young infants will frequently take 1 to 3 years for complete removal. The vascular-specific (585 nm) pulsed (450 μsec) dye laser is very safe, and side effects are minimal. Treatment has been greatly improved by the introduction of topical EMLA cream, which significantly decreases the pain associated with the procedure.[19]

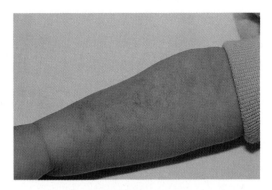

Fig. 13-29
Same patient shown in Fig. 13-27, after second laser treatment.

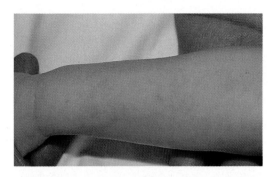

Fig. 13-30
Same patient shown in Fig. 13-27, 10 months following initial laser treatment. A total of only three laser treatments was required to achieve almost total clearing of the telangiectatic malformation.

Unlike port-wine stains, telangiectatic vascular malformations have a much smaller vessel load to destroy to return the skin to normal. Most of these lesions will be completely removed in 3 to 6 treatments[5] (Figs. 13-27 through 13-30).

Treatment of all other types of vascular malformations is difficult and must be handled on an individual basis. Referral to a multidiscipline specialty clinic with specific expertise in dealing with these types of birth defects is optimal.

Patient education

Parents of babies with capillary and telangiectatic malformations should be told about the possibility of treatment with the vascular-specific (585 nm) pulsed (450 μsec) dye laser. They should be referred to the nearest treatment center as soon as possible.

If a large facial port-wine stain is present, the possibility of the Sturge-Weber syndrome should be discussed, and the patient should be referred for neurologic and ophthalmologic consultation.

For other types of vascular malformations, the difficulty of treatment should be discussed, and, if possible, the child should be referred to a specialty clinic with expertise in managing these type of lesions.

Follow-up visits

The frequency of follow-up visits is determined by the degree of complications associated with a given malformation.

References

1. Mulliken JB, Glowacki B: Hemangiomas and vascular malformations in infants and children: a classification based on endothelial characteristics, *Plast Reconstr Surg* 69:412, 1982.

2. Mulliken JB, Young A: *Vascular birthmarks: hemangiomas and malformations,* Philadelphia, 1988, WB Saunders, p 24.

3. Mulliken JB, Young A: *Vascular birthmarks: hemangiomas and malformations,* Philadelphia, 1988, WB Saunders, p 41

4. Morelli JG, Tan OT, Yohn JJ, Weston WL: Treatment of ulcerated hemangiomas in infancy, *Arch Pediatr Adol Med* 148:1104, 1994.

5. Morelli JG, Huff JC, Weston WL: The treatment of congenital telangiectatic vascular malformations with the vascular specific pulsed dye laser, *Pediatrics* 92:603, 1993.

6. Mulliken JB, Young A: *Vascular birthmarks: hemangiomas and malformations,* Philadelphia, 1988, WB Saunders, p 63.

7. Mulliken JB, Young A: *Vascular birthmarks: hemangiomas and malformations,* Philadelphia, 1988, WB Saunders, p 77.

8. Eskowitz RAB, Mulliken JB, Folkman J: Interferon α-2a therapy for life threatening hemangiomas in infancy, *N Engl J Med* 326:1456, 1992.

9. Garden JM, Bakus AD, Paller AS: Treatment of cuta-

neous hemangiomas by the flashlamp-pumped pulsed dye laser: prospective analysis, *J Pediatr* 120:555, 1992.

10. Mulliken JB, Young A: *Vascular birthmarks: hemangiomas and malformations,* Philadelphia, 1988, WB Saunders, p 114.

11. Geronemus RG, Ashinoff R: The medical necessity of evaluation and treatment of port-wine stains, *J Dermatol Surg Oncol* 117:76, 1991.

12. Tallman B, Tan OT, Morelli JG, et al: Location of port wine stains and the likelihood of ophthalmic and/or CNS complications, *Pediatrics* 87:323, 1991.

13. Mulliken JB, Young A: *Vascular birthmarks: hemangiomas and malformations,* Philadelphia, 1988, WB Saunders, p 124.

14. Mulliken JB, Young A: *Vascular birthmarks: hemangiomas and malformations,* Philadelphia, 1988, WB Saunders, p 107.

15. Tan OT, Sherwood K, Gilchrest BA: Treatment of children with port-wine stains using the flashlamp-pulsed tunable dye laser, *N Engl J Med* 320:416, 1989.

16. Reyes BA, Geronemus R: Treatment of port-wine stains during childhood with the flashlamp-pulsed tunable dye laser, *J Am Acad Dermatol* 23:1142, 1990.

17. Goldman MP, Fitzpatrick RE, Ruiz-Esparza J: Treatment of port-wine stains (capillary malformations) with the flashlamp-pumped pulsed tunable dye laser, *J Pediatrics* 122:71-77, 1993.

18. Ashinoff RA, Geronemus RG: Flashlamp-pumped pulsed tunable dye laser for port-wine stains in infancy: earlier versus later treatment, *J Am Acad Dermatol* 24:467, 1991.

19. Tan OT, Stafford TJ: EMLA for laser treatment of port-wine stains in children, *Laser Surg Med* 12:543, 1992.

14

Vascular Reactions: Urticaria, Erythemas, and Purpuras

U rticaria, erythemas, and purpuras are considered together in a single chapter because they
represent a spectrum of disease characterized
by progressive signs of injury to cutaneous blood vessels. All are accompanied by vasodilation (erythema)
and leakage of fluid from blood vessels (edema).
Leakage of red blood cells also occurs in the purpuras
as a further sign of vascular insult. A complex interplay of chemical mediators may be involved.
Histamine is certainly involved in the urticarias, as are
complement fragments with vasoactive properties,
such as C3a and C5a. Eicosanoids and certain
cytokines may also participate. In addition, other
immunoreactants may be involved, such as
immunoglobulin E (IgE) and circulating antigen-
antibody complexes, particularly in the initial stages
of vascular injury. Immune complex disease seems to
be particularly important in the reactive erythemas
and the purpuras. Included because they mimic vas-

cular reactions are acquired angiomas, including vascular spiders, cherry angiomas, and angiokeratomas.

URTICARIA

Urticarial states are common in infancy and childhood, although the exact incidence is not known.
Several large studies indicate that 3% of preschool
children and about 2% of older children suffer from
urticaria.[1-5] This high incidence undoubtedly accounts
for a number with a single episode of short-lived
urticaria rather than persistent urticaria. Interestingly,
of all children with urticaria, only 3% to 5% have what
can be documented as immunoglobulin E (IgE) mediated allergic urticaria.[1-5] In contrast, approximately
15% of children with urticaria have a physical
urticaria, with the bulk of the patients in a large "idiopathic" group.[1-3] Some children with persistent idio-

pathic urticaria may have urticarial vasculitis. For purposes of presenting a clinical approach to urticaria, transient urticaria and persistent urticaria are discussed separately.

Transient urticaria and angioedema
Clinical features

Transient urticaria in children often follows infection,[1,2,6] encounters with stinging or biting insects,[7] ingestion of medications[8] (Chapter 22) or certain foods, or occurs with inflammatory systemic diseases such as collagen vascular disease or thyroiditis (see Box 14-1). The eruption is sudden in onset and pruritic, with erythematous raised wheals scattered over the body. The wheals are usually 2 to 15 mm in diameter, flat-topped, and have tense edema (Fig. 14-1). The edema can be appreciated by stretching the skin slightly to demonstrate whitish centers. The erythematous borders with pale centers can be quite large and mistaken for target lesions of erythema multiforme.[9] Occasionally, giant urticarial lesions up to 30 cm in diameter and with polycyclic borders will appear (Figs. 14-2 and 14-3). Such wheals commonly last from 20 minutes to 3 hours, disappear, then reappear in other areas. The entire episode of transient urticaria often lasts 24 to 48 hours; rarely, it lasts as long as 3 weeks. Transient urticaria, as it resolves, may leave flat dusky areas lasting several days (Fig. 14-4).

Subcutaneous extension of lesions, called *angioedema*, may occur. They appear as large swellings with indistinct borders around the eyelids and lips. They may also appear on the face, trunk, genitalia, and extremities (Fig. 14-5). The face, hands, and feet are involved in 85% of patients and are involved in other areas in 15%.[1-5] Up to half of patients with transient urticaria may have angioedema, with swelling of the hands and feet commonly seen.[1-5] All the persistent urticarias when examined within the first 4 weeks of illness may be indistinguishable from transient urticaria.

Hereditary angioedema accounts for only 0.4% of cases of urticaria, but its specific diagnostic tests and high mortality deserve special mention.[10] It is an autosomal dominant condition with repeated attacks of swelling of the extremities, face, and throat, accom-

---

Box 14-1   Transient urticaria

Infectious associations
- *Streptococcus*
- Infectious mononucleosis (Epstein-Barr virus)
- Hepatitis
- Adenovirus
- Enterovirus
- Parasites

Bites and stings
- Bees
- Wasps
- Scorpions
- Spiders
- Jellyfish

Drugs
- Penicillin
- Cephalosporins
- Salicylates
- Morphine, codeine, and other opiates
- Nonsteroidal anti-inflammatory drugs
- Barbiturates
- Amphetamines
- Atropine
- Hydralazine
- Insulin
- Blood and blood products

Foods
- Nuts
- Eggs
- Shellfish
- Strawberries
- Tomatoes

Systemic diseases
- Collagen vascular diseases
    - Lupus erythematosus
    - Juvenile rheumatoid arthritis
    - Polyarteritis nodosa
    - Dermatomyositis
    - Neonatal lupus syndrome
    - Sjögren's syndrome
    - Rheumatic fever

Box 14-1—cont'd   Transient urticaria

Inflammatory bowel diseases
  Crohn's disease
  Ulcerative colitis
Miscellaneous
  Aphthous stomatitis
  Behçet's disease
  Thyroiditis

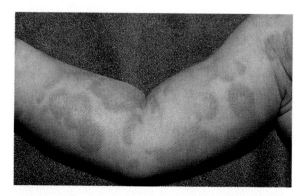

Fig. 14-2
Multiple polycyclic red wheals of different sizes in a child with urticaria. Commonly mistaken for erythema multiforme.

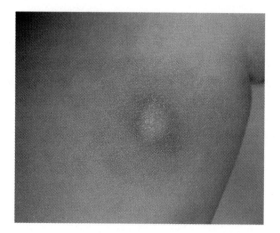

Fig. 14-1
Central wheal with red border in acute urticaria.

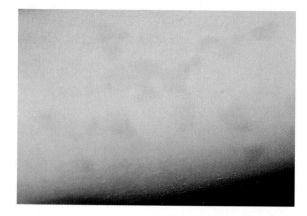

Fig. 14-3
Multiple shapes of urticarial lesions in a child.

panied by abdominal pain.[10] The onset usually follows trauma such as surgery, dental manipulation, or accidents. It presents as a diffuse, brawny swelling of the extremities in 75% of patients, abdominal pain in 52%, and swelling of the face and throat in 30%.[10] Its onset is usually in adolescence, with the more severe symptoms associated with the menses.[10] Abdominal pain eventually becomes a major complaint in 93% of patients. They do not have urticarial wheals, but 26% have erythema multiforme-like lesions.[10] Severe airway edema accounts for the mortality of almost 30% in untreated patients. Only 25% of patients give a positive family history. The diagnosis should be suspect-

ed if the serum C4 level is persistently low. It is confirmed by functional assay of the Cl esterase inhibitor. In some children hereditary angioedema is associated with lupus erythematosus or other collagen vascular diseases.[10,11]

Differential diagnosis
The conditions to be considered in the differential diagnosis of urticaria are listed in Box 14-2. Urticaria, especially giant urticaria, is frequently confused with erythema multiforme.[9] Urticarial lesions may blanch in the center, showing a red border and thus concentric zones of color change, as is seen in erythema multiforme. However, it should be remembered that indi-

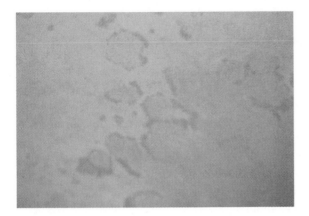

Fig. 14-4
Dusky centers with red borders in resolving childhood urticaria.

Box 14-2 Differential diagnosis of urticaria

Erythema multiforme
Mastocytosis
Flushing
Reactive erythemas
Juvenile rheumatoid arthritis
Vasculitis
Guttate psoriasis
Pityriasis rosea (early lesions)

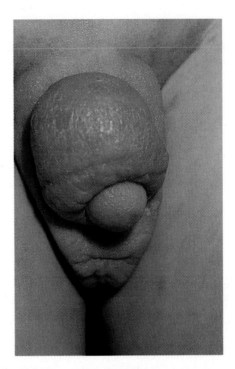

Fig. 14-5
Angioedema of the scrotum in an infant.

vidual urticarial lesions are transient, usually lasting less than 3 hours, whereas erythema multiforme lesions are fixed and stay in place at least 7 to 14 days. Also, the target lesions of erythema multiforme are dusky in the center, not lighter. Frequently—when polycyclic urticarial wheals of different sizes and shapes accompany edema of the hands and feet—erythema multiforme is incorrectly diagnosed. Urticarial lesions often clear with the administration of subcutaneous epinephrine; erythema multiforme does not.[9] A skin biopsy will also distinguish the two. Urticaria can be differentiated from mastocytosis by a skin biopsy, since increased numbers of mast cells are seen in mastocytosis. Flushing states are flat rather than elevated. In juvenile rheumatoid arthritis, faint erythe-matous macules with a clear center are present and are associated with a spiking fever. Vasculitis lesions have purpuric centers, whereas psoriasis and pityriasis rosea demonstrate scaling overlying the erythematous papules.

Angioedema (deep hives) (see Box 14-3) should be differentiated from cellulitis and erysipelas, which are tender, warm red lesions. Chronic thickening of tissues occurs in lymphedema, in contrast to the acute stretching of tissue seen in angioedema. Angioedema of the hands and feet, which accompanies urticaria, may be confused with erythema multiforme.[9] A skin biopsy will distinguish. Persistent angioedema of the face or lip should bring to mind lupus erythematosus or other collagen vascular diseases.[10,11]

Considerable deep edema can develop in acute contact dermatitis, but vesiculation of the overlying epidermis and epidermal papules will help distinguish it from angioedema. Idiopathic scrotal edema of children and the Melkersson-Rosenthal syndrome are rare and can be distinguished from angioedema by the furrowed

---

Box 14-3   Differential diagnosis of angioedema

Cellulitis and erysipelas
Lymphedema
Acute contact dermatitis
Idiopathic scrotal edema of children
Melkersson-Rosenthal syndrome

---

tongue and cranial nerve palsies of Melkersson-Rosenthal syndrome and the limitation of angioedema to the scrotum in idiopathic scrotal edema.

Pathogenesis

Histamine is undoubtedly the major chemical mediator of transient urticaria, and the mast cell is central in all forms of transient urticaria and angioedema. Histamine may be directly released from cutaneous mast cells in the case of certain foods or opiate drugs. Specific IgE antibodies bound to mast cell surfaces that "recognize" certain antigens, such as penicillin and other drugs, foods, and venom of certain stinging insects, result in the release of histamine after combination with antigen. Complement fragments, activated by immune complexes, may activate mast cells to release histamine or exert vasoactive effects of their own on cutaneous blood vessels. The latter mechanism is most often associated with infection, but careful documentation of the mechanism of histamine release involved with each inciting substance is not available. Eicosanoids may induce mast cell mediator release, and other cytokines have been implicated in urticaria.

In hereditary angioedema, a deficiency of the Cl esterase inhibitor permits unregulated cleavage of complement proteins once the complement system is activated, with particular consumption of C4. A C2 kinin activates the clotting system via the Hageman factor in hereditary angioedema.[10] Complement cleavage products may be responsible for the edema and erythema.

Treatment

Oral antihistamines are valuable in symptomatic control of urticaria. Hydroxyzine hydrochloride, 2 to 4 mg/kg/day in four divided doses, or diphenhydramine hydrochloride, 5 mg/kg/day in four divided doses, is the most helpful. If urticaria at night is the problem, administration of hydroxyzine 1 hour before bedtime may allow a single treatment per day. Nonsedating antihistamines are less effective in controlling urticaria. In angioedema not controlled by antihistamines, the addition of pseudoephedrine, 4 mg/kg/day in four divided doses, is useful. The same drugs may be used to treat chronic angioedema. In acute angioedema of the airway, epinephrine 1:1000, 0.01 ml/kg/dose to a maximum dose of 0.5 ml, may be used. There is no evidence to support the use of systemic glucocorticosteroids in urticaria or angioedema. It is unclear whether the addition of H_2 blocking drugs to H_1 antihistamines is of any additional benefit. Cromolyn sodium preparations, which may be efficacious in treatment of airway or bowel reactions, have not been particularly useful in skin. Allergen avoidance is an important strategy if the allergen can be identified. Virtually any drug may produce urticaria, but certain drugs are more frequently implicated. Drugs such as penicillin and aspirin account for most drug-induced urticaria, and they should be specifically questioned in review of the patient's history. Cephalosporins produce an urticarial serum-sickness–like reaction. Foods suspected of causing the urticaria could be avoided if nutrition is not compromised. Restriction diets are of little value if a suspected food factor has not been identified.

In hereditary angioedema, acute attacks are managed by intravenous fluid replacement and airway maintenance.[10] Administration of danazol or stanozolol, synthetic attenuated testosterones, increases Clq esterase inhibitor levels and prevents the attacks of angioedema. Fresh-frozen plasma or ε-aminocaproic acid may be useful before surgical procedures.[10]

Patient education

It should be explained that cause-and-effect relationships often cannot be found in transient urticaria and angioedema, but that lesions can be expected to resolve by 1 month in most instances. One should emphasize that control of symptoms is possible with the use of antihistamines. An extensive and expensive allergy workup is not indicated in children who have had urticaria less than 6 weeks, and workup of chronic urticaria should be guided by history.

Patients with angioedema should have an adrenergic agent available for airway attacks, and patients with hereditary angioedema should be advised of the high mortality and the need to continue taking prophylactic drugs.

Follow-up visits

In transient urticaria and angioedema a visit 1 week after the initial evaluation is useful for monitoring the course of the disease. In chronic urticaria it is useful to reevaluate precipitating factors periodically if a factor has not been identified. Patients with hereditary angioedema should be seen after 1 month of therapy to remeasure the Cl esterase inhibitor and adjust the drug dosage.

Persistent urticaria: the physical urticarias

Urticaria that persists for over 4 weeks may be simply prolonged common urticaria or due to one of the physical urticarias, urticarial vasculitis, or mastocytosis. The physical urticarias, which account for 15% of this group, consist of dermatographism, heat and exercise urticaria, delayed-pressure urticaria, cold urticaria, and familial cold urticaria.[1,12-14]

Clinical features

Dermatographism   Dermatographism occurs in 1% of adolescents[12] and is characterized by wheal and erythema following minor stroking of or pressure on the skin[13,14] (Fig. 14-6). It often results in mild itching. The wheal reaches maximal size in 6 to 7 minutes and persists for 10 to 15 minutes. Wheals are commonly found around the belt area and may follow widespread insect bites and transient episodes of urticaria. The wheal is seen in comatose children (e.g., in encephalitis, meningitis, drug overdose) and has been termed *tache cérébrale*. Dermatographism is also seen in about half of children with mastocytosis.[13]

Dermatographism may persist for years, but most patients can expect spontaneous regression within 2 years.[13]

Heat and exercise urticaria   Heat and exercise urticaria (cholinergic urticaria) is characterized by a large (10 to 20 mm) blotchy erythema surrounding tiny (1 to 3 mm) central wheals (Fig. 14-7).[12] It occurs in up to 3% of adolescents.[12] Heating of the skin or exercise sufficient to raise the body temperature 0.5° C will induce attacks of multiple wheals with itching.[14] Hot or spicy foods, febrile illnesses, and hot

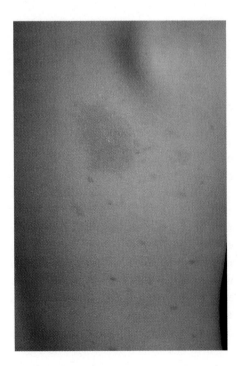

Fig. 14-6
Dermatographism. Light stroking of the skin evokes intense wheal and flare reaction.

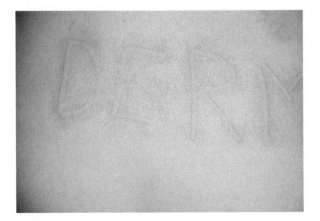

Fig. 14-7
Heat and exercise urticaria. Pinpoint central wheal surrounded by large, blotchy erythema.

baths may also initiate attacks. The onset is characteristically in adolescence, but the condition tends to persist into young adult years.[12]

Delayed-pressure urticaria Delayed-pressure urticaria, which occurs primarily in adolescents, appears after prolonged pressure with a heavy weight.[14,15] A 7-kg weight suspended from an extremity by a strap for 15 minutes will reproduce the disease.[14] Painful, deep swellings begin 4 to 6 hours after pressure and last up to 24 hours. Spontaneous remissions have been reported, but the natural history is unknown.[15]

Cold urticaria Cold urticaria appears in three forms: it may be associated with cryoglobulins and immune complex disease; it may appear as an acquired form not associated with cryoproteins, or it may occur as autosomal dominant familial cold urticaria. In the form associated with cryoglobulins the signs and symptoms of collagen vascular disease are often present. This disease is uncommon in children. The acquired form occurs after rewarming an area of skin exposed to cold. Wheals appear, and itching is severe. Cooling the entire body may result in widespread wheals and fainting. To test for acquired cold urticaria, an ice cube is applied to the patient's skin for 2 to 10 minutes, and the skin is allowed to rewarm. The wheal appears during the rewarming. There may be a spontaneous remission, but the natural history is not known.

Familial cold urticaria Familial cold urticaria is an autosomal dominant condition beginning shortly after birth. Erythematous macules appear in exposed areas 30 minutes following exposure to a cold wind, but not after ingestion of iced drinks or ice. Older children complain of burning in the skin. Fever and chills, arthralgias, and headaches appear and last up to 48 hours. A leukocytosis occurs during the attacks. The patient tends to suffer these attacks throughout life.

Differential diagnosis

The physical urticarias are often confused with other forms of urticaria (see Box 14-2). The role of light pressure in dermatographism and deep pressure in delayed-pressure urticaria should help distinguish these disorders from the other forms of urticaria. Heat and exercise urticaria may be distinguished from other types of urticaria by the characteristic tiny central wheal with a large rim of erythema. The cold urticarias may be distinguished by the history of cold exposure, and in the familial form, by the systemic symptoms accompanying the skin lesions. Box 14-4 lists the conditions to be considered in the differential diagnosis of cold urticaria.

Pathogenesis

The physical urticarias differ from other urticarial states in that histamine does not appear to be the chemical mediator of the disease. Histamine skin levels are normal in dermatographism, heat and exercise urticaria, cold urticaria with cryoglobulins, urticarial states, and familial cold urticaria. Histamine has been implicated in acquired cold urticaria and delayed-pressure urticaria. In dermatographism, as well as in heat and exercise urticaria, mediation through cholinergic fibers of the autonomic nervous system has been implicated. The vasoactive split products of the complement system may be involved in the cryoglobulinemic and familial cold urticarial forms.

Treatment

Many patients with physical urticaria require no therapy. If symptoms are severe enough to require therapy, hydroxyzine hydrochloride, 2 to 4 mg/kg/day in

---

Box 14-4   Differential diagnosis of cold urticaria

Cryoglobulinemia and immune complex diseases
Systemic lupus erythematosus and other collagen vascular diseases
Macroglobulinemia
Mycoplasma infections (cold hemagglutinins)
Syphilis
Cold urticaria
    Familial
    Acquired

four divided doses, may reduce the symptoms in dermatographism as well as in heat and exercise urticaria.[13,14] There is little additional benefit from adding an H_2 blocking agent.[16] A new H_1 blocking agent, cetirizine, is also efficacious.[17] Delayed-pressure urticaria may respond to prednisone, 1 mg/kg/day for 4 to 5 days, but prednisone is generally not required. There is no satisfactory treatment for cold urticaria other than cold avoidance, although cyproheptadine, 2 to 4 mg three times a day, has been reported to provide relief in some patients.[14] A combination of terbutaline and aminophylline-containing agents used three times weekly may be useful.[18]

Patient education

Patients with the physical urticarias must be instructed to reduce their exposure to the precipitating factors. Patients with dermatographism and delayed-pressure urticaria should not wear backpacks or carry other heavy weights and should avoid tight-fitting clothing and excessive friction or pressure on the skin. Patients with heat and exercise urticaria need to avoid excessive heating of the skin, vigorous exercise, hot baths, and other factors resulting in increased body heat. Patients with cold urticaria should avoid ice-cold food or drinks, dress warmly in cold weather, and avoid swimming in cold water.

Follow-up visits

A visit 2 weeks after the initial evaluation will be useful to monitor the progress of the disease and the therapeutic response.

Persistent urticaria: urticarial vasculitis
Clinical features

Urticarial vasculitis is characterized by fixed wheals distributed symmetrically over the extremities.[19] It is usually seen in adolescents and young adults. The true incidence is unknown, but it has been reported in up to 10% of patients with persistent urticaria. Lesions remain fixed in the same area for 24 to 72 hours and may be accompanied by mild arthralgias or malaise.[19] Most patients have an elevated erythrocyte sedimentation rate and depressed serum complement levels. Systemic signs and symptoms are uncommon but may be severe.[19] The natural history is not known. Although the findings are similar to those in necrotizing vasculitis with palpable purpura, most patients do not progress to palpable purpura.

Differential diagnosis

Urticarial vasculitis may be distinguished from other conditions (see Box 14-2) by the elevated erythrocyte sedimentation rate, depressed serum complement levels, the finding of small-vessel vasculitis on skin biopsy, and the associated arthralgias.

Pathogenesis

Urticarial vasculitis has been associated with circulating immune complexes, resulting in injury to postcapillary venules in the upper dermis. Immunofluorescence has demonstrated immunoglobulins and complement split products around inflamed venules.[19] Neutrophils and degenerating neutrophil nuclei are seen around the venules on skin biopsy, with swelling of the venule wall and fibrin deposition. The inflammatory events are most probably mediated through the interaction of immune complexes with the complement and clotting systems.

Treatment

If a cause for immune complex disease, such as streptococcal infection, can be determined, it can be eliminated, but such associations are difficult to document. There is no known effective treatment. Both antihistamines and low-dose prednisone therapy have been utilized, with variable success.[19]

Patient education

Patients should be advised of the difference between urticarial vasculitis and IgE-mediated urticaria.

Follow-up visits

Monthly visits are advisable to determine whether the disorder has progressed to involve vessels of other organs. Urinalysis, erythrocyte sedimentation rate, and complement levels may be used to follow the course of the disease.

Persistent urticaria: mastocytosis (including urticaria pigmentosa)
Clinical features

There are three distinct forms of mastocytosis observed in childhood.[20] The most common is the solitary mastocytoma (see Chapter 12), the second most common is urticaria pigmentosa,[21] and, uncommonly, diffuse cutaneous mastocytosis (bullous mastocytosis).[22] The macular and nodular pigmented lesions of urticaria pigmentosa appear in the first 8 months of life[20,21] (Fig. 14-8). One or two lesions are noted initially, but numerous lesions accumulate during the next

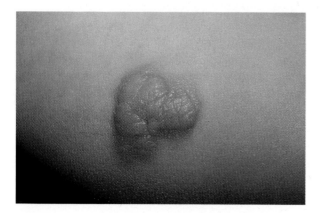

Fig. 14-8
Mastocytoma. Pink plaque on the skin of an infant.

few months (Fig. 14-9). The majority of lesions appear on the trunk, although some may appear on the face and extremities. Individual lesions are often red at first and may easily become blistered[20,21] (Fig. 14-10). Brown pigmentation may not appear until 6 months after the onset of the lesions. Stroking the pigmented lesion will result in tense edema within the lesion and an erythematous flare surrounding the area (Darier's sign).[20,21] Half the patients with mastocytosis will demonstrate dermatographism in uninvolved areas. Skin biopsy will confirm the diagnosis.[20,21]

Spontaneous bulla formation within lesions may occur or may be induced by a variety of drugs (see Box 14-5). These drugs or rubbing of the skin may induce enough histamine release to produce systemic symptoms, such as flushing, tachycardia, hypotension with fainting, diarrhea, and vomiting.[20,21] As the child ages, it becomes more difficult to urticate the lesions, or to induce blisters, or both. Often by age 5 they are asymptomatic, and by adolescence only residual flat pigmentation remains.[20]

Enlargement of the liver and spleen, systemic flushing episodes, and peptic ulcer symptoms should suggest systemic mastocytosis.[20] Systemic mastocytosis occurs in up to 2% of infants with urticaria pigmentosa.[20,21] Bony involvement can be documented by x-ray examination, and bone marrow examination will reveal increased numbers of mast cells. Extreme

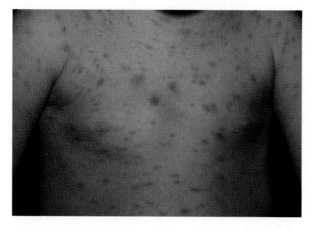

Fig. 14-9
Urticaria pigmentosa. Multiple, blotchy, brown macules on the chest of an infant.

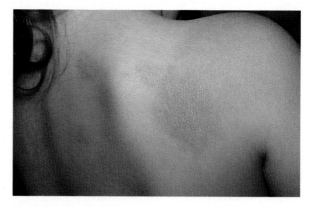

Fig. 14-10
Tense edema within tan macule of urticaria pigmentosa after stroking.

Box 14-5   Drugs producing histamine release in mastocytosis

Opiates (codeine, meperidine [Demerol], morphine)
Polymyxin B
Acetylsalicylic acid

---

infiltration of the liver sufficient to produce cirrhosis may occur. In the infant who has urticaria pigmentosa without systemic symptoms, skeletal surveys and bone marrow examinations are not warranted.[20]

Diffuse cutaneous mastocytosis presents as blisters in the neonatal period, often accompanied by flushing episodes.[20,22] The blisters are often large and peel, leaving large, eroded bases. After a severe blistering episode, 5 to 10 days may be required to regranulate mast cells, and the baby experiences recurrent episodes.[22] When the baby is evaluated, marked dermatographism is present. A leathery thickening with yellow-tan skin usually does not appear until 3 to 8 months of age. Severe syncopal episodes and death from prolonged hypotension have been reported.[20,22] Gastrointestinal symptoms are seen as the child becomes older, including chronic diarrhea states and recurrent episodes of vomiting associated with abdominal pain.[22] In addition to gastrointestinal involvement, bone marrow involvement is more likely.[22] It is an autosomal dominant disorder.

Differential diagnosis
Mastocytosis can be differentiated from other conditions (see Box 14-1) by skin biopsy.[20] The bullous lesions must be differentiated from other bullous diseases of infancy. Diffuse cutaneous mastocytosis has been confused with the scalded skin syndrome, especially "recurrent scalded skin syndrome," and with epidermolysis bullosa.

Pathogenesis
Excessive numbers of mast cells accumulate with the dermis in mastocytosis.[20,22,23] It is believed that mas-tocytosis may represent reactive mast cell hyperplasia in response to excessive mast cell growth factor.[23] Excessive histamine release from these mast cells results in whealing or blister formation. The blister is subepidermal and may bleed. Histamine is undoubtedly responsible for the local and systemic effects. Flushing and syncopal episodes are due to prostaglandin D_2 release, and bleeding to heparin release by cutaneous mast cells.[20]

Treatment
Most infants require no treatment. Flushing episodes or other systemic symptoms may be controlled by the use of hydroxyzine hydrochloride, 2 to 4 mg/kg/day divided into four doses.[20] Solitary mastocytomas may be treated with 2 weeks of superpotent topical steroids. Oral cromolyn sodium has been reported to be valuable in infants with gastrointestinal involvement. Diffuse cutaneous mastocytosis may respond to psoralen ultraviolet A-range (PUVA) therapy.[24]

Patient education
It is essential that the child not be given cough syrups with codeine or other medications with opiates. If surgery is contemplated, preoperative medications should be carefully selected. Substitution of other antipyretics for aspirin is also advised. The natural course should be emphasized and parents provided with lists of drugs to avoid. Genetic counseling is valuable for diffuse cutaneous mastocytosis.

Follow-up visits
A visit in 2 weeks is useful in determining the presence or absence of systemic symptoms. If treatment is given, monthly visits are advisable.

ERYTHEMAS

Erythemas of the skin without wheal production are uncommon in infants and children. Often called the reactive erythemas, they include the annular erythemas (including erythema chronicum migrans, erythema marginatum, and erythema annulare), erythema multiforme, and erythema nodosum. Erythema multiforme is covered in detail in Chapter 11 and erythema chronicum migrans in Chapter 5.

Annular erythemas
Clinical features
Annular, polycyclic, and partially marginated lesions are called *annular erythemas*. One should remember that giant urticaria can assume annular shapes.

Erythema annulare In erythema annulare the lesions have erythematous borders, a trailing scale, and a dusky center (Fig. 14-11). They may occur anywhere on the skin.[25,26] Multiple lesions are usually present, and they slowly enlarge. They last for several months and tend to recur. In infants the lesions may be associated with a maternal collagen vascular disorder, particularly with Sjögren's syndrome.[25]

Erythema marginatum Erythema marginatum is a transient eruption consisting of curvilinear, migrating areas of erythema that form incomplete circles (Fig. 14-12). The marginated lesions may move rapidly over the skin within several hours and disappear.[27] Inducing cutaneous vasodilation may make the lesions more visible. It is found in only 10% of children with acute rheumatic fever, despite being one of the Jones criteria for diagnosis, and is associated with the fever and well-established carditis.[27] A thorough evaluation for acute rheumatic fever is indicated. It may also be seen following streptococcal infections without evidence of acute rheumatic fever.

Differential diagnosis
Conditions to be considered in the differential diagnosis of annular erythemas are given in Box 14-6. Dermatophyte lesions have a scaly border and may be diagnosed by potassium hydroxide (KOH) examination and fungal cultures. Granuloma annulare lesions have a distinct nodular and papular border. The lesions of pityriasis rosea may be annular on occasion and have central clearing. Lupus erythematosus, sarcoidosis, and syphilis may also present with annular lesions. The transient urticarial lesions of juvenile rheumatoid arthritis tend to be limited to the abdomen, and clear slightly in the center.

Pathogenesis
Two of the erythemas demonstrate infectious agents within the skin lesions with an attendant host response. In erythema chronicum migrans, *Borrelia burgdorferi* is found (see Chapter 5) and in erythema multiforme, herpes simplex virus (see Chapter 11). In erythema annulare and in erythema marginatum, the

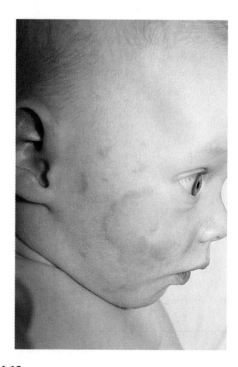

Fig. 14-12
Erythema marginatum. Fleeting, semiannular erythema on the face of an infant with acute rheumatic fever.

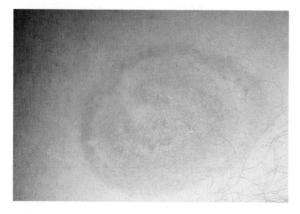

Fig. 14-11
Erythema annulare. Concentric zones of red and dusky skin.

Box 14-6 Differential diagnosis of annular erythemas

Erythema annulare
Erythema chronicum migrans
Erythema marginatum
Tinea corporis
Pityriasis rosea
Subacute cutaneous lupus erythematosus
Neonatal lupus syndrome
Sarcoidosis
Syphilis
Juvenile rheumatoid arthritis

---

mechanism of disease is unknown. Dense accumulation of lymphocytes that surround superficial dermal blood vessels is seen on skin biopsy, which helps distinguish annular erythemas from urticaria.

Treatment
No treatment is useful for erythema annulare. Children with erythema marginatum are treated with penicillin.

Patient education
It should be emphasized that such eruptions are skin reactions that do not require treatment but serve as a clue to a systemic disorder.

Follow-up visits
A visit 1 week after the initial evaluation is useful to discuss the results of laboratory evaluation for systemic disorders. The need for follow-up care is determined by the nature of the associated systemic disorder.

Erythema nodosum
Clinical features
Erythema nodosum is characterized by the abrupt onset of symmetric, very tender, erythematous nodules on the extensor surface of the extremities[28-31] (Fig. 14-13). Occasionally, lesions will involve other areas of skin such as the soles of the feet, hands, or trunk.[28] Widespread involvement is more characteristic of infants (Fig. 14-14). The nodules have indistinct borders. Occasionally, it will be unilateral at presentation. The lesions may be so painful that the patient will limp. A prodrome of cough, sore throat, and fever will occur in about 25% of children. It occurs most commonly in adolescents and is uncommon before age 2 years. Females predominate at a ratio of 1.7:1. Lesions last from 2 to 6 weeks. Recurrences are reported in 4% of children. Lesions resolve as a bruise, with a color change to purple, then yellow-brown. Infectious causes, such as streptococci, tuberculosis, histoplasmosis, tularemia, and coccidioidomycosis, are the most common associations.[29-31] A careful history should be obtained for preceding infections. Drugs may uncommonly produce erythema nodosum, particularly oral contraceptives in adolescent females.

Differential diagnosis
Erythema nodosum may be confused with many other processes involving the subcutaneous fat. In contrast to erythema nodosum, thrombophlebitis usually occurs on the lateral or flexor surface of the lower legs and heals with fibrosis. The nodose lesions of polyarteritis nodosa are associated with an exaggerated dusky, mot-

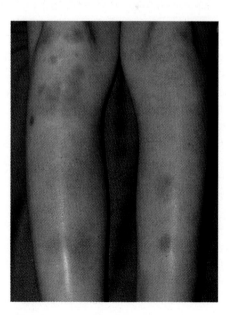

Fig. 14-13
Tender red nodules with indistinct borders in a teenage girl with erythema nodosum.

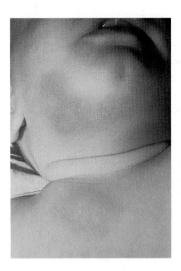

Fig. 14-14
Atypical location of erythema nodosum in an infant.

tling pattern called *livedo reticularis*. Giant insect bite reactions may be confused with erythema nodosum, but a central punctum will help differentiate. Panniculitis can be distinguished on biopsy of skin to include subcutaneous fat. The lesions of erythema nodosum are usually so characteristic that they are seldom confused with those of other disorders.

Pathogenesis

Erythema nodosum is a chronic injury of the blood vessels of the lower dermis and subcutaneous fat.[31] Initially the perivascular inflammation is neutrophilic, then lymphocytic, then granulomatous as the lesions age.[31] There is increasing evidence to implicate circulating immune complexes in the pathogenesis of erythema nodosum as a part of the host immune response to an infectious agent. Fat cell destruction usually does not occur in erythema nodosum, so it is not a true panniculitis.

Treatment

Symptomatic treatment with acetylsalicylic acid or antihistamines may suffice, because in many cases the erythema nodosum resolves within 3 weeks. In patients with acutely tender lesions that interfere with walking, nonsteroidal anti-inflammatory agents, such as indomethacin, may be tried. Although some relief can be obtained with prednisone, oral steroids are not generally recommended and should not be used chronically.

Patient education

It should be emphasized that erythema nodosum is a response to infection or to certain drugs. A search for such associations should be guided by the history and should not involve expensive laboratory tests. Parents should be reassured that most children recover within 3 weeks.

Follow-up visits

A return visit in 1 week is useful to ascertain the need for, or response to, therapy.

Gustatory flushing
Clinical features

Gustatory flushing usually develops in early infancy and may first present when solid foods are introduced.[32] An erythematous flush of one cheek occurs during or just after eating, lasting from 5 to 60 minutes.[32-34] Sweating may develop within the flushed area, and tearing of the adjacent eye may occur.[33] Frequently the infant is misdiagnosed as having food allergy.[34] Spontaneous remission has been reported after several years.

Differential diagnosis

Urticaria and food allergy are often considered in the diagnosis. However, gustatory flushing always occurs in the same site and does not move from skin area to skin area as urticaria would. Food allergy reactions should occur with specific foods and be widespread and not localized. Gustatory flushing occurs with any foods that stimulate the taste buds. Herpes facialis may be considered, but it presents with persistent erythema that lasts for at least 3 days and usually evolves to vesicle formation. Contact dermatitis also produces a persistent erythema on the cheek.

Pathogenesis

Gustatory flushing is caused by cross-linking of the parasympathetic nerve fibers innervating the parotid gland to the sympathetic fibers supplying the sweat glands and cutaneous vessels along the distribution of the auriculotemporal nerve. Foods that would ordinarily stimulate salivation instead produce flushing and sweating. In infancy, cases are believed to be due to a congenital malformation resulting in cross-linking of nerve fibers. It may result from nerve regeneration following parotid surgery or injury in older children.

Treatment
There is no known effective treatment. Topical antiperspirants will control the sweating.

Patient education
It should be emphasized that the condition does not represent allergy, and that spontaneous remission can be expected in most infants. Allergy evaluation should be discouraged.

Follow-up visits
Routine follow-up visits are unnecessary.

PURPURAS

Purpuric lesions always prompt investigation into bleeding states. They may involve small areas (e.g., petechiae) or large areas (e.g., ecchymoses). Palpable purpura (purpuric papules), dissecting purpura, and chronic pigmented purpura are presented in this section. Neonatal purpura (see Box 14-7), acral petechiae and purpura (see Box 14-8), and flat generalized petechiae and purpura (see Box 14-9) are not discussed, but are presented to aid the reader in making a differential diagnosis of these lesions.

Palpable purpura (purpuric papules)
Clinical features
Discrete 1- to 5-mm papules with petechial centers or those that are completely purpuric characterize palpable purpura[35-37] (Fig. 14-15). They are usually found on the extremities and are symmetric and numerous (Fig. 14-16). Palpable purpura should immediately

bring to mind vasculitis or septicemia.[35-37] The vasculitis that occurs is called *cutaneous necrotizing venulitis* (anaphylactoid purpura, Henoch-Schönlein purpura [HSP]) and may be associated with vasculitis of renal, gastrointestinal, joint, or cerebral vessels.[35-37] The lesions may begin as discrete urticarial wheals,

---

Box 14-7 Differential diagnosis of neonatal purpura

Congenital infection
Toxoplasma
Enterovirus
Rubella
Cytomegalovirus
Herpes simplex
Syphilis
Coagulation defects
Autoimmune disorders (systemic lupus erythematosus and erythroblastosis fetalis)
Hemangioma with platelet trapping syndrome

Box 14-8 Differential diagnosis of flat acral purpura

Rocky Mountain spotted fever
Meningococcemia
Atypical measles
Coagulation disorders
Progressive pigmentary purpura

Box 14-9 Differential diagnosis of flat generalized purpura

Thrombocytopenic states (idiopathic thrombocytopenic purpura, leukemia)
Coagulation disorders
Trauma (including child abuse)

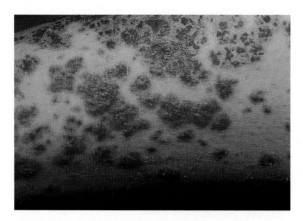

Fig. 14-15
Papules with petechial centers on the leg of a child with necrotizing vasculitis (Henoch-Schönlein purpura).

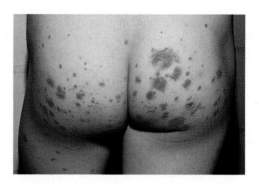

Fig. 14-16
Numerous purpuric macules and papules on the buttocks of a child with necrotizing vasculitis.

then progress to papular purpura and pustular purpura. Occasionally, cutaneous infarcts and gangrene with subsequent ulceration and scarring will occur.[35-37] Arthralgia or arthritis of the knees and ankles is found in 80% of patients.[35-37] Cramping abdominal pain, vomiting, hematemesis, and melena signal gastrointestinal involvement. Abdominal pain is common but in most children lasts less than 24 hours. The kidney is involved in 70% of children.[35-38] Most have asymptomatic microscopic hematuria, but only 25% on the first visit. Some children may present with a nephrotic syndrome. Up to 10% of children may progress to chronic renal failure.[38] Rarely, seizures, paresis, or coma occur with involvement of the central nervous system vessels.

Most episodes of necrotizing venulitis have skin changes that last from 4 to 6 weeks and then resolve.[35-37] In addition to necrotizing vasculitis, septicemic states also present with palpable purpura, which may evolve to pustules. Lesions are acral, symmetric, and few in number. Palpable purpura is seen in chronic meningococcemia, gonococcemia, and subacute bacterial endocarditis and is frequently associated with arthritis or arthralgias of the large joints.[39] Blood cultures or genital cultures will confirm the diagnosis. It is difficult to culture organisms from lesions, but they may be identified by specific immunofluorescence from smears of lesions. Rarely,

---

> **Box 14-10   Differential diagnosis of palpable purpura**
>
> Necrotizing venulitis (anaphylactoid purpura)
> Meningococcemia
> Gonococcemia
> Staphylococcal sepsis
> *Pseudomonas* sepsis
> Subacute bacterial endocarditis

Pseudomonas, staphylococcal, deep fungal, or gram-negative septicemia is responsible. Palpable purpura is also seen in collagen vascular diseases of childhood, especially juvenile rheumatoid arthritis and lupus erythematosus.[40] It occurs in long-standing disease, often years after the diagnosis was confirmed.

Differential diagnosis
Biopsy plus bacterial and fungal culture will distinguish infectious causes of palpable purpura from one another (see Box 14-10). Immunofluorescent examination of a skin biopsy will reveal immunoglobulin A (IgA) deposits surrounding superficial cutaneous blood vessels in HSP.[38] Antineutrophil cytoplasmic antibodies (ANCAs) may help in the diagnosis.[41] Associated collagen vascular disease is usually already established, and diagnostic serologies are not required.

Pathogenesis

In necrotizing venulitis and in septicemic states, circulating immune complexes have been implicated in the production of lesions through their interaction with the complement and clotting systems. The prodrome of upper respiratory tract infection, and sometimes positive streptococcal throat cultures, has implicated infectious agents as likely triggers of immune complex formation in HSP. An association with parvovirus B19 in childhood HSP may also be found.[42] Fibrinoid necrosis of venule walls in the upper dermis, with perivascular accumulation of neutrophils, nuclear fragments, and extravasation of red blood cells, is seen on skin biopsy. Organisms may also be detected with tissue Gram stains of skin biopsies in the septicemic states.

Treatment

In necrotizing venulitis with skin involvement only, no treatment is required. Prednisone, 2 mg/kg/day, may be indicated with internal organ involvement. The administration of systemic antibiotics, with the choice of agent based on appropriate cultures, is indicated for septicemic states. In severe prolonged necrotizing venulitis, pulse therapy with intravenous methylprednisolone and plasmapheresis may be useful.[36,37]

Patient education

The serious nature of vasculitis of internal organs and septicemic states should be emphasized. Future upper respiratory tract illnesses should be brought to the physician's attention promptly and appropriate cultures taken. Early treatment of an associated streptococcal infection may be required.

Follow-up visits

In necrotizing venulitis weekly follow-up visits are recommended for the first 4 weeks to monitor internal involvement, particularly of the kidney. Microscopic examination of the urinary sediment and protein determination are required. Thereafter, evaluations of renal function every 3 months are valuable to identify the children at risk of renal failure.

Nodular purpura with livedo: polyarteritis nodosa (periarteritis nodosa)

Clinical features

There are three polyarteritis syndromes in childhood: infantile polyarteritis nodosa, Kawasaki disease, and chronic cutaneous polyarteritis nodosa. The infantile form may represent Kawasaki disease without cutaneous findings and is considered with Kawasaki disease in Chapter 11.

The cutaneous findings of livedo reticularis plus palpable tender linear purple nodules are found in children with chronic cutaneous polyarteritis nodosa[43,44] (Fig. 14-17). Typically, older children rather than toddlers are affected.[36] Fever, myalgias, arthralgias, and gastrointestinal symptoms are observed in 70%.[35,36,40,43,44] Hypertension,[35] renal disease,[36] pulmonary involvement,[45] and localized neuropathy (mononeuritis multiplex)[46] may be observed. The skin lesions are usually located symmetrically on the proximal extremities and persist for weeks, with recurrent crops of new nodules appearing (Fig. 14-18). Exacerbations may occur on cold exposure. Focal areas of skin infarction and ulceration may accompany the nodules.[43,44] The course is quite chronic and may last for years.[35,36,43,44] Newborns of mothers with long-standing polyarteritis nodosa may develop a transient polyarteritis nodosa with lesions lasting 3 months.[48] ANCAs may be present, and the affected child may have a positive antinu-

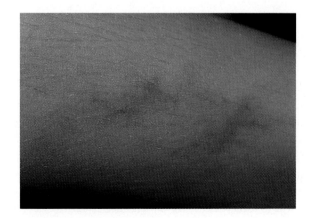

Fig. 14-17
Livedo pattern of purple lacy macules in childhood polyarteritis nodosa.

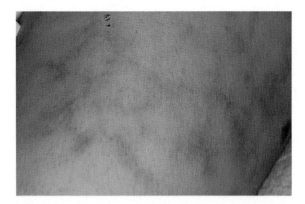

Fig. 14-18
Linear tender red nodules and livedo reticularis in childhood polyarteritis nodosa.

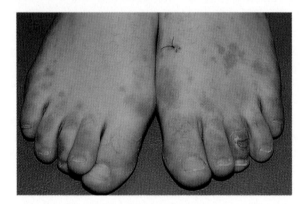

Fig. 14-19
Purple oval nodules on the toes in a child with pernio.

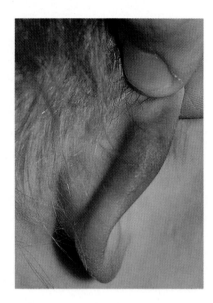

Fig. 14-20
Purple nodule on the ear of toddler with pernio.

clear antibody test.[41] The erythrocyte sedimentation rate is virtually always elevated.[35,36,40,43,44]

Differential diagnosis
Livedo patterns must be distinguished from mottling, which may be seen transiently with cold exposure—mottling disappears on rewarming and livedo do not. Careful palpation of the skin within the livedo area may be required to detect the linear nodules. Selection of a site for skin biopsy is critical. One must biopsy a linear nodule, including subcutaneous fat, to detect the characteristic pathology because artery involvement is segmental.[35,36,43,44] Biopsy of the livedo area or a shallow biopsy may miss the pathology.

Pathogenesis
Polyarteritis nodosa is an inflammatory segmental disease of the walls of cutaneous arteries. Neutrophilic infiltration of the arterial wall and adjacent periarterial tissue is seen. Thrombosis of vessels may be found. In children there is an association with parvovirus B19,[42] hepatitis B, and with streptococcal infection.[48]

Treatment
Most children respond well to low-dose oral steroids (0.5 mg/kg prednisone).[35,36,43,44] In children who require high-dose oral steroids, low-dose once-weekly methotrexate has been used successfully.[49]

Patient education
Avoiding cold exposure is advisable. The child and the family should be informed about the chronic and persistent nature of this condition, and advised of potential systemic complications and the need for monitoring of renal, gastrointestinal, and pulmonary involvement.

Follow-up visits
Initially follow-up visits should be every 2 weeks until disease control is established. After the disease is sta-

bilized, evaluation of renal status and other systemic complications should be performed every 4 to 6 weeks.

Nodular purpura: pernio

Clinical features

Pernio is characterized by asymptomatic purple to purple-red nodules, several days to weeks following exposure to wetness and cold.[50] The nodules are usually on the digits and may be accompanied by a livedo pattern of the adjacent skin[50,51] (Fig. 14-19). Other acral areas such as the ears may also be involved (Fig. 14-20). The livedo pattern slowly fades and the nodules remain for weeks. The cold exposure may seem trivial rather than severe, and associated wetness is required. Pernio has been associated with anorexia nervosa in adolescent girls.[51]

Differential diagnosis

The nodules of pernio must be differentiated from lymphoma or leukemia states, which also produce red-purple nodules. Pernio lesions have an insidious onset rather than the abrupt onset of lymphomas, and, once established, do not grow but remain stable. Polyarteritis nodosa nodules are linear rather than oval and tender rather than nontender. A skin biopsy will distinguish the two conditions.

Pathogenesis

The exact mechanism of the response to cold injury is not known. Pathology shows middermal inflammation including a lymphohistiocytic infiltrate around blood vessels but is not specific.[50]

Treatment

In most circumstances no treatment is required.

Patient education

Protection against cold and wetness is critical.

Follow-up visits

A follow-up visit in 2 weeks may be useful to ascertain the course of the condition and to reinforce the cold and wetness avoidance.

Dissecting purpura (disseminated intravascular coagulation)

Clinical features

Dissecting purpura, or disseminated intravascular coagulation, has an acute onset, with high fever and extensive, large, dissecting purpuric areas on the extremities.[52,53] The purpuric "lakes" are large and are not associated with petechiae (Fig. 14-21). The condition has been associated with overwhelming infections, such as meningococcemia,[53] *Escherichia coli* septicemia, and Rocky Mountain spotted fever, or it may follow common childhood infections, such as streptococcal pharyngitis or varicella, by 5 to 10 days.[52] Vascular collapse is common, and mortality is high in untreated patients. Even in those who survive, large areas of infarcted skin require long-term management.

Differential diagnosis

The large purpuric lakes are so characteristic that they are not confused with other purpuric diseases.

Pathogenesis

The syndrome is triggered by the massive release of tissue thromboplastin with widespread fibrin deposition in the blood vessels of skin, lungs, and kidneys; fibrinolysis; and consumption of coagulation factors,

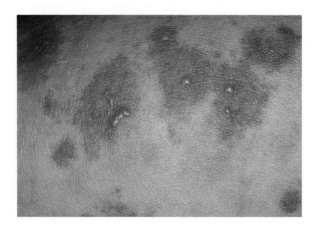

Fig. 14-21
Purpuric lakes with hemorrhagic blisters in a child with disseminated intravascular coagulation.

leading to secondary bleeding.[52] Protein C and protein S are particularly consumed by the infections as well.[52,53] Protein C is a vitamin K–dependent plasma serine protease that acts as an anticoagulant by inactivating clotting factors Va and VIIIa after clotting is initiated. Protein S acts as a cofactor for protein C in the inactivation of clotting factor Va. When protein C or protein S is deficient, intravascular hypercoagulability results, with widespread thrombosis.

Treatment

Replacement of consumable clotting factors with fresh plasma, protein C concentrate,[54] or platelet concentrates is the treatment of choice.[52,53] Most children require hospitalization. With persistent disseminated intravascular coagulation, heparin, 100 U/kg intravenously every 4 to 6 hours, may be given. Antibiotic treatment of the triggering bacterial infection is necessary. With extensive areas of skin necrosis, admission to a burn unit with appropriate debridement, prevention of secondary infection, and biologic dressings may be useful.[55]

Patient education

Advice depends on the nature of the triggering disease. Counseling regarding the grave prognosis and need for long-term care should be provided.

Follow-up visits

Follow-up visits daily, while the child is hospitalized, to reevaluate clotting by laboratory assays are useful.

Chronic pigmented purpura
Clinical features

Chronic pigmented purpura is characterized by an insidious onset and slow progression of grouped nonpalpable petechiae over the extremities, trunk, or neck (Fig. 14-22) in adolescents.[56,57] Individual lesions show fresh and old petechiae intermixed and an interplay of red, brown, and yellow spots. Lesions are usually flat (Fig. 14-23), but a lichenified epidermis may overlie the lesions. The grouped petechiae are oval and may begin unilaterally,[58] but progress to become symmetric (Fig. 14-24). The lower extremities are most commonly involved, with more lesions in dependent areas.[56,57] Lesions may progress to involve the entire trunk and upper extremities. Itching is usually mild or absent, and no systemic symptoms are associated with chronic pigmented purpura. Spontaneous remission occurs within 1 to 2 years, but the natural course of the disease is not well documented.

Differential diagnosis

The lesions of grouped petechiae of multiple ages is so characteristic that this type of purpura is seldom

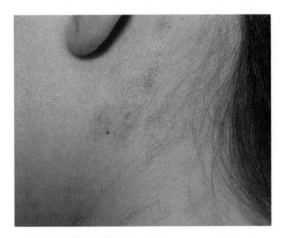

Fig. 14-22
Golden-brown and cayenne-pepper macules on the neck of a child with progressive pigmentary purpura.

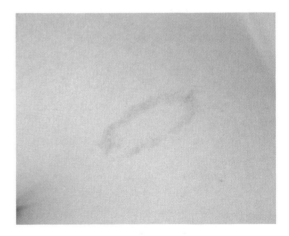

Fig. 14-23
Annular pigmented macules in progressive pigmentary purpura.

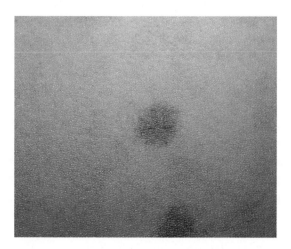

Fig. 14-24
Pigmented macule in progressive pigmentary purpura.

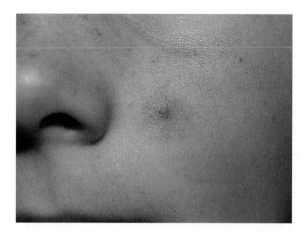

Fig. 14-25
Vascular spider with prominent central feeding vessel on the cheek of a child.

confused with other disorders. Occasionally trauma (e.g., child abuse) or a mild bleeding disorder is suspected.

Pathogenesis
A mild capillaritis is seen in these disorders, with extravasation of red blood cells, hemosiderin deposits, and a mild perivascular lymphocytic infiltration of superficial dermal blood vessels.[59] The vascular injury is mild, and its cause is unknown.

Treatment
There is no specific therapy. Reduction of venous stasis may be helpful.

Patient education
The expected remission and the mild nature of this disorder should be emphasized.

Follow-up visits
Follow-up visits are unnecessary.

Spider angioma (nevus araneus)
Clinical features
A spider nevus is a small, telangiectatic lesion consisting of a central arteriole from which superficial blood vessels radiate peripherally (Fig. 14-25). They usual-

ly appear between ages 2 and 6 years and are located in sun-exposed areas, usually on the cheeks, nose, dorsa of the hands, and forearms.[60] Sometimes the central arteriole is prominent and may be pulsatile on diascopy. Approximately 40% of light-skinned children will have these lesions.

Differential diagnosis
Spider angiomas must be differentiated from the telangiectatic mats of the autosomal dominant Osler-Weber-Rendu syndrome, in which confluent telangiectasia compose each lesion and multiple lesions are seen over the dorsum of the hands, lips, and face. Associated epistaxis, or peptic ulcer–like symptoms, or both may be important systemic symptoms to help differentiate the two conditions. Spider angiomas may be confused with the telangiectatic mats seen in collagen vascular diseases such as scleroderma and lupus erythematosus.

Pathogenesis
The cause of these lesions is unknown.

Treatment
If the cosmetic appearance is a concern to the child, lesions may be removed without scarring using the pulsed dye laser at 585 nm.[60]

Patient education
The common and nonserious nature of these lesions should be emphasized.

Follow-up visits
Follow-up visits are unnecessary.

Cherry angiomas and diffuse angiokeratomas
Clinical features
True cherry angiomas are rare in childhood and usually appear as 1- to 3-mm solid-red, dome-shaped, blanching papules (Fig. 14-26). The appearance of multiple cherry angiomas around the umbilicus and scrotum, which increases progressively with age, should bring to mind two diagnoses: Fabry's disease and α-fucosidosis. In Fabry's disease, attacks of pain, numbness, and tingling of the hands and feet often accompany the eruption. The usual onset of the eruption is between 4 and 12 years of age. In α-fucosidosis, severe mental retardation and neuromuscular spasticity accompany the disorder. Localized angiokeratomas are discussed in Chapter 13.

Differential diagnosis
Cherry angiomas and angiokeratomas must be differentiated from small pyogenic granulomas and small superficial hemangiomas. Usually the differentiation is quite simple. Cherry angiomas are small (2 to 5 mm) and dome-shaped with a normal epithelium over them. Pyogenic granulomas (see Chapter 12) have a friable and often crusted surface. When they first appear, angiokeratomas have a smooth surface but later will develop a rough scaly surface.

Pathogenesis
Fabry's disease is an X-linked recessive disorder in which activity of a specific lysosomal hydrolase, α-galactosidase A, is deficient.[52] The glycosphingolipid, ceramide trihexoside, accumulates within endothelial cells and produces the cutaneous vascular lesions. Rearrangements or point mutations in the gene encoding α-galactosidase have been found.[52] On electron microscopy the endothelial cells of the affected vessels are shown to contain multiple laminated inclusions diagnostic of the disease. In α-fucosidosis the lysosomes of the endothelial cells are widely dilated, but the material is washed out during fixation so the cells appear empty. Fibroblast culture and analysis of α-galactosidase A activity may be performed to confirm the diagnosis of Fabry's disease. In α-fucosidosis, an autosomal recessive trait, fibroblast cultures may also be useful in confirming the diagnosis.

Treatment
There is no effective treatment for either Fabry's disease or α-fucosidosis. Renal transplantation has resulted in improvement in some patients with Fabry's disease. Angiokeratomas and cherry angiomas may be easily treated with the pulsed dye laser at 585 nm, if desired.[60]

Patient education
The patient should be informed about the seriousness of each of these conditions and referred for genetic counseling. They should be advised that prenatal diagnosis is possible for future pregnancies, and that molecular probes are available to screen carrier females.[62] Pediatric neurologic care is usually advisable. Since the condition of patients with Fabry's disease progresses to severe renal disease, and they may succumb to renal failure, evaluation of renal function with appropriate consultation should be recommended to the parents.

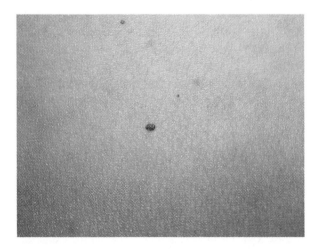

Fig. 14-26
Cherry angioma on the trunk of a child.

Follow-up visits

Follow-up visits should be arranged with the appropriate pediatric care specialists.

References

1. Ghosh S, Kanwar AJ, Kaur S: Urticaria in children, *Pediatr Dermatol* 10:107, 1993.

2. Legrain V, Taieb A, Sagi T, et al: Urticaria in infants: a study of forty patients, *Pediatr Dermatol* 7:101, 1990.

3. Aoki T, Kojima M, Horiko T: Acute urticaria: history and natural course of 50 cases, *J Dermatol* 21:73, 1994.

4. Quaranta J, Rohr AS, Rachelefsky GS, et al: The etiology and natural history of chronic urticaria and angioedema, *J Allergy Clin Immunol* 79:182, 1987.

5. Aberg N, Engstrom I, Lindberg U: Allergic diseases in Swedish school children, *Acta Paediatr Scand* 78:246, 1989.

6. Schuller DE, Elvey SM: Urticaria with streptococcal infection, *Pediatrics* 65:592, 1980.

7. Janniger CK, Schutzer SE, Schwartz RA: Childhood insect bite reactions to ants, wasps, and bees, *Cutis* 54:14, 1994.

8. Lowery N, Kerans GL, Young RA, et al: Serum sickness-like reaction associated with cefprozil therapy, *J Pediatr* 125:325, 1994

9. Weston JA, Weston WL: The overdiagnosis of erythema multiforme, *Pediatrics* 89:802, 1992.

10. Ruddy S: Hereditary angioedema. Undersuspected, underdiagnosed, *Hosp Pract* 8:91, 1988.

11. Perkins W, Stables GI, Lever RS: Protein S deficiency in lupus erythematosus secondary to hereditary angioedema, *Br J Dermatol* 130:381, 1994.

12. Zuberbier T, Althaus C, Chantraine-Hess S, et al: Prevalence of cholinergic urticaria in young adults, *J Am Acad Dermatol* 31:978, 1994.

13. Breathnach SM, Allen R, Milford Ward A, et al: Symptomatic dermatographism: natural history, clinical features, laboratory investigation and response to therapy, *Clin Exp Dermatol* 8:463, 1983.

14. Casale TB, Sampson HA, Hanifin J, et al: Guide to the physical urticarias, *J Allerg Clin Immunol* 82:758, 1988.

15. Lawlor F, Black AK, Ward AM, et al: Delayed pressure urticaria; objective evaluation of a variable disease using a dermographometer and assessment of treatment using colchicine, *Br J Dermatol* 120:403, 1989.

16. Sharpe GR, Shuster S: In dermographic urticaria H_2 receptor antagonists have a small but therapeutically irrelevant additional effect compared with H_1 antagonists alone, *Br J Dermatol* 129:575, 1993.

17. Sharpe GR, Shuster S: The effect of cetirizine on symptoms and wealing in dermographic urticaria, *Br J Dermatol* 129:580, 1993.

18. Husz S, Toth-Kasa J, Kiss M, et al: Treatment of cold urticaria, *Int J Dermatol* 33:210, 1994.

19. Martini A, Ravelli A, Albani S, et al: Hypocomplementemic urticarial vasculitis with severe systemic manifestations, *J Pediatr* 124:742, 1994.

20. Kettlehut BV, Metcalfe DD: Pediatric mastocytosis, *Ann Allergy* 73:197, 1994.

21. Azana JM, Torrelo A, Mediero IG, et al: Urticaria pigmentosa: a review of 67 pediatric cases, *Pediatr Dermatol* 11:102, 1994.

22. Olgun N, Oren H, Irken G, et al: Diffuse erythrodermic cutaneous mastocytosis with bone marrow infiltration, *Dermatology* 187:127, 1993.

23. Longley J: Is mastocytosis a mast cell neoplasia or a reactive hyperplasia? Clues from the study of mast cell growth factor, *Ann Med* 26:115, 1994.

24. Smith MB, Orton P, Chu H, et al: Photochemotherapy of dominant diffuse cutaneous mastocytosis, *Pediatr Dermatol* 7:251, 1990.

25. Helm TN, Bass J, Chang LW, et al: Persistent annular erythema of infancy, *Pediatr Dermatol* 10:46, 1993.

26. Katayama I, Yamamoto T, Otoyama K, et al: Clinical and immunological analysis of annular erythema associated with Sjögren's syndrome, *Dermatology* 189 (suppl) 1:14, 1994.

27. Bisno AL, Shulman ST, Dajani AS: The rise and fall (and rise?) of rheumatic fever, *JAMA* 259:728, 1988.

28. Suarez SM, Paller AS: Plantar erythema nodosum: cases in two children, *Arch Dermatol* 129:1064, 1993.

29. Ozols II, Wheat LJ: Erythema nodosum in an epidemic of histoplasmosis in Indianapolis, *Arch Dermatol* 117:709, 1981.

30. Akdis AC, Kilicturgay K, Helvaci S, et al: Immunological evaluation of erythema nodosum in tularemia, *Br J Dermatol* 129:275, 1993.

31. Sanz Vico MD, De Diego V, Sanchez Yus E: Erythema nodosum versus nodular vasculitis, *Int J Dermatol* 32: 108, 1993.

32. Kozma C, Gabriel S: Gustatory flushing syndrome. A pediatric case report and review of the literature, *Clin Pediatr* 32:629, 1993.

33. Schuen WD: Recognizing the signs and symptoms of the auriculotemporal syndrome, *Cutis* 7:37, 1994.

34. Beck SZ: Auriculotemporal syndrome seen clinically as food allergy, *Pediatrics* 83:601, 1989.

35. Raimer SS, Sanchez RL: Vasculitis in children, *Semin Dermatol* 11:46, 1992.

36. Dillon MJ: Diagnosis and management of vasculitides in childhood, *Br J Rheumatol* 33:187, 1993.

37. Szer IS: Henoch-Schönlein purpura, *Curr Opin Rheumatol* 6:25, 1994.

38. Wyatt RJ: The complement system in IgA nephropathy and Henoch-Schoenlein purpura: functional and genetic aspects, *Contrib Nephrol* 104:82, 1993.

39. Tuysuz B, Ozlu I, Aji DY, et al: Prognostic factors in meningococcal disease and a new scoring system, *Acta Paediatr* 82:1053, 1993.

40. Ilowite NT: Childhood systemic lupus erythematosus, dermatomyositis, scleroderma and systemic vasculitis, *Curr Opin Rheumatol* 5:644, 1993.

41. Goecken JA: Antineutrophil cytoplasmic and anti-endothelial cell antibodies: new mechanisms for vasculitis, *Curr Opin Dermatol* 1:75, 1995.

42. Finkel TH, Torok TJ, Ferguson PJ, et al: Chronic parvovirus B19 infection and systemic necrotizing vasculitis: opportunistic infection or causative agent? *Lancet* 343:1255, 1994.

43. Ozen S, Besbas N, Saatci U, et al: Diagnostic criteria for polyarteritis nodosa in childhood, *J Pediatr* 12:206, 1992.

44. Jones SK, Lane AL, Golitz LE, et al: Cutaneous periarteritis nodosa in childhood, *Am J Dis Child* 139:920, 1985.

45. Matsumoto T, Homma S, Okada M, et al: The lung in polyarteritis nodosa, *Hum Pathol* 24:717, 1993.

46. Draalsma JM, Fiseller JW, Mullaart RA: Mononeuritis multiplex in a child with cutaneous polyarteritis, *Neuropediatrics* 23:28, 1992.

47. Stone MS, Olson RR, Weisman DN, et al: Cutaneous vasculitis in the newborn of a mother with cutaneous polyarteritis nodosa, *J Am Acad Dermatol* 28:101, 1993.

48. Fink CW: The role of streptococcus in post-streptococcal reactive arthritis and childhood polyarteritis nodosa, *J Rheumatol* 29(suppl)18:14, 1991.

49. Jorizzo JL, White WL, Wise CM, et al: Low-dose weekly methotrexate for unusual neutrophilic vascular reactions: cutaneous polyarteritis nodosa and Behçet's disease, *J Am Acad Dermatol* 24:973, 1991.

50. Goette DK: Chilblains (perniosis), *J Am Acad Dermatol* 23:257, 1990.

51. White KP, Rothe MJ, Milanese A, et al: Perniosis in association with anorexia nervosa, *Pediatr Dermatol* 11:1, 1994.

52. Auletta MJ, Headington JT: Purpura fulminans: a cutaneous manifestation of severe Protein C deficiency, *Arch Dermatol* 124:1387, 1988.

53. Powars D, Larsen R, Johnson J, et al: Epidemic meningococcemia and purpura fulminans with induced protein C deficiency, *Clin Infect Dis.* 17:254, 1993.

54. Carson WT, Dickerman JD, Bovill EG, et al: Severe acquired Protein C deficiency in purpura fulminans associated with disseminated intravascular coagulation. Treatment with protein C concentrate, *Pediatrics* 91:418, 1993.

55. Chasen PE, Hansbrough JF, Cooper ML: Management of cutaneous manifestations of extensive purpura fulminans in a burn unit, *J Burn Care Rehabil* 13:410, 1992.

56. Ratnam KV, Su WD, Peters MS: Purpura simplex (inflammatory purpura without vasculitis): a clinicopathologic study of 174 cases, *J Am Acad Dermatol* 25:642, 1991.

57. Petruzzellis V: Idiopathic chronic pigmentary purpura: findings in 22 cases and proposal of a new classification, *VSA* 23:114, 1994.

58. Riordan CA: Unilateral linear capillaritis, *Clin Exp Dermatol* 17:182, 1992.

59. Simon M Jr., Heese A, Gotz A: Immunopathological investigations in purpura pigmentosa chronica, *Acta Derm Venereol (Stockh)* 69:101, 1989.

60. Tan OT, Kurban AK: *Noncongenital benign cutaneous vascular lesions: pulsed dye laser treatment.* In Tan OT, editor: *Management of benign cutaneous vascular lesions,* Philadelphia, 1992, p 158.

61. Bernstein HS, Bishop DF, Astrin CH, et al: Fabry's disease: six gene rearrangements and an exonic point mutation in the α-galactosidase gene, *J Clin Invest* 83:1390, 1989.

15

Hair Disorders

Children more commonly seek medical attention because of hair loss, rather than for excessive hair. This chapter is divided into two sections: hair loss and excessive hair.

HAIR LOSS

When evaluating hair loss in children, one should determine whether it is congenital or acquired, circumscribed or diffuse. This results in four diagnostic categories of hair loss (see Box 15-1). Hair loss (alopecia) accounts for approximately 3% of children's visits to a dermatologist. It causes the parents and the child considerable anxiety and the health team considerable frustration. Three types among the numerous causes of hair loss in children account for the great majority of health visits for alopecia: alopecia areata, tinea capitis (see Chapter 6), and traumatic alopecia. All three are forms of acquired, circumscribed hair loss (see Box 15-2). These three conditions should always be considered in the differential diagnosis of hair loss.

Alopecia areata
Clinical features
Alopecia areata is characterized by complete or almost complete hair loss in circumscribed areas (Fig. 15-1). Usually from one to three areas are involved. It is most commonly seen (in 90% of patients) in the frontal or parietal scalp, but body hair, sexual hair, eyelashes, and eyebrows may be involved. The appearance of a circumscribed area that is completely devoid of hair without any scalp change is a constant feature. Scalp erythema or scaling may occur in alopecia areata following sunburn. A positive family history for alopecia areata is found in 10% to 20% of the patients.

Nail disease occurs in 46% of children with alopecia areata.[1] Nail pitting is the most common change and appears as shallow, wide (1 to 2 mm) depressions in the nail plate. The pits are wider than those seen in psoriasis (Fig. 15-2).

The prognosis for most children is excellent. Complete regrowth of the hair occurs within a year in 95% of children with alopecia areata. Spontaneous remission is the rule. Approximately 30% will have a future episode of alopecia areata.

> **Box 15-1   Diagnostic categories of hair loss in children**
>
> Congenital circumscribed alopecia
> Acquired circumscribed alopecia
> Congenital diffuse alopecia
> Acquired diffuse alopecia

> **Box 15-2   Major types of acquired, circumscribed alopecia in childhood**
>
> Alopecia areata
> Tinea capitis
> Traction alopecia (including trichotillomania)

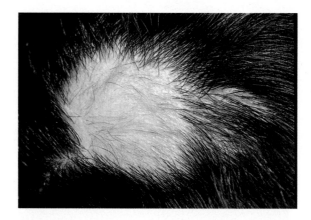

Fig. 15-1
Alopecia areata. Circumscribed patch of completely bald scalp.

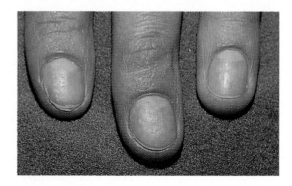

Fig. 15-2
Nail pitting in a child with alopecia areata.

Ophiasis, an unusual subtype involving less than 5% of all patients with alopecia areata, begins in the occiput or along the frontal scalp (Fig. 15-3) and spreads, with many patches of alopecia along the hair margins. Ophiasis is likely to eventuate in loss of all the scalp hair (alopecia totalis) (Fig. 15-4) or all the scalp and body hair (alopecia universalis). When this occurs, the prognosis for regrowth is extremely poor.

Differential diagnosis

Trichotillomania or other forms of traction alopecia may mimic alopecia areata. Broken-off hairs, scalp petechiae, and a history of trauma are features that help distinguish these conditions. Tinea capitis, particularly the black-dot form, may be confused with alopecia areata. Careful examination of the scalp will reveal broken-off hairs within the follicle, and microscopic examination of these hairs in potassium hydroxide (KOH) 10% will reveal hyphae within the hair shaft. A fungal culture will help confirm the diagnosis. Much has been made of the importance of exclamation point hairs in the differential diagnosis of circumscribed hair loss, but this change is not specific.[2] Although a scalp biopsy may be helpful in difficult cases, it is only rarely necessary.

The scarring alopecias may present circumscribed areas of hair loss, but the scalp thickening and color change seen in these conditions will help distinguish them from alopecia areata.

Circumscribed alopecia may be congenital and present from birth. It is characteristic of certain birthmarks in the scalp, particularly sebaceous nevus and aplasia cutis congenita. These alopecias are usually not difficult to differentiate from alopecia areata. The history of onset at birth, and the yellow plaques or scarred areas in the scalp, will differentiate congenital circumscribed alopecias from alopecia areata.

Pathogenesis

It has been presumed that alopecia areata represents an immune mechanism, since a dense perifollicular

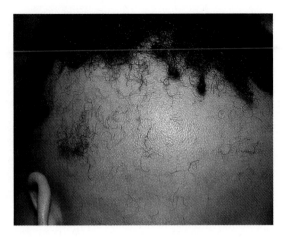

Fig. 15-3
Ophiasis pattern of alopecia areata, with hair loss starting in occiput.

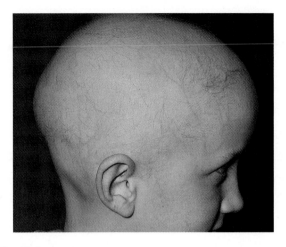

Fig. 15-4
Alopecia totalis. Ophiasis progressing to a completely bald scalp.

accumulation of lymphocytes precedes the hair loss. The exact mechanism of hair loss is not understood, but direct lymphocyte injury to the hair matrix has been postulated, and 100% of alopecia areata patients compared with 44% of controls have autoantibodies to as yet unidentified hair follicle antigens.[3]

The injury to the growing hair results in premature conversion of growing hairs to resting hairs that are shed. Evaluation of clinically normal scalp hairs to determine the anagen (growing) to telogen (resting) ratio can be used to predict the likelihood of short-term hair regrowth.[4]

Treatment

There is no reliable treatment for alopecia areata. Since spontaneous regrowth occurs in 95% of cases, the prognosis is good in most patients. Many forms of local therapy, including intralesional or superpotent topical steroids, anthralin, minoxidil, contact sensitizers, and combinations of the above, have demonstrated short-term hair regrowth, but they do not alter the long-term course of alopecia areata.[5-8] The administration of systemic glucocorticosteroids or cyclosporine has been advocated for their antiinflammatory effect. However, the suppression of inflammation and hair regrowth is temporary and variable. Withdrawal of steroids or cyclosporine results in prompt loss of

the hair that has grown back. Thus the risks of side effects outweigh the benefits of temporary hair growth.

In complete hair loss, referral to a dermatologist may be useful, and prompt attention should be given to obtaining a wig for the child. Excellent children's wigs are manufactured, and a physician's prescription may allow the family to obtain a wig at reduced prices. A support group, the National Alopecia Areata Foundation, has a number of North American chapters that provide excellent psychological support and the latest treatment information for persons with alopecia areata.

Patient education

Parents should be informed that there is no reliable treatment of alopecia areata. However, in children with the usual type of alopecia areata, with one to three circumscribed patches of complete scalp hair loss, it is important to emphasize the excellent prognosis even without treatment. Explaining the proposed mechanism of the disease, and the excellent chances for spontaneous recovery, will greatly aid understanding of the problem. Ophiasis patients should be told of the poor prognosis. Considerable effort should be devoted at the first visit to answering questions for the child and the family. The risks and benefits of all current therapy should be explained in detail, and the psychological benefits of wearing a wig should be discussed.

Patients should be informed about the National Alopecia Areata Foundation, 710 C Street, Suite 11, San Rafael, CA 94901.

Follow-up visits

In the usual type of alopecia areata, a visit every 3 months is useful to check on progress and the chances for spontaneous regression.

In the ophiasis type, a visit in 2 weeks to reexplain the illness and encourage the use of a wig is most helpful. Frequent visits may be necessary to establish the proper physician-patient relationship.

Tinea capitis

Tinea capitis is a major cause of acquired, circumscribed hair loss in children. It is covered in detail in Chapter 6.

Traumatic alopecia

Traumatic alopecia results from hair injury produced by traction, friction, chemical, or other injury to hair. The common types seen in childhood include trichotillomania (hair pulling) and the traction alopecia seen with various popular hairstyles.

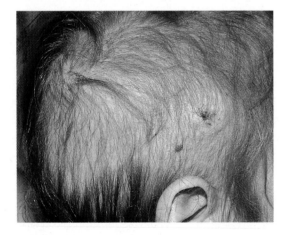

Fig. 15-5
Trichotillomania. Hair broken at many different lengths associated with scalp excoriations.

Trichotillomania
Clinical features

Circumscribed areas of hair loss with irregular borders and hairs broken off at different lengths are seen in trichotillomania (Fig. 15-5). Frequently scalp excoriations and perifollicular petechiae are present (Fig. 15-5). Commonly, only one area of the scalp is involved, with the frontoparietal and frontotemporal scalp being the most usual sites. Rarely, the eyebrows or eyelashes (Fig. 15-6) may be plucked. The estimated lifetime prevalence is 0.5% to 1% or higher, with the majority of patients exhibiting onset of trichotillomania before the age of 18 years.[9] The mean age of onset is 8 years for males and 12 years for females.[10] The condition is more common in females but is not rare in males.[10] Children with trichotillomania may exhibit personality disorders, including obsessive-compulsive behavior. In a study of 48 females with trichotillomania, 42% exhibited personality disorders, but there were no particular personality disorders that separated this group from controls.[11] In emotionally disturbed children extensive areas of the scalp may be involved.

Differential diagnosis

The diseases considered in the differential diagnosis of trichotillomania are the same as those for alopecia areata and tinea capitis (see Box 15-2). One should

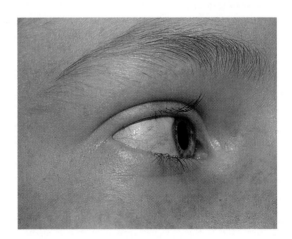

Fig. 15-6
Trichotillomania of the eyelashes.

also consider the possibility that someone other than the affected child, such as a sibling, playmate, parent, or baby-sitter, is doing the hair pulling.

Pathogenesis

Traumatic events, such as the death of a family member or close friend, separation or divorce of parents, or difficulties in school, precipitate trichotillomania in 5% to 10% of cases.[10] Otherwise, trichotillomania is associated with a large variety of psychiatric diagnoses and symptoms. Some authorites believe that trichotillomania should not be considered a specific disease, but that it is a symptom with many different psychiatric origins and meanings.[10] Parents often vehemently deny such hair pulling, since they have not personally observed it.

Treatment

The search for antecedent traumatic events is helpful. In children in whom a precipitating event can be identified, relief of stress will result in ending the nervous habit. Application of oils to the hair makes it more difficult to pull. Psychodynamic therapy, chemical treatments with antidepressants, and behavior modification have all been used to treat trichotillomania. However, it is difficult to evaluate which therapy is most effective and which patients will benefit most from whatever form of therapy is chosen. Some children persist with trichotillomania into adult life. In severe forms that are associated with other signs of emotional stress, psychiatric referral may be indicated.

Patient education

A careful search for a precipitating event, and an explanation of the complex nature of the process, are crucial to patient and parent education. One should avoid blaming the child or one or more family members. If a precipitating event can be identified, suggest that remedying the circumstances surrounding that event will likely lead to cessation of the hair pulling. If no precipitating event can be demonstrated, explain that this habit is often a difficult one to break. Emphasize that hair pulling may just be a nervous habit; however, it may be a sign of significant stress or

other emotional problems, and if the child is having other psychosocial difficulties, counseling may be useful.

Follow-up visits

A follow-up visit in 1 to 2 months is useful in evaluating progress. Continued reassurance should be given. If the problem persists, referral to a child psychologist or psychiatrist is indicated.

Traction alopecia

Clinical features

Thinning of hair in particular areas of the scalp may result from constant traction or friction. Very few fractured hairs are found in the involved areas, although the hairs may be smaller in diameter than those found in adjacent areas (Fig. 15-7). The thinning is often patchy, depending on the nature of the trauma. The history of methods of hair care and types of hairstyle is crucial for the diagnosis.

Differential diagnosis

The differential diagnosis is the same as for alopecia areata and tinea capitis (see Box 15-2).

Pathogenesis

Several different sources of traction or friction have been identified as responsible for traction alopecia.

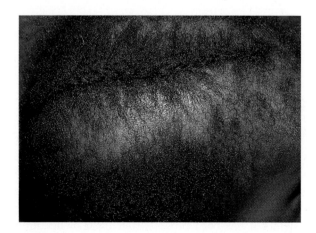

Fig. 15-7
Traction alopecia. Hair loss due to tight braiding.

The hairstyle or chemical or thermal treatment or friction produces incomplete and complete fractures of hair. One should always consider child abuse (e.g., pulling the child by the hair). Neonatal occipital alopecia is physiologic hair loss exacerbated by the rubbing of the baby's head on the sheet or mattress. Massage alopecia may occur from vigorous scalp massage and frequent shampooing. Marginal alopecia is seen with hair straightening or tight hair curlers. Cornrow alopecia, ponytail alopecia, and braid alopecia are all related to tight hairstyles. Hot-comb alopecia occurs on the vertex of the scalp and may involve scarring. It is the result of use of a hot comb to straighten or style hair. Marginal alopecia is sometimes seen in hot-comb alopecia.

Treatment

Discontinuation of the trauma to the hair is the obvious treatment of choice. The use of mild shampoos and wide-toothed combs with rounded ends, infrequent shampooing, and gentle brushing are all important components of therapy. Recovery may take 3 to 6 months.

Patient education

The susceptibility of certain hair types to such trauma should be explained and the benefits of being gentle with the hair emphasized.

Follow-up visits

A follow-up visit in 3 to 6 months is useful to assess hair regrowth.

OTHER FORMS OF HAIR LOSS

The remaining types of hair loss are uncommon or rare. No attempt is made to consider these numerous conditions in detail, but an orderly approach to them is presented. One should first determine whether the hair loss is circumscribed or diffuse, then determine whether it has been present from birth or acquired later in life. This results in four diagnostic categories: congenital circumscribed alopecia, acquired circumscribed alopecia, congenital diffuse alopecia, and acquired diffuse alopecia (see Box 15-1). In congenital diffuse alopecia, a further diagnostic step, the hair mount examination, is necessary. Only the general clinical features of each group and the differential diagnoses are given. Telogen effluvium is discussed in more detail later in this chapter.

The mechanisms of hair loss in most of these unusual forms of alopecia have not been uncovered. However, certain associations are of therapeutic importance. An extraordinary number of clinical conditions are associated with hair loss, and one should characterize hair loss into one of the preceding four types to permit proper diagnosis and therapy.

Congenital circumscribed alopecia
Clinical features

Localized areas of scalp hair loss present from birth usually overlie a birthmark, such as a sebaceous or epidermal nevus. The scalp surface is smooth, particularly in newborns or infants with circumscribed hair loss, and yellow to tan (Fig. 15-8). As the child gets older, a plaque is noted. A congenital circumscribed alopecia may also occur in aplasia cutis congenita (Fig. 15-9). Aplasia cutis congenita occurs most commonly as an isolated defect, but it may be associated with other malformations or genetic syndromes.[12]

Differential diagnosis

A scalp biopsy will help to identify and characterize these birthmarks, which represent hyperplasia of epidermal cells or sebaceous structures. Aplasia cutis congenita demonstrates scarring of the scalp in a circumscribed area and represents failure of formation of one or more layers of the scalp. In the other rare forms, circumscribed patches of hair loss without scalp changes are present. The differential diagnosis of this type of alopecia is given in Box 15-3.

Acquired circumscribed alopecia: scarring forms
Clinical features

Circumscribed hair loss acquired during childhood, other than alopecia areata, tinea capitis, and traction

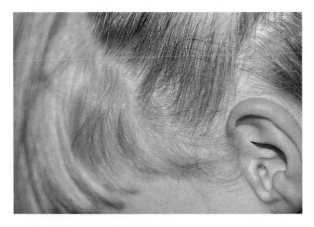

Fig. 15-8
Nevus sebaceous. Absence of hair in the area of yellow-orange plaque of a birthmark.

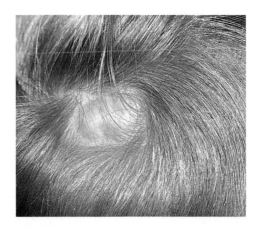

Fig. 15-9
Localized scarring of the scalp in aplasia cutis congenita.

Box 15-3   Differential diagnosis of congenital circumscribed hair loss

Birthmarks
Sebaceous nevus
Epidermal nevus
Hair follicle hamartomas
Aplasia cutis congenita (scarlike)
Conradi's disease
Incontinentia pigmenti
Sutural alopecia in Hallermann-Streiff syndrome
Triangular alopecia of the frontal scalp

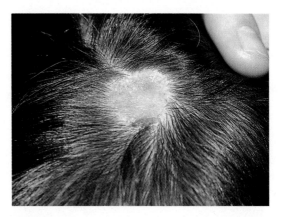

Fig. 15-10
Aquired circumscribed inflammatory scarring alopecia.

alopecia, is usually scarring in nature (Fig. 15-10)—that is, the hair follicles are replaced by fibrous tissue following injury to the hair follicles after infection, trauma, or inflammatory skin disease.

Differential diagnosis
Box 15-4 presents the conditions to be considered in the differential diagnosis.

Congenital diffuse alopecia
Clinical features
Diffuse scalp hair loss present from birth usually results in the complaint that the child's hair simply will not grow. Such children never require haircuts. Included in this group are hair shaft defects in which the failure of hair growth is the result of structural defects that cause the breaking off of hairs[13] (Figs. 15-11 through 15-16). The child has short, broken hairs of equal length. In many forms of ectodermal dysplasia, reduced numbers or absence of hair follicles produce the clinical picture of congenital diffuse alopecia (Fig. 15-17).

Differential diagnosis
Removing hairs and placing them on a microscope slide with mounting fluid will allow demonstration of

Box 15-4 Differential diagnosis of acquired, scarring, circumscribed hair loss

Postinfectious
   Kerion due to tinea capitis
   Pyoderma
   Varicella
Postinflammatory
   Lichen planus
   Lupus erythematosus
   Darier's disease
   Porokeratosis of Mibelli
Postinjury
   Physical trauma (abrasions, cuts)
   Chemical or thermal burns
   Radiation injury

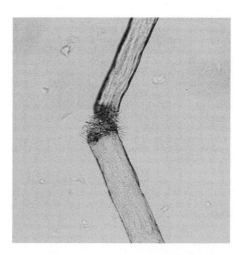

Fig. 15-12
Photomicrograph of hair mount demonstrates broomstick fracture of trichorrhexis nodosa.

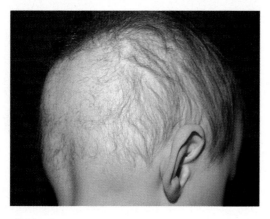

Fig. 15-11
Three-year-old male with congenital trichorrhexis nodosa.

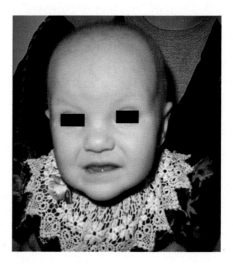

Fig. 15-13
Two-year-old female with monilethrix.

the particular type of structural hair defect. Many rare forms of diffuse congenital hair loss are associated with syndromes, and complete examination of the child is necessary for accurate diagnosis. The differential diagnosis of this type of hair loss is given in Box 15-5.

Acquired diffuse alopecia

Hair loss with onset in childhood after a period of normal hair growth usually results from an underlying systemic disorder. In these children a careful search for endocrine, metabolic, and chemical abnormalities is warranted (see Box 15-6). A rigorous and detailed history should be taken and appropriate laboratory studies ordered if the clinical data so indicate. Since most of the endocrine, metabolic, and nutritional causes are correctable, one should consider undertaking a thorough laboratory evaluation in such children.

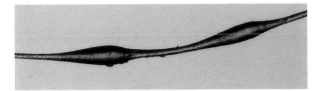

Fig. 15-14
Photomicrograph of hair mount demonstrates beading of the hair in monilethrix.

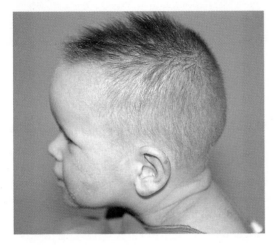

Fig. 15-15
Child suffering from trichorrhexis invaginata in Netherton's syndrome.

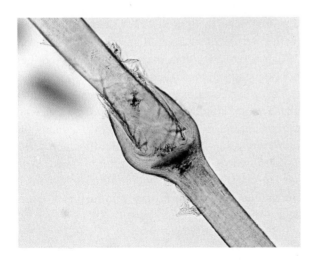

Fig. 15-16
Photomicrograph of hair mount demonstrates bamboo hair in trichorrhexis nodosa.

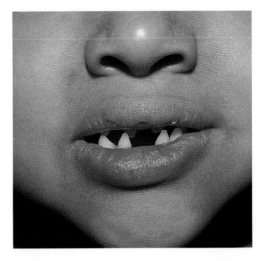

Fig. 15-17
Cone-shaped teeth in a child with hypohidrotic ectodermal dysplasia.

Box 15-5   Differential diagnosis of congenital diffuse hair loss

Hair shaft defects
   Trichorrhexis nodosa (broomstick fractures)
      Familial form
      Argininosuccinic aciduria
   Pili torti (twisted hair)
      Classic form
      Menkes' syndrome
   Monilethrix (beaded hair)
   Trichorrhexis invaginata (bamboo hair)
      Netherton's syndrome
Congenital hypothyroidism ectodermal dysplasias
      Hidrotic ectodermal dysplasia
      Hypohidrotic ectodermal dysplasia
      Trichothiodystrophy
      Atrichia congenita
      Cartilage-hair hypoplasia
      Follicular atrophoderma
Progeria
Marinesco-Sjögren's syndrome

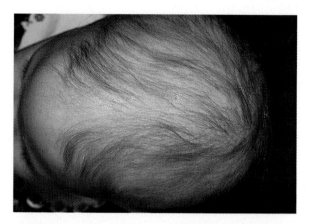

Fig. 15-18
Acquired diffuse nonscarring alopecia in telogen effluvium.

Box 15-6   Differential diagnosis of acquired diffuse hair loss

Endocrine
   Hypothyroidism
   Hypopituitarism
   Hypoparathyroidism
   Diabetes mellitus
   Androgenetic alopecia (male pattern) in
      adolescents
Chemical
   Thallium poisoning (rat poison)
   Antithyroid drugs
   Heparin
   Coumarin
   Antimetabolites (e.g., cyclophosphamide)
Nutritional
   Hypervitaminosis A
   Acrodermatitis enteropathica (zinc deficiency)
   Marasmus

Telogen effluvium

Telogen effluvium is the name given to the acquired diffuse alopecia that results from rapid conversion of scalp hairs from the growing state to the resting state[14] (Fig. 15-18). In physiologic circumstances an infant or child has 88% of scalp hair in a growing, or anagen, state and only 12% of hair in a resting, or telogen, state. Each individual scalp hair grows for 3 years, then regresses over 2 or 3 weeks, and rests for 3 months. This growth throughout the scalp is asynchronous in that the majority of hairs are growing at any time of observation. Acutely stressful events, such as birth, auto accidents, illnesses with high fever, and acute psychiatric problems, may result in a rapid conversion of growing hairs to resting hairs. Following the event by 2 to 4 months, the hairs are shed and usually continue to shed over 3 to 4 months. Each hair shed is a resting hair and will be replaced by a normal growing hair. In the newborn the hairs are shed in two phases from the frontal scalp to the occipital scalp and are not asynchronous in growth phase until about 12 months of age.

Diagnosis of telogen effluvium can be made by plucking at least 50 hairs from a child's scalp and examining the roots to determine whether they are growing or resting. This is best done by cutting away the remainder of the hairs and mounting the roots in a commercial slide-mounting medium. A growing, or anagen, hair will have a pigmented core and a bulbous root that is larger in diameter than the hair shaft. Often the external root sheath is present. In a telogen, or resting, hair, the external root sheath is absent or fragmented, pigment is often absent, and the root of the hair is narrower than the caliber of the other hair and frequently curved. One can reassure the patient with telogen effluvium that complete regrowth is possible. Telogen effluvium has been reported following surgery, crash diets, and the use of anticoagulants and antithyroid drugs. Anagen effluvium, in which growing hairs are lost, is an expected result of cancer treatment in children in which the antimetabolites interfere with hair growth or radiation to the head injures the growing hair.

EXCESSIVE HAIR

Excessive hair may be congenital or acquired.

Congenital hypertrichosis
Clinical features

Excessive hair may be generalized (hypertrichosis lanuginosa) or circumscribed (nevoid hypertrichosis). Excessive body hair in the newborn may be a transient problem, especially in premature infants, and resolves by 6 months of age, or may represent the rare hypertrichosis lanuginosa in which long, fine lanugo hairs cover the entire glabrous skin (Fig. 15-19). Hypertrichosis lanuginosa is thought to be autosomal dominant, but most cases are sporadic.[15] Congenital hypothyroidism may also demonstrate excessive body hair. Circumscribed hypertrichosis may be seen as one to six patches of excessive, long hair over various body regions. It is persistent.[16] Circumscribed hypertrichosis, when in the midline, may be associated with nervous system abnormalities. Hypertrichosis over the lumbosacral spine (the "human tail") may be a clue to spina bifida; over the occiput, to meningocele or encephalocele. Facial hypertrichosis may be seen in a number of syndromes listed in Box 15-7.

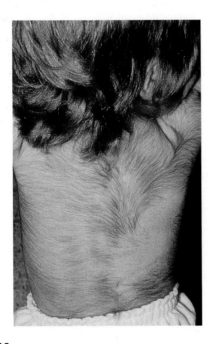

Fig. 15-19
Hypertrichosis lanuginosa.

Differential diagnosis

Circumscribed areas of hypertrichosis must be differentiated from congenital smooth muscle and pilar nevus and congenital pigmented nevi (see Box 15-8). Differentiating hypertrichosis lanuginosa from the transient lanugo overgrowth may be difficult in the first few months of life, although the body and facial hairs in hypertrichosis lanuginosa are longer, often reaching 2 inches in length.

Pathogenesis

In nevoid hypertrichosis, excessive numbers of hair follicles are found. In hypertrichosis lanuginosa, body hairs appear as terminal hairs. Endocrine evaluations are normal.

Treatment

There is no satisfactory treatment for either diffuse or circumscribed hypertrichosis. Cutting or shaving hair

---

Box 15-7   Syndromes with hypertrichosis

Cornelia de Lange's syndrome
Rubinstein-Taybi syndrome
Gingival hyperplasia with hypertrichosis
Winchester syndrome
Recessive dystrophic epidermolysis bullosa
Fetal hydantoin syndrome
Erythrohepatic porphyria

Box 15-8   Differential diagnosis of circumscribed congenital hypertrichosis

Congenital pigmented nevus
Pilar and smooth muscle hamartoma
Nevoid hypertrichosis
Midline nevoid hypertrichosis with spinal or
    central nervous system malformations

may be considered. Hair removal chemicals may be too irritating for the skin of an infant or child.

Patient education

In circumscribed hypertrichosis, an explanation of a malformation with excessive follicular structures in that segment of skin should be given. In hypertrichosis lanuginosa, genetic counseling may be useful.

Follow-up visits

Support and counseling are very useful for parents and children, and regularly scheduled visits are useful.

Acquired excessive hair (hirsutism)

Clinical features

Hirsutism is the growth of terminal hair in part or all of the male sexual pattern. It is observed predominantly in adolescent females. In Mediterranean races, females may have some male pattern hair, and it may be impossible to distinguish clinically from true hirsutism. Asian females, in contrast, have no racial pattern of hirsutism. Excessive facial hair in the beard or moustache area may or may not be accompanied by excessively long body hairs. Other features of virilization may be seen, such as increased muscle mass, clitoral hypertrophy, and deepening of the voice. A history of abnormal menses is often obtained.

Differential diagnosis

Racial forms that mimic hirsutism lack other signs of virilization, have female family members with similar

---

findings, and lack endocrine abnormalities (see Box 15-9). Porphyrias may have facial hirsutism, but have a history of photosensitivity and scars from previous skin lesions.

Pathogenesis

Hirsutism is androgen dependent, and a careful gynecologic and endocrine evaluation will detect underlying disease.[17,18] Hyperandrogenism should be considered in any female with hirsutism[19] (see Box 15-9). Normal testosterone production by the female is 50% adrenal and 50% ovarian. Although the skin does not produce androgens from cholesterol, it is capable of metabolizing weaker androgens to more potent androgens such as dihydrotestosterone. Most patients with moderate to severe hirsutism, and 50% of those with mild hirsutism, will demonstrate elevated levels of plasma free testosterone.[19]

Treatment

Screening evaluation for hyperandrogenism should include measurements of free testosterone, androstenedione, and dehydroepiandrosterone.[19] Treatment depends on the underlying endocrine abnormality and whether it is of ovarian or adrenal origin. Spironolactone is an effective treatment in some adolescent females with ovarian hyperandrogenism.

Patient education

It should be explained that hirsutism is just one feature of a endocrine disorder, and correcting the underlying endocrine disease is required.

Follow-up visits

Follow-up 2 weeks after gynecologic or endocrine consultation is obtained is useful.

Unmanageable hair

The uncombable hair syndrome, woolly hair, and woolly hair nevus result in hair that is difficult to comb. In the uncombable hair syndrome, an autosomal dominant condition, the entire scalp hair is blond

---

> **Box 15-9 Conditions resulting in hirsutism**
>
> Racial hirsutism
> Polycystic ovaries
> Ovarian tumors
> Congenital adrenal hyperplasia
> Cushing's syndrome
> Exogenous androgens

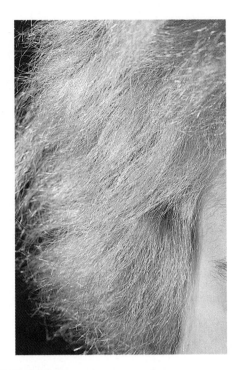

Fig. 15-20
Unmanageable hair.

or silvery and does not lay flat when combed (Fig. 15-20). Generalized woolly hair is tightly curled hair differing considerably from that of other family members. In woolly hair nevus there are one to three patches of scalp hair that are curly and coarse, different from the remaining hair.[20] Also, the cowlick of long, straight hairs over the scalp vertex is seen in 7% of children.

Scalp whorls

A single whorl in the parietal scalp is found in 98% of children. In 45% it is in the midline, in 40% to the right of midline, and to the left in the remainder. Abnormal locations of scalp whorls may be clues to central nervous system disease. For example, Down syndrome, trisomy 13, Prader-Willi syndrome, and Rubinstein-Taybi syndrome show anterior scalp whorls, while malformations of cranial bones often display widely spaced biparietal whorls.

References

1. Tosti A, Morelli R, Bardazzi F, Peluso AM: Prevalence of nail abnormalities in children with alopecia areata, *Pediatr Dermatol* 11:112, 1994.
2. Ihm CW, Han JH: Diagnostic value of exclamation point hairs, *Dermatology* 186:99, 1993.
3. Tobin DJ, Orentreich N, Fenton DA, Bystryn JC: Antibodies to hair follicles in alopecia areata, *J Invest Dermatol* 5:721, 1994.
4. Peereboom-Wynia JD, Beek CH, Mulder PG, Stolz E: The trichogram as a prognostic tool in alopecia areata, *Acta Derm Venereol* 73:280, 1993.
5. Orecchia G, Malagoli P, Santagostino L: Treatment of alopecia areata with squaric acid dibutylester in pediatric patients, *Pediatr Dermatol* 11:65, 1994.
6. Hull SM, Pepall L, Cunliffe WJ: Alopecia areata in children: response to treatment with diphencyprone, *Br J Dermatol* 125:164, 1991.
7. Fiedler VC, Wendrow A, Szpunar GJ, et al: Treatment-resistant alopecia areata. Response to combination therapy with minoxidil plus anthralin, *Arch Dermatol* 126:756, 1990.
8. Olsen EA, Carson SC, Turney EA: Systemic steroids with or without 2% topical minoxidil in the treatment of alopecia areata, *Arch Dermatol* 128:1467, 1992.
9. Christenson GA, Pyle RL, Mitchell JE: Estimated lifetime prevalence of trichotillomania in college students, *J Clin Psychiatry* 10:415, 1991.
10. Grabe J, Arndt WM: Trichotillomania, *Compr Psychiatry* 34:340, 1993.
11. Christenson GA, Chernoff-Clementz E, Clementz BA: Personality and clinical characteristics in patients with trichotillomania, *J Clin Psychiatry* 11:407, 1992.
12. Blunt K, Quan V, Carr D, Paes BA: Aplasia cutis congenita: a clinical review and associated defects, *Neonatal Netw* 11:17, 1992.
13. Price VH: *Structural abnormalities of the hair shaft.* In Orfanos C, Happle R, editors: *Hair and hair diseases,* 1990, Springer-Verlag.
14. Headington JT: Telogen effluvium. New concepts and review, *Arch Dermatol* 129:356, 1993.
15. Lee IJ, Im SB, Kim DK: Hypertrichosis universalis

congenita: a separate entity, or the same disease as gingival fibromatosis, *Pediatr Dermatol* 10:263, 1993.

16. Rupert LS, Bechtel M, Pellegrini A: Nevoid hypertrichosis: multiple patches associated with premature graying of lesional hair, *Pediatr Dermatol* 11:49, 1994.

17. Balducci R, Toscano V: Bioactive and peripheral androgens in prepubertal simple hypertrichosis. *Clin Endocrinol* 33:407, 1990.

18. Berta L, Fortunati N, Fazzari A, et al: Hormonal and clinic evaluation of patients with moderate body hair growth, *Contraception* 48:47, 1993.

19. Rosenfield RL, Lucky AW: Acne, hirsutism, and alopecia in adolescent girls, *Endocrinol Metab Clin North Am* 22:507, 1993.

20. Redo AR, Rogers RS, Peters MS: Woolly hair nevus, *J Am Acad Dermatol* 22:377, 1990.

16

Nail Disease

Nail disorders are uncommon in children. However, nail changes may be useful in the clinical identification of systemic disorders. Normal variations are important to recognize and distinguish from nail disease. Concave nail shapes are normal from birth to 3 years of age.[1] Normal nails may have a few small pits in the nail plate. Scattered white spots are common in the nail plate and are caused by minor trauma.[1,2] Longitudinal ridging is also common in normal nails and worsens with age.[1,2]

DISRUPTION OF THE NAIL SURFACE

Clinical features

Changes in the surface of the nail, including pitting, scaling, longitudinal ridging, transverse ridges, or splitting, occur in childhood[1,2] (Fig. 16-1). Pitting is predominantly seen in psoriasis and alopecia areata.[1-4] At least 50% of children with alopecia areata[1,2,4] will have pitting, whereas 15% of children with psoriasis may demonstrate pitting.[1-3] Pits are more numerous in alopecia areata, but it is often

difficult to distinguish between the nail pitting of alopecia areata and psoriasis. Roughening and splitting of the nail surface (trachyonychia) is seen in 20-nail dystrophy,[1,2,5,6] psoriasis,[1,2,3] alopecia areata,[1,2,4] lichen planus,[1,2,7] trauma[1,2,8] (Fig. 16-2), dermatitis of the digits,[1,2] and in some of the ectodermal dysplasias.[1,2] Transverse ridges (Beau's lines) are seen after a severe illness[1,2] or toxic event such as cancer chemotherapy[8] or from a nervous habit of nail-picking.[9] Multiple transverse ridges from repeated nail self-trauma (Fig. 16-3) may weaken the nail plate and lead to central splitting[1,2,9,10] (Fig. 16-4). This is particularly seen on the thumbnails of children and is associated with disruption of the cuticle.

Differential diagnosis

When a disturbance of the nail surface is seen, onychomycosis is often considered in the differential diagnosis. Onychomycosis is quite uncommon in children and usually affects nails by producing thickening as well as surface roughening.[1,2] A potassium hydroxide (KOH) examination and fungal culture will help differentiate.

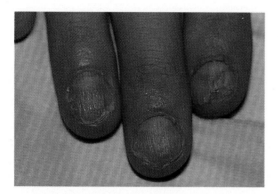

Fig. 16-1
Trachyonychia. Disruption of the nail surface.

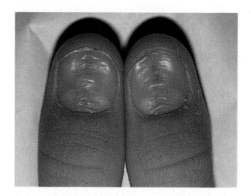

Fig. 16-3
Multiple medial transverse grooves from repeated self-trauma.

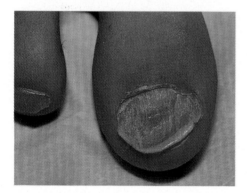

Fig. 16-2
Trachyonychia. Scaling and grooving of the nail in childhood 20-nail dystrophy.

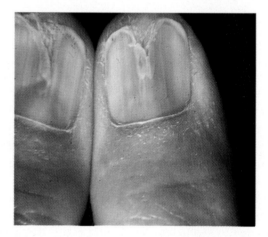

Fig. 16-4
Central splitting of the nail from repeated self-trauma.

Pathogenesis

Injury to the germinative cells of the nail is the cause of disturbances of the nail surface, whether from inflammation, trauma, toxins, or chemotherapeutic agents.

Treatment

Treatment is difficult. If trauma is identified, behavior modification may help. Recovery is likely from all causes.

Patient education

If self-trauma is the cause, open discussion with the patient regarding alternative habits is recommended. Reassurance that eventual recovery will occur should be given.

Follow-up visits

A follow-up visit in 4 to 6 weeks may be useful in determining the course of disease.

THICK NAILS

Clinical features

Nails thicken in proliferative epidermal disease. In psoriasis and lichen planus of children, all 20 nails may be involved.[1-4] In psoriasis, thickening begins distally and is associated with distal nail separation (onycholysis), giving a yellow color to the nails[1-3]

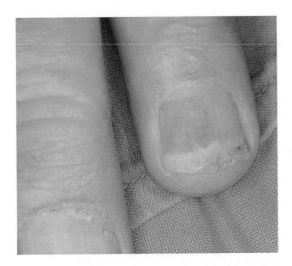

Fig. 16-5
Psoriasis of the nail. Yellowing within nail represents separation of the nail plate from the nail bed.

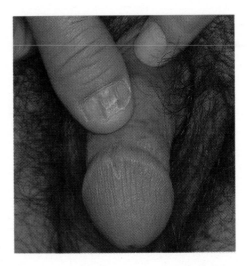

Fig. 16-7
Lichen planus of the nail. "Pincer" deformity with lichen planus lesion of the penis.

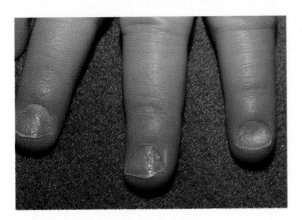

Fig. 16-6.
Nail pitting in a child with psoriasis.

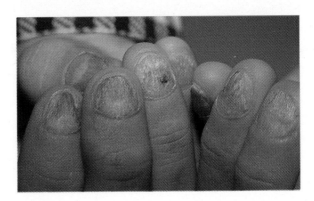

Fig. 16-8
Twenty-nail dystrophy. Exaggerated longitudinal ridging and rough surface of all 20 nails.

(Fig. 16-5). The entire nail plate may then be involved. Pitting of the nail surface also occurs (Fig. 16-6). In lichen planus there is thickening of the nails, with a pinched-up central ridge and synechia formation over the nail surface[1,2,4] (Fig. 16-7).

The so-called 20-nail dystrophy of childhood also presents with thickened nails with exaggerated longitudinal ridges (Fig. 16-8). At least in some children, this disease may be a hereditary disorder. Twenty-nail dystrophy may be the presenting sign of alopecia areata, lichen planus, or psoriasis. Long-term follow-up is required to determine the development of associated features.[1,2]

Psoriasis, lichen planus, and 20-nail dystrophy account for most cases of thick nails.[1-4] Nails may be thickened, shiny, and contain horizontal ridges in dermatitis that involves the hands and cuticular skin.[1,2] Pachyonychia congenita, an autosomal dominant disorder, presents with thickened nails at birth that will become more thickened by age 2 or 3

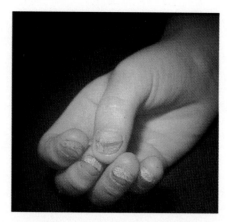

Fig. 16-9
Pachyonychia congenita type I. Distal thickening and elevation of the nails.

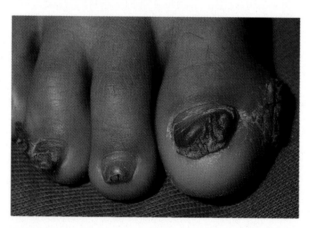

Fig. 16-10
Pachyonychia congenita type II. Distal thickening of the nails associated with painful circumscribed keratoses of the feet.

years (Fig. 16-9). Dermatophyte infections of the nail (onychomycosis) will also thicken the nails but are unusual in children with a prevalence of 0.2% and will usually involve only one or two nails[1,2] (Fig. 16-10).

Differential diagnosis

Conditions to be considered in the differential diagnosis of thick nails are listed in Box 16-1. Longitudinal nail biopsy may be useful in differenti-

---

> **Box 16-1   Differential diagnosis of thick nails**
>
> Psoriasis
> Lichen planus
> Onychomycosis
> Twenty-nail dystrophy
> Dermatitis
> Pachyonychia congenita
> Ectodermal dysplasia
> Palmoplantar keratodermas (Unna-Thost, mal de Meleda, Papillon-Lefèvre) focal dermal hypoplasia
> Dyskeratosis congenita
> Norwegian scabies

ating nail disorders. Involvement of all 20 nails should suggest psoriasis, lichen planus, or 20-nail dystrophy, but not fungal infection. Finding characteristic papulosquamous skin lesions will help in the diagnosis of psoriasis and lichen planus. Thickened nails may be seen in children with scabies who cannot scratch.

Pathogenesis

The increased turnover time in the nail matrix results in a thickened, often dystrophic nail.[11] This occurs primarily in psoriasis and lichen planus.

Treatment

There is no satisfactory treatment for hypertrophic disorders of the nail. In dermatophyte infection, griseofulvin, 20 mg/kg/day for 3 months, is effective in only about 30% of cases.

Patient education

One must be careful to explain that nail thickening merely reflects overgrowth of nail cells and that it does not represent a specific disease.

Follow-up visits

Visits every 6 months may be useful in following the course of these conditions.

THIN OR ATROPHIC NAILS

Clinical features

Poorly developed or absent nails are characteristic of a wide variety of congenital syndromes.[1,2,12] These nail plate abnormalities generally reflect nail matrix disorders. Most often this is the result of ectodermal dysplasia (Figs. 16-11 and 16-12), but intrauterine injury to the nail, such as that caused by epidermolysis bullosa, may be responsible. Usually most or all the nails are affected. The nails are often narrow and the nail plate thin and fragile.

Congenital anonychia, or complete absence of some or all nails, has been described as an isolated dominant or sometimes recessive condition or associated with other congenital ectodermal defects.[12] With anonychia, neither the nail plate nor the nail bed is present.

The nail-patella syndrome deserves special comment. It is thought to be an autosomal dominant syndrome with both ectodermal and mesodermal manifestations.[1,2,12] The nail matrix of, usually, the thumb, index fingers, and great toes is hypoplastic (Fig. 16-13). Occasionally it is absent. Other nails may be involved. The lunula is often characteristically triangular. In addition, there are multiple bone abnormalities: rudimentary or absent patellas, bony spurs on the posterior iliac crest, subluxation of the elbows, and thickening of the scapulae are seen. Other anomalies described include skin laxity, heterochromia irides, and proteinuria. Periodic shedding of one or more nails is inherited as an autosomal dominant trait. This is a rare problem, and during the period of regrowth the nails may be dystrophic.

The more important causes of acquired thin or atrophic nails include trauma, infection, lichen planus, erythema multiforme, and bullous drug eruptions. Poor acral circulation, such as in Raynaud's disease or vascular malformations, may also contribute.

Differential diagnosis

One must first determine whether the nail disorder is congenital or acquired. Most often the associated

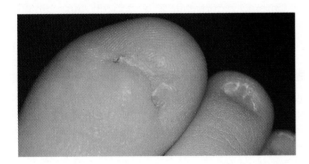

Fig. 16-11
Thin, hypoplastic nail in ectodermal dysplasia.

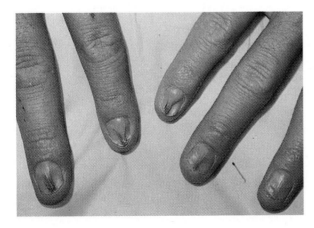

Fig. 16-12
Thin nails with "pincer" nail deformity in a child with hidrotic ectodermal dysplasia.

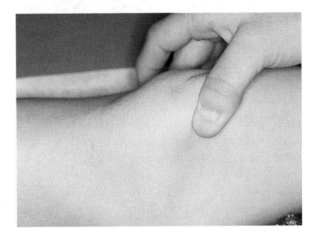

Fig. 16-13
Thin, hypoplastic thumbnail and dislocated patella in nail-patella syndrome.

Box 16-2 Differential diagnosis of thin, absent, or atrophic nails

Congenital
Ectodermal dysplasia (anhidrotic, hidrotic)*
Epidermolysis bullosa
Incontinentia pigmenti
Nail-patella syndrome*
Acrodermatitis enteropathica
Anonychia with or without ectrodactyly*
Coffin-Siris syndrome*
Hallermann-Streiff syndrome*
Progeria

Acquired
Trauma
Infection
Lichen planus
Erythema multiforme
Focal dermal hypoplasia
Ellis–van Creveld syndrome
     (chondroectodermal dysplasia)
Turner's syndrome
Dyskeratosis congenita
Trisomy 13
Periodic shedding
Severe Raynaud's phenomenon
Vascular disease
Bullous drug eruptions

*May be absent from birth.

clinical features are very useful in distinguishing one cause of nail disease or atrophy from another. Box 16-2 lists the conditions to be considered in the differential diagnosis of thin or atrophic nails.

Treatment
There is no treatment.

Patient education
It should be emphasized that the cells responsible for nail growth are poorly formed or injured.

Follow-up visits
Follow-up visits are unnecessary.

PARONYCHIA

Clinical features
Acute paronychia is most often due to *Staphylococcus aureus* or *Candida albicans*.[1,2] Occasionally, gram-negative organisms such as *Pseudomonas* and *Proteus* are implicated. This is a common, painful infection of the nail fold in which the red, inflamed, swollen periungual tissue has a purulent exudate. Herpes simplex infection may also occur in the paronychial area (herpetic whitlow) and is distinguished by grouped vesicles on an erythematous base.[1,2]

Chronic paronychia is a difficult but common problem, primarily in thumb-suckers, nail-biters, and nail-pickers.[9] It appears as dull-red swelling of the cuticle area that is usually not tender. Hobbies and habits that recurrently traumatize the nail fold are important causes. Chronic or recurrent dermatitis often occurs around the nail folds and may be the underlying cause. The nail fold is red, indurated, and raised, and the cuticle margin is lost (Fig. 16-14). Often there is proximal separation of the nail plate from the nail bed. *C. albicans* is the most important causative organism.[2]

Differential diagnosis
Paronychia is so characteristic that it is not easily confused with other conditions.

Pathogenesis
Alterations in the integrity of the cuticle area, such as maceration and trauma, alter the epidermal barrier and allow microbial invasion.

Treatment
Treatment is complicated by the fact that avoiding the underlying cause may be extremely difficult. Systemic antibiotics are required in acute bacterial paronychia. Treatment with nystatin (Mycostatin) is useful in *Candida* infection, and good success may be achieved

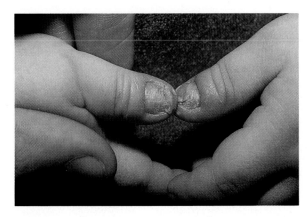

Fig. 16-14
Candida paronychia. Swelling and redness of the proximal nail fold in a thumb-sucker.

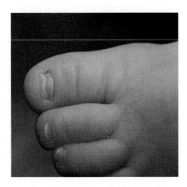

Fig. 16-15
Ingrown toenails with lateral nail fold hypertrophy.

with the nightly application of nystatin cream followed by airtight occlusion. One must avoid the aspiration of occluding material in thumb-suckers by covering the thumb with a cotton sock taped around the wrist. Imidazole antiyeast agents will also be effective.[2] Other topical agents, such as gentamicin cream, sulfonamide solutions, and gentian violet, have limited efficacy.

Patient education
Elimination or reduction of the causes of maceration and trauma should be emphasized.

Follow-up visits
A visit in 1 month will be useful to determine the response to therapy.

INGROWN TOENAILS

Clinical features
The large toes have a particular predilection for penetration of their nails into the lateral nail fold, producing a tender and sometimes erythematous swelling[1,2,13,14] (Fig. 16-15). Limping and discomfort on walking are frequent complaints. Purulence is sometimes seen secondary to bacterial invasion, usually due to *S. aureus*.[1,2]

This may proceed to cellulitis. In infants this may appear at 1 to 2 months of age with hypertrophy of the lateral nail folds.[13,14]

Differential diagnosis
An ingrown toenail is usually so characteristic that it is not confused with other processes.

Pathogenesis
Ingrown toenails are caused by the penetration of ragged edges of the nail plate into the lateral nail fold, giving rise to a foreign body inflammatory response with eventual formation of granulation tissue.[1,2] Tight-fitting shoes and improper nail cutting promote crowding of the nail plate. In infants asynchronous growth of the nail plate and the lateral nail folds may produce the penetration of the edge of the nail plate within the nail fold.[13,14]

Treatment
The majority of cases resolve with simple local measures. The foreign body, namely, the ragged lateral spicules of the nail plate, must be removed. This can be done by excising the lateral portion of the nail plate and inserting a small cotton wad to keep the nail plate separated from the inflamed area. Frequent soaking softens the indurated area. Systemic antibiotics should be used in infected lesions. When granulation tissue is present, it can be surgically curetted, then cauterized. Occasionally, surgical removal of the later-

---

Box 16-3   Causes of specific color changes in nails

Black
Peutz-Jeghers syndrome
Vitamin B deficiency
Pinta
Ammoniated mercuric sulfide
Hair dyes
Film developer
Irradiation
Junctional nevus
Malignant melanoma
Fungus

Blue lunulae
Antimalarials
Wilson's disease
Purpura
Cyanosis
Antimalarials
Argyria

Green
Pseudomonas
Aspergillus

Red
Resorcinol (nail lacquer)
Hemorrhage
Half-and-half nail of renal disease

Red lunulae
Collagen vascular diseases
Systemic lupus erythematosus
Rheumatoid arthritis
Carbon monoxide poisoning
Cardiac failure
Cirrhosis
Psoriasis
Twenty-nail dystrophy

Yellow
Yellow nail syndrome
Onycholysis

Gray
Silver salts
Phenolphthalein
Malignant melanoma

White
Arsenic (Mees' lines)
Partial onycholysis
Leukonychia (hereditary, traumatic, idiopathic)
Hypoalbuminemia

Brown
Resorcinol (nail lacquer)
Film developer
Fungus infection
Tobacco staining

---

al one fourth of the nail plate is necessary to reduce the size of the nail plate. Avulsion of the complete nail is unnecessary.

Patient education

Instructions in cutting the toenails are invaluable. The lateral margins must remain smooth. One should not cut the toenail until it grows beyond the distal end of the lateral nail fold. Trimming the nail straight across rather than in an arc is required. Patients should be instructed to avoid tight-fitting shoes. In infants an explanation of a slow-growing nail plate penetrating a rapidly growing lateral nail fold may be given.

Follow-up visits

A visit in 1 month is useful in evaluating therapy and reemphasizing toenail care.

COLOR CHANGES IN THE NAIL

It is beyond the scope of this chapter to discuss nail color changes in detail, but Box 16-3 lists the disorders to be considered when specific color changes in the nail are encountered.

References

1. Barth JH, Dawber RPR: Diseases of the nails in children, *Pediatr Dermatol* 4:275, 1987.

2. Pappert AS, Scher RK, Cohen JL: Nail disorders in children, *Pediatr Clin North Am* 38:921, 1991.

3. Akinduro OM, Venning VA, Burge SM: Psoriatic nail pitting in infancy, *Br J Dermatol* 130:800, 1994.

4. Tosti A, Morelli R, Bardazzi F, et al: Prevalence of nail abnormalities in children with alopecia areata, *Pediatr Dermatol* 11:112, 1994.

5. Tosti A, Bardazzi F, Piraccini BM, et al: Idiopathic trachyonychia (twenty-nail dystrophy): a pathological study of 23 patients, *Br J Dermatol* 131:866, 1994.

6. Commens CA: Twenty nail dystrophy in identical twins, *Pediatr Dermatol* 5:117, 1988.

7. Tosti A, Peluso AM, Fanti PA, et al: Nail lichen planus: clinical and pathologic study of twenty-four patients, *J Am Acad Dermatol* 28:714, 1993.

8. Ben-Dayan D, Mittelman M, Floru S, et al: Transverse nail ridgings (Beau's lines) induced by chemotherapy, *Acta Haematol* 91:89, 1994.

9. Lubitz L: Nail biting, thumb sucking and other irritating behaviours in childhood, *Aust Fam Physician* 21:1090, 1992.

10. Kechijian P: Traumatic split nail dystrophy, *JAMA* 265:912, 1991.

11. Johnson M, Shuster S: Determinants of nail thickness and length, *Br J Dermatol* 130:195, 1994.

12. Telfer NR: Congenital and hereditary nail disorders, *Semin Dermatol* 10:2, 1991.

13. Rufli T, von Schulthess A, Itin P: Congenital hypertrophy of the lateral nail folds of the hallux, *Dermatology* 184:296, 1992.

14. Hammerton MD, Shrank AB: Congenital hypertrophy of the lateral nail folds of the hallux, *Pediatr Dermatol* 5:243, 1988.

17

Disorders of Pigmentation: the White Lesions and the Brown Lesions

Infants' skin color is always light at birth and becomes darker with age. Hyperpigmentation of the scrotum and of the linea alba is common in dark-skinned infants. Pigmentary changes are very common in infants and children. Loss of skin color or increase in skin color in an infant or child may cause concern in parents. Mongolian spots are expected in dark-skinned newborns and café-au-lait spots are very common. Hypopigmented lesions, in contrast, are uncommon in infants, with piebaldism or ash-leaf macules occurring in less than 1% of babies. Alterations in skin color in an infant or child are often the earliest clues to genetic diseases, such as the hypopigmented macules in tuberous sclerosis and café-au-lait spots in neurofibromatosis.

Acquired pigmentary changes are also common. The prevalence of vitiligo is estimated to be 5.5 per 1000 school-age children, whereas the average number of acquired benign pigmented nevi is 3 per prepubertal child. This chapter is divided into discussions of white lesions and brown lesions.

WHITE LESIONS: CONGENITAL CIRCUMSCRIBED FLAT HYPOPIGMENTATION OR DEPIGMENTATION

Localized areas of hypopigmented skin are uncommon in infants and newborns. A hypopigmented area of the skin is found in approximately 8 per 1000 live births, and a hypopigmented tuft of hair is found in 3 per 1000 live births[1] (Fig. 17-1).

Piebaldism and Waardenburg's syndrome
Clinical features
Piebaldism is the name designated to circumscribed areas of absence of pigment in the newborn. This disorder is transmitted in an autosomal dominant pattern. Although completely devoid of melanocytes, the white patches of skin may be difficult to detect at birth because of the light color of most newborn skin. The use of a Wood's lamp to examine the infant's skin may accentuate differences in color. A depigmented tuft of hair, usually in the frontal region, may

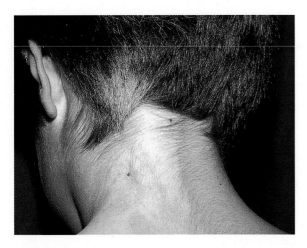

Fig. 17-1
Piebaldism. Segmental white patch on the neck with a tuft of white hair present from birth.

also be seen. Waardenburg's syndrome is an autosomal dominant syndrome that exhibits a white forelock, white patches on the skin, heterochromia of the irises, sensorineural deafness in one or both ears, and other defects.

Differential diagnosis

The differential diagnosis of congenital circumscribed depigmentation includes piebaldism, Waardenburg's syndrome, ash-leaf or hypopigmented macules, nevus depigmentosus, and nevus anemicus. It is at times difficult in the newborn to distinguish hypopigmented macules from totally depigmented macules. Examination of the skin with a Wood's lamp will help accentuate the color differences. Biopsy of a depigmented lesion will reveal a total lack of melanocytes, whereas melanocytes will be present in a hypopigmented macule. A family history of piebaldism, Waardenburg's syndrome, or tuberous sclerosis is very helpful. Nevus depigmentosus is a congenital localized area of hypopigmentation secondary to hypofunctional melanocytes, whereas nevus anemicus is a hypopigmented macule caused by alterations in vascular tone. Nevus anemicus can be differentiated by loss of the borders by pressing with a glass microscope slide.

Pathogenesis

Piebaldism is due to mutations in the *kit* protooncogene, which encodes for a cell surface receptor transmembrane tyrosine kinase for stem cell factor.[2] Waardenburg's syndrome is caused by mutations in the *pax*-3 gene.[3]

Treatment

There is no treatment for the depigmentation of skin or hair in piebaldism or Waardenburg's syndrome. Patients with Waardenburg's syndrome should be referred to the appropriate specialists, depending on their associated problems.

Patient education

The genetic nature of these diseases should be explained to the families. Patients with Waardenburg's syndrome should be told of the associated difficulties.

Follow-up visits

No follow-up visits are necessary for the skin changes. Follow-up of a patient with Waardenburg's syndrome depends on the associated features.

White patches of tuberous sclerosis (ash-leaf macules)
Clinical features

The white spots of tuberous sclerosis appear as hypopigmented macules, which may be lance-ovate (ash-leaf macules), polygonal (thumbprint), or confetti-shaped[4] (Fig. 17-2). The macules range in size from 0.1 to 12 cm at their greatest diameter.[4] In the newborn period they may be the only sign of tuberous sclerosis, and in families in which this condition occurs, involvement of the newborn infant may be first suspected by the presence of these lesions. A Wood's lamp examination is often necessary to detect the lesions in the newborn. They may be found anywhere on the skin but are most predominant on the posterior trunk and the extremities. Hypopigmented macules by themselves are not diagnostic of tuberous sclerosis because 2 to 3 per 1000 otherwise normal newborns will also demonstrate these patches.[5]

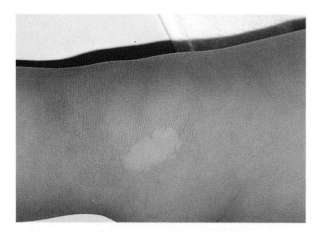

Fig. 17-2
Ash-leaf white macule of tuberous sclerosis.

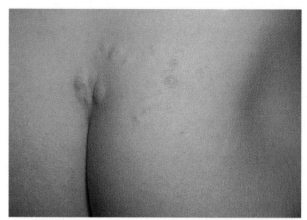

Fig. 17-4
Shagreen patch on sacral skin (tuberous sclerosis).

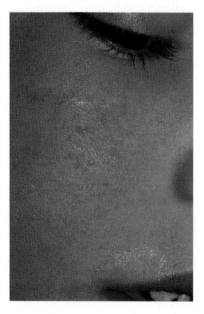

Fig. 17-3
Facial angiofibromas of tuberous sclerosis that mimic acne.

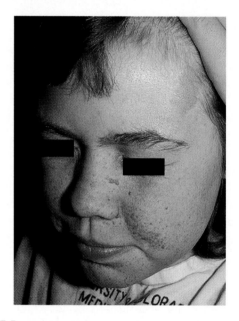

Fig. 17-5
Red forehead plaque of tuberous sclerosis.

The other signs and symptoms of tuberous sclerosis do not appear until later in life.[6] The angiofibromas found on the nose and face, which may mimic acne, usually begin to appear between the ages of 5 and 10 years (Fig. 17-3). Seizure disorders may appear within the first 10 years of life, but renal tumors and periungual fibromas usually appear after adolescence. A large connective tissue nevus, designated as a shagreen patch, may be present at birth or may become more apparent as the child becomes older. It is skin-colored to ivory-colored and feels thickened (Fig. 17-4). The red fibrous forehead plaque (Fig. 17-5) is one of the secondary features of tuberous sclerosis[7] (see Box 17-1).

Box 17-1 Diagnostic criteria for tuberous sclerosis

Primary features
- Facial angiofibromas
- Multiple ungual fibromas
- Cortical tuber (histologic confirmation)
- Subependymal nodule or giant cell astrocytoma (histologic confirmation)
- Multiple calcified subependymal nodule protruding in the ventricle (radiographic evidence)
- Multiple retinal astrocytomas

Secondary features
- Affected first-degree relative
- Cardiac rhabdomyoma (histologic confirmation or radiographic evidence)
- Other retinal hamartoma or achromic patch
- Cerebral tubers (radiographic evidence)
- Noncalcified subependymal nodule (radiographic evidence)
- Shagreen patch
- Forehead plaque
- Pulmonary lymphangiomatosis (histologic confirmation)
- Renal angiomyolipoma (histologic confirmation)
- Renal cysts (histologic confirmation)

Tertiary features
- Hypomelanotic macules
- "Confetti" skin lesions
- Renal cysts (radiographic evidence)
- Randomly distributed enamel pits in deciduous and/or permanent teeth
- Hamartomatous rectal polyps (histologic confirmation)
- Bone cysts (radiographic evidence)
- Pulmonary lymphangiomatosis (radiographic evidence)
- Cerebral white matter "migration tracts" or heterotopias (radiographic evidence)
- Gingival fibromas
- Hamartoma of other organs (histologic confirmation)
- Infantile spasms

Definite tuberous sclerosis: Either one primary feature or two secondary features, or one secondary plus two tertiary features
Probable tuberous sclerosis: Either one secondary feature plus one tertiary feature or 3 tertiary features
Suspect tuberous sclerosis: Either one secondary feature or two tertiary features

---

Differential diagnosis

The differential diagnosis of hypopigmented macules in the newborn includes nevus depigmentosus, nevus anemicus, piebaldism, and hypomelanosis of Ito. Nevus depigmentosus is generally a larger segmental area of hypopigmentation. The involved skin in piebaldism is totally depigmented. The areas of hypopigmentation in hypomelanosis of Ito are swirled and may cover a large portion of the body. In an infant without a family history of tuberous sclerosis, other criteria must be present to establish the diagnosis[7] (see Box 17-1).

Pathogenesis

Tuberous sclerosis is an autosomal dominant condition with variable penetrance. Often a family history is difficult to obtain. The spontaneous mutation rate is as high as 60% to 70%.[6,8] Tuberous sclerosis has been linked to two separate chromosomal loci on 9q34 and 16p13.[9]

Treatment

There is no effective treatment for the hypopigmented macules. Although these lesions do contain melanocytes, they are hypofunctional[4]; therefore they are more susceptible to ultraviolet radiation (UVR) and should be protected from excess sunlight. Children in whom the diagnosis of tuberous sclerosis has been documented are best managed in an appropriate multispecialty clinic.

Patient education

For those children with a family history of tuberous sclerosis and hypopigmented macules, the family should be told that it is highly likely that the child has tuberous sclerosis. In families without a history of tuberous sclerosis, discussion should be based on the number of hypopigmented macules present. A child with multiple hypopigmented macules is likely to have tuberous sclerosis and should be referred to the appropriate multispecialty clinic for evaluation for other stigmata of the disease. A child with one or two hypopigmented macules is unlikely to have tuberous sclerosis. The parents should be told about the other findings associated with tuberous sclerosis.

Follow-up visits

Infants likely to have tuberous sclerosis should be followed in a multispecialty clinic. Infants with one or two hypopigmented macules should be evaluated on a yearly basis.

Nevus depigmentosus
Clinical features

Nevus depigmentosus generally presents at birth as a unilateral, localized, quasi-dermatomal patch of hypopigmentation[10] (Fig. 17-6). The borders may be regular or irregular and at times the lesions may be whorled. A negative family history for hypopigmented birthmarks is usually obtained.

Differential diagnosis

The differential diagnosis of nevus depigmentosus is the same as that for hypopigmented macules (see Box 17-2).

Pathogenesis

Nevus depigmentosus should be considered a birthmark consisting of hypofunctional melanocytes.[11] In

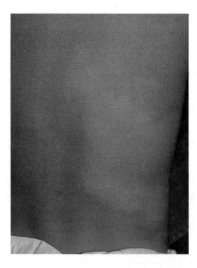

Fig. 17-6
Nevus depigmentosus. Quasi-dermatomal hypopigmentation.

Box 17-2 Differential diagnosis of patchy pigment loss in children

Postinflammatory hypopigmentation
Pityriasis alba
Tinea versicolor
Vitiligo
White spots (ash-leaf macules) with or without tuberous sclerosis
Halo nevus
Piebaldism
Scleroderma
Lichen sclerosus et atrophicus
Hypomelanosis of Ito
Waardenburg's syndrome
Chediak-Higashi syndrome

---

general, hypofunctioning melanocytes produce and transfer less melanin to the surrounding keratinocytes. Therefore the skin supplied by these melanocytes appears lighter than normal skin.

Treatment

As with the other forms of congenital hypopigmentation, there is no effective treatment. Due to the hypopigmentation in these areas, they should be chronically protected from excess UVR.

Patient education

Parents should be informed of the chronicity and benign nature of this birthmark. They should be told that the involved area of skin will be more sensitive to UVR than the child's normal skin, and that the area should be protected from excess sunlight.

Follow-up visits

Follow-up visits are not necessary.

Hypomelanosis of Ito

Clinical features

Newborns with hypomelanosis of Ito have bizarre hypopigmented swirls on their skin that follow Blaschko's lines (Figs. 17-7 and 17-8). The hypopigmentation may be quite extensive, involving an entire half of the body or, in some circumstances, it may even be found bilaterally. Approximately 50% of patients with hypomelanosis of Ito have associated neurologic, skeletal, and/or ocular abnormalities.[12]

Differential diagnosis

The differential diagnosis of hypomelanosis of Ito is the same as that for hypopigmented macules, but it is distinguished by the whorled pattern following Blaschko's lines and by involvement of an extensive portion of the body. Hypomelanosis of Ito is often confused with incontinentia pigmenti, linear and whorled hypermelanosis, or the linear hypermelanosis associated with the *Proteus* syndrome, all of which follow Blaschko's lines and have sharp midline demarcation of pigmentation. Hypomelanosis is lighter than normal skin color, rather than darker. Rarely patients with incontinentia pigmenti will also have whorled hypopigmentation, making differentiation from hypomelanosis of Ito difficult.

Pathogenesis

The hypopigmentation is secondary to a decreased number of melanosomes within the pigment cells and within keratinocytes. It is thought that a mishap early in embryogenesis is responsible, with two distinct genetically different melanocyte populations produced. The inheritance of hypomelanosis of Ito is not known. Some authorities consider hypomelanosis of

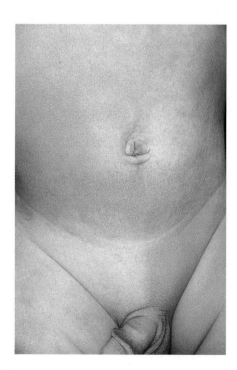

Fig. 17-7
Hypomelanosis of Ito. Whorls of hypopigmentation of the trunk with demarcation at midline.

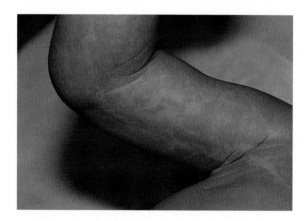

Fig. 17-8
Hypomelanosis of Ito. Whorls of hypoigmentation extending down an extremity.

Ito to be a nonspecific descriptive term applied to individuals with extensive areas of whorled pigmentation but without a consistent genetic defect.[12]

Treatment

As with the other hypopigmented and depigmented problems, no treatment is available for the pigmentary changes. Associated neurologic, skeletal, or ophthalmologic problems should be referred to the appropriate specialist.

Patient education

Parents should be informed that 50% of infants will have associated problems, and all children should be evaluated. The families should be told that no specific genetic defect has been identified.

Follow-up visits

Follow-up will depend on the associated abnormalities.

Nevus anemicus
Clinical features

Nevus anemicus presents as a solitary, localized, hypopigmented macule (Fig. 17-9).

Differential diagnosis

Nevus anemicus is separated from the other forms of congenital hypopigmentation by diascopy. This will cause blanching of the surrounding normal skin and obscure the original borders of the lesion.

Pathogenesis

Unlike the other congenital hypopigmented macules, nevus anemicus is a problem of vascular control and not of melanocytes. The defect is thought to be a localized vascular hypersensitivity to catecholamines via α-adrenergic receptors.[13] Injection of α-blocking agents will temporarily return the skin to normal color.

Treatment

No treatment is necessary.

Patient education

The benign nature of the disorder should be discussed.

Follow-up visits

No follow-up visits are necessary.

Acquired circumscribed flat hypopigmentation or depigmentation: vitiligo
Clinical features

Vitiligo is a patchy loss of skin pigment. The patches are flat, completely depigmented, and have distinct borders (Fig. 17-10). A small percentage of patients will have inflammatory vitiligo with raised erythema-

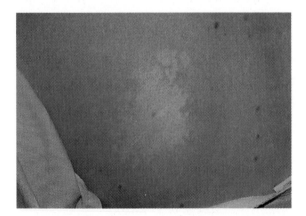

Fig. 17-9
Nevus anemicus. Hypopigmented macule that disappears with pressure on the surrounding skin.

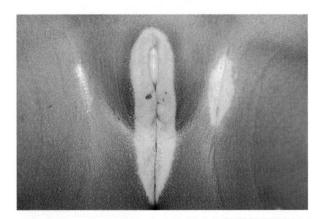

Fig. 17-10
Vitiligo type A. Involvement of perineal and inguinal skin. Note the distinct borders.

tous borders. In dark-skinned patients hypopigmented skin can be seen between the depigmented and normal skin (trichrome vitiligo). Hair within the patch of vitiligo is often depigmented as well. Fifty percent of cases of vitiligo start before the age of 18 years. The distribution of patches has been used to distinguish two types of vitiligo. In type A the distribution is generalized, acral, and roughly symmetric (Fig. 17-11), whereas in type B it is in a segmental, dermatomal distribution (Fig. 17-12). The extensor surface of the extremities and the face and neck are the areas most commonly involved in type A vitiligo. Although type A vitiligo is the most common form, segmental vitiligo is more common in children than in adults.[14,15] Type A continues to spread and develop new lesions for years, whereas type B vitiligo spreads rapidly, then stops spreading after 1 year. Uncommonly, type A vitiligo may be associated with diabetes mellitus, asthma, alopecia areata, pernicious anemia, Addison's disease, hypothyroidism, or hypoparathyroidism. Vitiligo of the face, eyelashes, and scalp hair in association with uveitis, dysacousis, and alopecia areata occurs in the rare Vogt-Koyanagi syndrome. Complete spontaneous repigmentation is unusual in vitiligo. Partial repigmentation occurs in about half of the affected children during the months when they are exposed to the sun. Pigmentation returns first around hair follicles. In black and other dark-skinned children, vitiligo produces great distress.

Differential diagnosis

The conditions to be considered in the differential diagnosis are listed in Box 17-2. In pityriasis alba and tinea versicolor, in contrast to vitiligo, the abnormally pigmented areas are hypopigmented rather than depigmented and often have scaling as well as indistinct borders. In postinflammatory hypopigmentation, irregular mottling of both hyperpigmented and hypopigmented areas is often seen. In piebaldism, lesions are present from birth and rarely have hyperpigmented borders. Scleroderma and lichen sclerosus et atrophicus present with immobilized skin as well as hypopigmentation.

Pathogenesis

It has long been presumed that vitiligo is an immune disorder because of the lymphocytic infiltrate that precedes the injury to melanocytes and the association with other autoimmune diseases. Long-standing inactive lesions of vitiligo always lack melanocytes.[16] Recently antibodies directed against melanocytes have been detected in patients with type A vitiligo, and antibody-dependent cellular cytotoxicity may be one method of destruction of melanocytes.[17,18]

Treatment

There is no entirely satisfactory treatment. Skin stains such as dyes and walnut oil may be used, but children generally will not comply. Psoralen, a furocoumarin

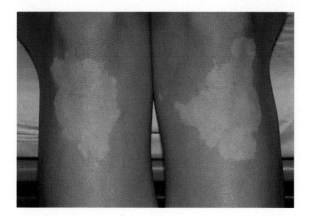

Fig. 17-11
Symmetric, acral vitiligo.

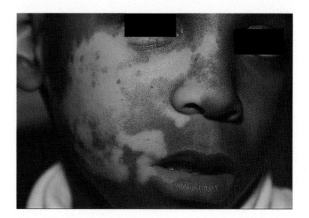

Fig. 17-12
Rapidly progressing segmental vitiligo.

derived from plants, is a potent stimulator of melanocytes. Psoralen, in combination with ultraviolet A radiation (PUVA [psoralen ultraviolet A-range]) has resulted in successful repigmentation in over half the patients treated.[19] Even in those patients with a good result, repigmentation is seldom complete (Fig. 17-13 *A* and *B*). It is best used by an experienced dermatologist, since it is easy to produce severe sunburns with this photosensitizing drug. Psoralens may be given either topically, if less than 20% of the body surface is involved, or orally. Topical psoralens must be used cautiously because of the high risk of phototoxic burns even when treatment is supervised by an experienced dermatologist. If systemic therapy is to be used, an ophthalmologic examination, complete blood cell count, liver function tests, and an antinuclear antibody test should be obtained before therapy. PUVA therapy requires 6 months of biweekly treatment to evaluate efficacy. If repigmentation occurs, treatments are often continued up to 1 year. Because the use of a photosensitizer combined with UVR enhances photoaging and increases the risk for the development of skin cancer, PUVA therapy is not recommended for children under 9 years of age.[19] Older, motivated children achieve the best results. Some repigmentation has been noted with topical steroids.

Patient education
The natural history of vitiligo should be discussed and the need to follow a strict regimen emphasized in those motivated to undergo therapy.

Follow-up visits
During therapy, monthly visits are advisable.

Pityriasis alba
Clinical features
Pityriasis alba is characterized by multiple oval, scaly, flat, hypopigmented patches on the face, extensor surface of arms, and upper trunk (Fig. 17-14). The lesions range from 5 to 20 mm in diameter, and 10 to 20 patches are often seen. The borders are indistinct.

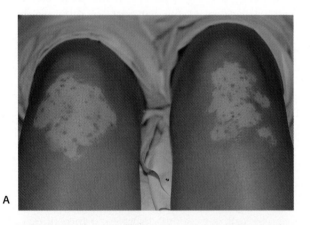
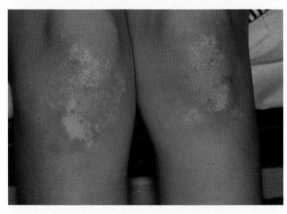

Fig. 17-13
Symmetric, acral vitiligo pre-PUVA treatment. Same patient shows perifollicular pattern of repigmentation during PUVA therapy.

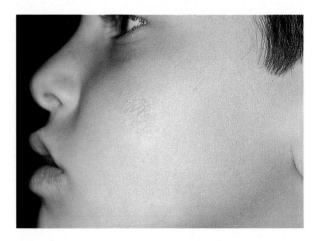

Fig. 17-14
Pityriasis alba. White, slightly scaly patches with indistinct borders on child's cheek.

It occurs predominantly between the ages of 3 and 16 years, and up to 30% of all children may be affected. The lesions do not itch, and medical help is sought because of the child's appearance. It is particularly distressing in dark-skinned children. It is a chronic dermatitis and often lasts several years.

Differential diagnosis
Pityriasis alba most closely mimics tinea versicolor, which can be excluded by findings in a negative potassium hydroxide (KOH) examination. (See Box 17-2 for the list of conditions to be considered in the differential diagnosis.)

Pathogenesis
On pathologic examination the lesion resembles that seen in chronic dermatitis. Hyperkeratosis, parakeratosis, spongiotic edema, and a lymphocytic infiltrate are seen. The cause of the hypopigmentation is not known, but is likely related to inflammatory mediators that inhibit melanocyte function. Some regard this as a form of atopic dermatitis, but in many children it occurs without the features of atopic dermatitis.

Treatment
There is no satisfactory treatment. Topical glucocorticosteroids have some influence on the disorder. Dyes or stains are occasionally useful.

Patient education
The natural history of this disorder should be emphasized.

Follow-up visits
Follow-up visits should be scheduled at monthly intervals if a treatment program is considered.

Postinflammatory hypopigmentation
Clinical features
Following any inflammatory skin disease or injury to the skin, irregular hypopigmented areas may appear. The hypopigmentation is most obvious in dark-skinned people. The hypopigmented blotches are usually in a mottled pattern and may be associated with hyperpigmented areas (Figs. 17-15 and 17-16). They resolve several months after the inflammatory disorder.

Differential diagnosis
Blotchy hypopigmentation associated with hyperpigmentation, and a history of a preceding inflammatory dermatosis, differentiate this form of hypopigmentation (see Box 17-2).

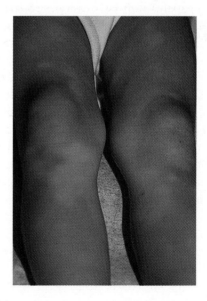

Fig. 17-16
Blotchy hypopigmentation following treatment for atopic dermatitis.

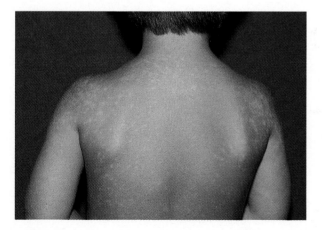

Fig. 17-15
Postinflammatory hypopigmentation with numerous hypopigmented patches on child's back.

Pathogenesis

Inflammatory injury to melanocytes, as well as to epidermal cells, results in decreased pigment production and transfer.

Treatment

Treatment is not necessary.

Patient education

The patient should be informed of the nature of the pigment loss and told that recovery is expected.

Follow-up visits

Follow-up visits are unnecessary.

Diffuse hypopigmentation albinism

Clinical features

Albinism can be separated into those individuals with only eye involvement (ocular albinism) and those with eye, skin, and hair abnormalities (ocular cutaneous albinism [OCA]). There are at least four classes of OCA, with multiple subsets within each class[20] (see Box 17-3). All variants of OCA have defects in melanin synthesis, resulting in reduction or total absence of pigmentation. Regardless of the pigment defect, all patients with OCA will have visual abnormalities.[21] All newborns with OCA1 have fine white hair, pink skin, blue irides, severe nystagmus, and photophobia. The skin and hair in patients with OCA1A will remain white their entire life. Patients with variants of OCA1 may develop darker hair, skin, and eyes, as well as freckles, lentigines, and nevi. In the other classes of OCA, hair and skin pigment may be present at birth and increase with age. Pigmented nevi and freckles commonly develop in these patients. The phenotypic expression of these forms of OCA is quite variable.

Differential diagnosis

The diagnosis of OCA1 in a child with white skin and hair and blue eyes is usually obvious. The other classes may be difficult to diagnose in light-skinned whites. The major differential is between the classes of OCA.

Pathogenesis

OCA1 is caused by mutations in the genes encoding for the protein tyrosinase.[20] OCA1A is due to complete lack of functional tyrosinase. In the variants of OCA1, partial tyrosinase function remains. Tyrosinase is the enzyme necessary for the final assembly of the pigment melanin. OCA2 is caused by defects in the human homologue to the mouse pink-eyed dilution (*p*) gene.[20] The function of this gene product has not yet been determined. The genetic defects in the other classes of OCA remain unknown.

Treatment

No treatment is available for the pigmentary changes. Due to the lack of pigmentation, sun protection is required for all children with albinism.

Patient education

The families should be referred to the appropriate specialists for genetic counseling and identification of the class of OCA expressed, as well as referral to an ophthalmologist. The need for photoprotection should be stressed.

Box 17-3 Classification of oculocutaneous albinism

Tyrosinase related OCA1
    No tyrosinase activity OCA1A
Residual tyrosinase activity
    Yellow OCA1B
    Minimal pigment OCA1MP
Unusual tyrosinase activity
    Temperature-sensitive OCA1TS
Tyrosinase-positive OCA2
    Prader Willi/Angelman syndrome
Unclassified
    Brown OCA
    Rufous OCA
Defects in melanocytes and other cells
    Hermansky-Pudlak syndrome
    Chediak-Higashi syndrome

Follow-up visits

Follow-up visits are determined by the type of OCA and the degree of ocular involvement.

BROWN LESIONS

In considering a hyperpigmented state, one should first determine whether the hyperpigmentation is circumscribed or diffuse.

Circumscribed flat hyperpigmentation
Clinical features

Freckles   Freckles are small, 1- to 5-mm, light brown, pigmented macules that are UVR responsive and occur in sun-exposed skin (Fig. 17-17). They are autosomal dominant and first appear at age 3 to 5 years, predominantly on the face and extensor surface of the extremities. They are most frequent in fair-skinned, light-haired, blue-eyed children.

Lentigines   Lentigines are brown or brown-black, 1- to 2-mm macules found sparsely scattered over the body, including the mucous membranes (Fig. 17-18). They do not change with sun exposure. They usually first appear during school age. Lentigines on the lips (Fig. 17-19) are also seen in the autosomal dominant Peutz-Jeghers syndrome associated with multiple

bowel polyps and an increase risk of gastrointestinal and genitourinary carcinomas.[22,23] Multiple lentigines are associated with cardiac abnormalities in the so-called LEOPARD syndrome[24] (*l*entigines, *e*lectrocardiograph abnormalities, *o*cular hypertelorism, *p*ulmonary stenosis, *a*bnormalities of the genitalia, growth *r*etardation, *d*eafness) (Fig. 17-20). Central facial lentigines have been described in association with cardiac defects and malignancies in the NAME syndrome[25] (*n*evi, *a*trial myxomas, *m*yxoid neurofibroma, *e*phelides).

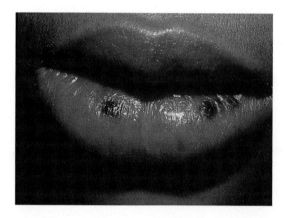

Fig. 17-18
Lip lentigines not associated with the Peutz-Jeghers syndrome.

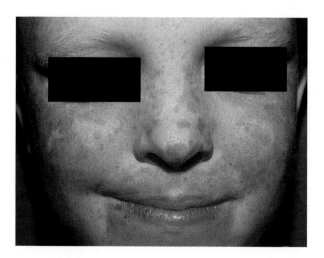

Fig. 17-17
Freckles. Note the sunburn between freckled areas.

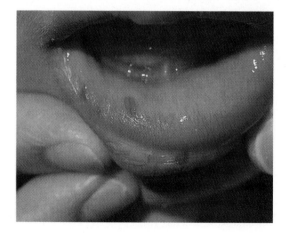

Fig. 17-19
Lip lentigines in an adolescent with the Peutz-Jeghers syndrome.

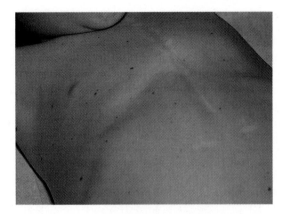

Fig. 17-20
Infant with multiple lentingines and the LEOPARD syndrome. Note scars from repair of pulmonary stenosis.

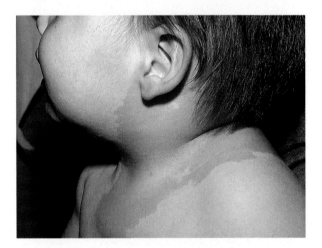

Fig. 17-21
Café-au-lait spot. Large lesion on a child's neck.

Café-au-lait spots Café-au-lait spots are tan, flat, oval macules with distinct borders (Fig. 17-21). They frequently have a diameter greater than 0.5 cm. One café-au-lait spot larger than 0.5 cm is found in 10% of white children and 22% of black children. Multiple café-au-lait spots occur in type 1 neurofibromatosis (NF-1) (see Box 17-4). In children six or more café-au-lait macules over 0.5 cm are a major criterion for NF-1[26] (see Box 17-4) (Figs. 17-22 and 17-23). Some families have autosomal dominant multiple café-au-lait macules without other stigmata of neurofibromatosis.[27] Café-au-lait spots are rarely present at birth (in 19 of 1000 live births), but appear

Box 17-4 Diagnostic criteria for neurofibromatosis type 1 (two or more must be found)

Six or more café-au-lait spots greater than 5 mm in diameter in prepubertal children; greater than 1.5 mm in postpubertal children
Two or more neurofibromas of any type
One plexiform neurofibroma
Axillary freckling
Inguinal freckling
Two or more Lisch nodules (iris hamartomas)
Distinctive osseous lesion, such as sphenoid dysplasia or thinning of a long bone with or without pseudoarthrosis
A first-degree relative with NF-1

between the ages of 2 and 16 years and tend to persist until age 60 to 70. They are also seen in Albright's syndrome, tuberous sclerosis, and the *Proteus* syndrome. The *Proteus* syndrome can be mistaken for NF-1 because of the skeletal overgrowth and large hamartomas that are confused with plexiform neurofibromas. In NF-1, more café-au-lait spots appear with age, and may be accompanied by soft cutaneous neurofibromas (Fig. 17-24).

Mongolian spots The mongolian spot is a blue-black macule found over the lumbosacral area in up to 90% of Asian, black, and American Indian babies.[28] They are occasionally noted over the shoulders and back and may extend over the buttocks and extremities (Fig. 17-25). The difference in the pigmentation from normal skin pigment becomes less obvious as a newborn's skin darkens in color. Some traces of mongolian spots may persist into adult life.

Nevus of Ota, nevus of Ito Flat, blue-black, speckled pigmentary discoloration may be noted in the skin surrounding the eye (nevus of Ota) (Fig. 17-26) or around the chest and shoulder (nevus of Ito). Most cases are present at birth, but some are acquired.[29] The sclera may be involved in nevus of Ota.

Linear and whorled nevoid hypermelanosis Hypermelanotic macules arranged in streaks corre-

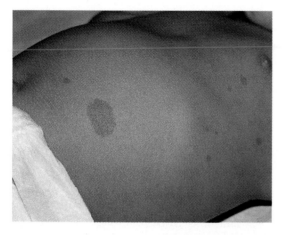

Fig. 17-22
Numerous café-au-lait spots on the abdomen and chest of a child with neurofibromatosis type 1.

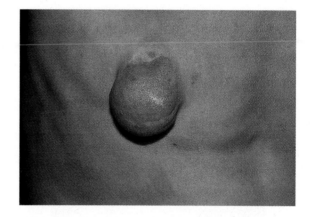

Fig. 17-24
Soft cutaneous neurofibroma surrounded by café-au-lait spots in an adolescent with neurofibromatosis type 1.

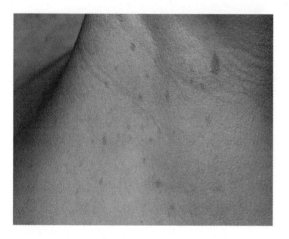

Fig. 17-23
Numerous café-au-lait spots in a child's axilla in neurofibromatosis type 1.

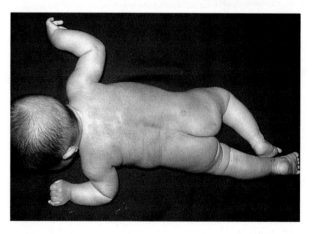

Fig. 17-25
Mongolian spots. Extensive lesions over the back and buttocks.

sponding to Blaschko's lines, with sharp demarcation at the midline, characterize linear and whorled nevoid hypermelanosis[30] (Fig. 17-27).

Postinflammatory hyperpigmentation In children with dark skin, any inflammatory skin disorder may heal with hyperpigmentation. Often the pigmentation persists for months.

Differential diagnosis
Freckles are small, acquired, sun-responsive macules, whereas lentigos and café-au-lait macules are not related to sun exposure. Café-au-lait macules are larger and lighter brown than lentigos. Skin biopsy may differentiate the acquired flat pigmented lesions from one another, but should only be done if it will help delineate one of the associated genetic syndromes. Mongolian spots, nevus of Ota, and nevus of Ito are blue-black with location being used to differentiate. Linear and whorled nevoid hypermelanosis is obvious by the extent of the condition and the pigmentation occurring along the lines of Blaschko. Unlike incontinentia pigmenti, linear and whorled nevoid hyperme-

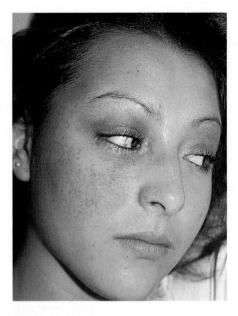

Fig. 17-26
Nevus of Ota. Speckled blue macules in the periorbital skin and sclera.

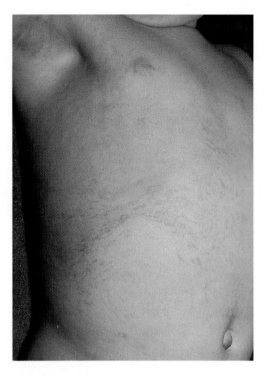

Fig. 17-27
Linear and whorled hypermelanosis. Brown whorls over the trunk of a child.

lanosis is not preceded by a vesicular or verrucous stage. The conditions to be included in the differential diagnosis are given in Box 17-5.

Pathogenesis

Freckles   Freckles are areas with increased pigment secondary to sun-induced hyperplasia of melanocytes.[31]

Lentigines   In lentigines, increased numbers of melanocytes are dispersed along the basal layer of the epidermis, and the epidermal rete ridges are elongated.

Café-au-lait spots   In café-au-lait spots, melanocyte activity is increased, as is the melanin in melanocytes and in epidermal cells. The number of melanocytes is not increased. Despite this in vivo increase in function, no differences have been demonstrated in vitro in melanocytes grown from café-au-lait macules compared with melanocytes from normal skin.[32] Neurofibromatosis is an autosomal dominant disease caused by mutations in the gene located on chromosome 17q11.2. This gene encodes a protein, neurofibromin, which acts as a tumor suppressor.[33]

Box 17-5 Differential diagnosis of circumscribed, flat pigmented lesions

Acquired
　Freckles
　Lentigo
　Café-au-lait spot
　Junctional melanocytic nevi
　Postinflammatory hyperpigmentation
Congenital
　Mongolian spot
　Nevus of Ota
　Linear and whorled nevoid hypermelanosis

Mongolian spots   The pathology of Mongolian spots consists of spindle-shaped cells that contain pigment and are located between collagen fibers deep within the dermis.

Nevus of Ota, nevus of Ito Similar to mongolian spots, spindle-shaped melanocytes are found within the dermis.

Linear and whorled nevoid hypermelanosis Epidermal melanocytes are increased in number, and keratinocytes have increased melanin in the affected area. It is thought that two genetically distinct populations of melanocytes are produced.

Postinflammatory hyperpigmentation The excess pigment is related to loss of pigment from damaged epidermal keratinocytes and melanocytes into the dermis, where the large polymer melanin sits free in the dermis or is engulfed by macrophages to form melanophages. Breakdown of the dermal pigment is slow.

Treatment

No treatment is necessary, but café-au-lait macules and lentigos may be treated with a pulsed-dye laser,[34] *q*-switched ruby laser, or *q*-switched alexandrite laser, whereas nevus of Ota and nevus of Ito respond only to the *q*-switched lasers.[35]

Patient education

The common and benign nature of these pigmented areas should be emphasized. Parents of children with multiple café-au-lait macules should be told of the possibility of NF-1.

Follow-up visits

Children with multiple café-au-lait macules should be referred for evaluation for NF-1, otherwise follow-up visits are unnecessary.

MELANOCYTIC NEVI

There are two distinct forms of melanocytic nevi with entirely different natural histories. These are congenital melanocytic nevi (CMN) and acquired nevi. They will be considered separately.

Congenital melanocytic nevi
Clinical features

Skin-colored to tan, or brown, solitary papules with smooth surfaces represent CMN. Most such nevi present at birth are small, measuring less than 1.5 cm at their greatest diameter[36] (Fig. 17-28). Large melanocytic nevi, which are defined as being greater than 10 cm at their greatest diameter, are very uncommon, occurring in 1 in 20,000 live births. Large melanocytic nevi are often not uniform in color and contain flat tan areas, brown areas, blue-black plaques, and pigmented, long, thick hair (Fig. 17-29). Numerous smaller nevi located at skin sites distant from the large nevi are found. These "satellite lesions" are more often uniform in color and may arise

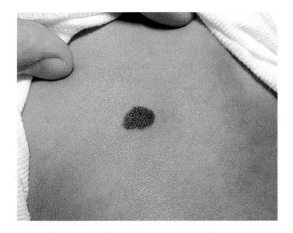

Fig. 17-28
Small congenital nevus.

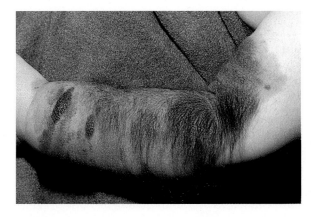

Fig. 17-29
Large congenital nevus with long, pigmented hair and a mixture of tan, brown, and blue within the lesion.

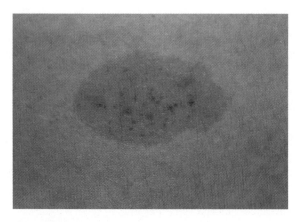

Fig. 17-30
Nevus spilus. Large flat, tan lesion containing numerous small, dark brown areas.

throughout childhood. A variant of CMN is the nevus spilus. Nevus spilus is a café-au-lait macule studded with small, dark, raised nevi (Fig. 17-30).

Differential diagnosis
Occasionally, a congenital melanocytic nevus will be flat at birth and will appear as a café-au-lait macule, but with time it becomes raised. Congenital smooth muscle and pilar hamartomas may also present as light brown plaques with fine hair and may be difficult to distinguish from CMN. Biopsy will differentiate.

Pathogenesis
Nests of pigment cells are found within the epidermis and dermis. Sometimes the pigment cells are large and unusually shaped, making it difficult to distinguish benign from malignant changes.[37,38] In giant CMN, pigment cells may populate the entire dermis and extend around hair and eccrine sweat structures. Most authorities consider congenital nevocellular nevi to be developmental errors in pigment cell proliferation and migration. The pathogenesis of CMN is unknown. There is a slightly increased frequency of large, congenital pigmented lesions in blacks and in those infants born to mothers with acute illnesses. There is no correlation of large pigmented nevi with sex, twins, parental consanguinity, parental age, birth order, radiation exposure, or drug intake.

Treatment
Many authorities recommend prophylactic removal of large CMN within the first year of life. This recommendation is controversial, based on the very small likelihood of malignant melanoma. Currently it is advisable to take into consideration the potential for cosmetic improvement and surgical risk before recommending removal of such lesions.[39-41] There is no compelling reason to remove these in the child's first year. For best cosmetic results the use of tissue expanders is preferred. Small lesions can be removed during adolescence. There is no urgency to remove small congenital nevi before puberty. There is a small risk of melanoma arising in a small congenital nevus in late adolescence or in young adults.

Patient education
Since there is no uniform agreement among authorities as to the best management for congenital nevi, this should be explained to the parents with the positive and negative reasons detailed. CMN will grow proportionately with the child, and this should not be a concern. Satellite lesions may continue to develop throughout childhood. Any change in one portion of the CMN should be evaluated for the need for biopsy.

Follow-up visits
Yearly visits are recommended for large CMN, as well as at any time there is a non-proportional change in the birthmark.

Acquired melanocytic nevi (common moles)
Clinical features
The development of acquired melanocytic nevi in white children is related to genetic susceptibility and sun exposure. This is not true for nonwhite children, who develop fewer nevi.[42] There are families in which members develop numerous, large, atypical nevi beginning in childhood. Members of these families are at markedly increased risk for the development of melanoma.[43] In white families not affected by the atypical mole syndrome, the development of moles is related to skin type, hair and eye color, freckles, and sun exposure. Those children with light skin, light hair and eye color, many freckles, and a history of numer-

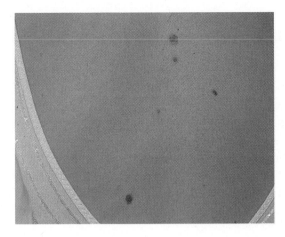

Fig. 17-31
Back of an adolescent with multiple benign junctional and compound nevi.

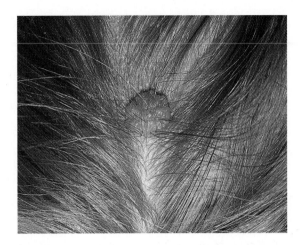

Fig. 17-33
Nonpigmented intradermal nevus of the scalp.

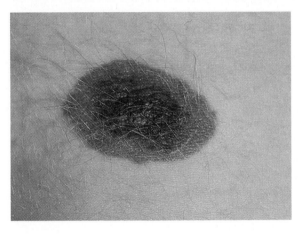

Fig. 17-32
Intradermal nevus darker in the center.

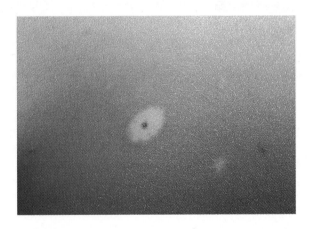

Fig. 17-34
Halo nevus. Loss of pigment around regressing central intradermal nevus.

ous sunburns develop the highest number of nevi.[44] Children with similar genetic backgrounds who are exposed to more UVR will develop more nevi.[45] The average number of nevi greater than 2 mm on an arm of a white adolescent will range from 4 to 10.[45]

Acquired melanocytic nevi begin as flat, well-demarcated, and brown to brown-black lesions (Fig. 17-31). These are called junctional melanocytic nevi. They characteristically have regular borders and may have a light brown rim and/or a dark brown center. They usually measure 2 to 5 mm but may occasionally be larger. Most nevi found in infants and children

are junctional nevi. If many nevi appear before age 5 years, the child is likely to have a large number of moles after puberty. After puberty the number of moles continues to increase. They may appear anywhere on the skin, but they are most common on sites of intermittent intense sun exposure.[46]

A few junctional melanocytic nevi will progress to compound melanocytic nevi, which appear as small, raised, dome-shaped, brown to brown-black papules (Fig. 17-31). It is common for the center to be darker than the periphery (Fig. 17-32). They may also appear skin-colored, with little melanin production

(Fig. 17-33). They frequently darken at puberty, with pregnancy, or with the use of oral contraceptives.

Dermal nevi are usually few in number before the preadolescent growth period, averaging one or two. More appear during adolescence.

Nevi typically regress after age 60, but a few will regress during childhood. A halo may appear around a nevus that is regressing in childhood (Fig. 17-34), producing the "halo nevus." Multiple halo nevi may be seen in an individual, and this is at times associated with vitiligo.

OTHER NEVI

Blue nevi, which are uncommon, are blue to blue-black, 4- to 10-mm solitary papules that begin in childhood (Fig. 17-35).

The Spitz, or spindle and epithelioid cell, nevus begins as a solitary red or red-brown nodule, usually on the extremities or face (Fig. 17-36). It appears in school-age children and tends to persist.

A large, pigmented, hairy nevus, called Becker's nevus, occurs most commonly over the shoulder and is often first noticed in adolescence (Fig. 17-37). Becker's nevus is considered a hamartoma of hair follicles and associated arrector pilae muscles. It may be seen in other locations.

Malignant melanoma

Malignant melanomas are rare in childhood and appear as pigmented nodules of variegated colors. Within a single lesion (Fig. 17-38) red, white, and blue may be seen, as well as brown and tan. The most important clinical feature is rapid, progressive growth of a pigmented lesion. Notching of the border of a pigmented nodule and a nonuniform irregular surface should also arouse suspicion of melanoma; ulceration and bleeding are far-advanced signs. In familial malignant melanoma, multiple primary melanomas may be found, usually first appearing in late adolescence or

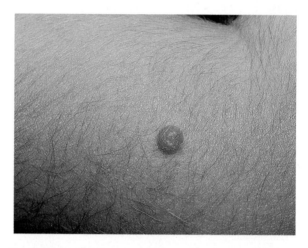

Fig. 17-36
Spitz nevus. Reddish-brown papule on a teenager's arm.

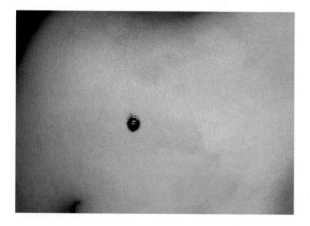

Fig. 17-35
Blue nevus. Blue-black papule on a child's shoulder.

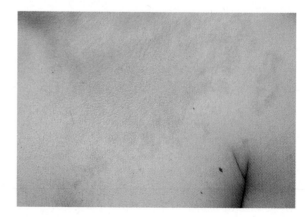

Fig. 17-37
Becker's nevus on the chest of an adolescent male.

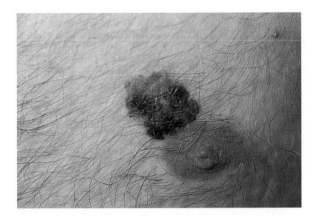

Fig. 17-38
Malignant melanoma on the chest of an adolescent male.

early adult life.[47] There is a correlation with skin type, large numbers of nevi, and a history of excess sun exposure in childhood and melanoma later in life.[48-50]

Differential diagnosis

The conditions to be considered in the differential diagnosis are listed in Box 17-6. Skin biopsy will differentiate these pigmented lesions from one another.

Pathogenesis

Junctional, compound, and dermal melanocytic nevi   Clumps of increased numbers of melanocytes are located at the dermal-epidermal junction in junctional nevi. Dermal melanocytic nevi represent accumulations of groups of immature melanocytes within the middermis to upper dermis. When associated with clumps of melanocytes at the dermal-epidermal junction, such a nevus is called a compound nevus. Development of these types of nevi is related to genetic background and amount of sun exposure.

Other nevi   A blue nevus represents clumps of mature melanocytes located in the deep dermis.

Spindle and epithelioid cell nevi (Spitz nevi) are composed of collections of melanocytes with irregular cytoplasmic and nuclear shapes and are located throughout the dermis. These nevi are associated with a proliferation of blood vessels. The bizarre nuclear shapes often result in confusion with melanoma. An

---

> **Box 17-6 Differential diagnosis of circumscribed, acquired pigmented lesions**
>
> Junctional melanocytic nevus
> Dermal melanocytic nevus
> Compound melanocytic nevus
> Pyogenic granuloma
> Mastocytoma
> Dermatofibroma
> Blue nevus
> Spindle and epithelioid cell nevus
> Juvenile xanthogranuloma
> Malignant melanoma

experienced dermatopathologist should review all pigmented lesions in which the diagnosis of melanoma is considered.

In Becker's nevus the number of melanocytes is slightly increased, and melanin is seen throughout the epidermis.

Malignant melanoma   In malignant melanomas the tumor originates at the dermal-epidermal junction and has a radial growth phase before it demonstrates a vertical growth phase. The tumor cells within a melanoma show great variation in size and shape and invade epidermal structures. The depth of invasion is an important prognostic factor and is the basis for histologic classifications of melanomas. Familial melanoma has been linked to the 9p21 gene.[47] There are compelling data to support a role of sunlight in melanomas arising from acquired nevi or nonpigmented skin.[51]

Treatment

In any raised pigmented lesion in which melanoma is suspected, surgical excision is the treatment of choice. Although malignant melanoma is rare in childhood, a high index of suspicion of malignant melanoma should be maintained for any rapidly growing pigmented skin lesion. Any excised skin lesion, particularly pigmented skin lesions, should be sent to the pathologist.

However, it is unnecessary to remove the common dermal melanocytic nevus that is uniform in color.

Patient education

Families with the atypical mole or familial melanoma traits must be counseled regarding the high risk for the development of melanoma and the importance of routine follow-up and the need for excision of any changing lesion. Parents of children with light skin, light hair, blue eyes, and freckles need to be told of the correlation between sun exposure in childhood and the increased risk of developing melanoma later in life. Proper sun protection programs should be discussed. If a lesion is removed, after confirmation by the pathologist, the nature of the lesion can be explained to the patient.

Follow-up visits

Children with the atypical mole or familial melanoma syndromes should be followed yearly. If a lesion has been excised, a visit 1 week after surgical removal is necessary to inform the patient of the diagnosis and suggested further treatment, if any.

Acanthosis nigricans
Clinical features

Acanthosis nigricans is characterized by hyperpigmentation and a velvety thickening of irregular folds of skin of the posterior neck and the axilla (Figs. 17-39 and 17-40). It is common in dark-skinned children and is found in as many as 7% of pubertal children.[52] Often parents complain that their child's skin is dirty and cannot be cleaned. Small papillomatous growths (skin tags) may be found within the irregular folds. Acanthosis nigricans can be found in other skin areas as well, such as elbows, inguinal creases, areolae, and knuckles. It is associated with obesity, and correlates well with hyperinsulinemia and insulin resistance.[53] With obesity the age of onset correlates with the onset of obesity. Less commonly it is associated with various lipodystrophies; hirsutism; hypogonadism syndromes such as Prader-Willi; Cushing's syndrome; estrogen therapy; acromegaly; Addison's disease; and hypothyroidism.[53]

Differential diagnosis

Acanthosis nigricans is so distinctive that it is seldom misdiagnosed. A lichenified chronic dermatitis may mimic.

Pathogenesis

The epidermis is papillomatous with no abnormality of pigmentation. The association with insulin resistance is so striking that a role for insulin, insulinlike growth factors, or insulinlike receptors in the papillomatous overgrowth is suspected.[52]

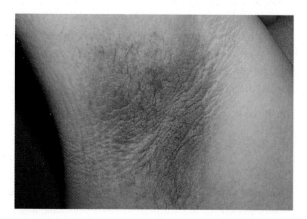

Fig. 17-39
Acanthosis nigricans of a child's axilla. Velvety, brown rows of hyperpigmentation.

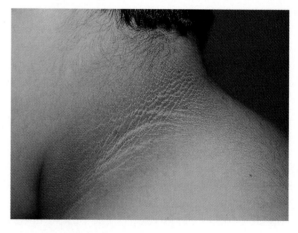

Fig. 17-40
Acanthosis nigricans of a child's neck.

Treatment

Weight loss has resulted in reversal of the acanthosis nigricans, as has stopping hormone therapy or treating the hypothyroidism.

Patient education

Parents should be told that this is not dirt and is unrelated to hygiene. If the child is obese, its relationship to obesity should be emphasized and the institution of a weight control program considered. Nonobese children with signs of associated hyperandrogenism should be referred for endocrine evaluation.

Follow-up visits

Follow-up visits should be determined by therapy.

Diffuse hyperpigmentation

Diffuse hyperpigmentation is rare in infancy and childhood but may occur as a result of endocrine disturbances. Adrenal insufficiency, with overproduction of adrenocorticotropic hormone (ACTH) and its melanocyte-stimulating fragments, or hyperfunction of the pituitary may result in diffuse hyperpigmentation. Pigmentation of the scrotum, linea alba, and palmar creases may occur. Box 17-7 lists the conditions

---

Box 17-7 Differential diagnosis of diffuse hyperpigmentation

Addison's disease
Acromegaly
Cushing's syndrome of pituitary origin
Thyrotoxicosis
ACTH administration
Subacute bacterial endocarditis
Lymphomas and leukemia
Scleroderma, dermatomyositis
Renal failure
Hemochromatosis
Familial progressive hyperpigmentation
Chronic arsenism
Argyria

---

to be included in the differential diagnosis of diffuse hyperpigmentation.

References

1. Alper JC, Holmes LB: The incidence and significance of birthmarks in a cohort of 4,641 newborns, *Pediatr Dermatol* 1:58, 1983.
2. Spritz RA: Molecular basis of human piebaldism, *J Invest Dermatol* 103:137S, 1994.
3. Baldwin CT, Lipsky NR, Hoth CF, et al: Mutations in PAX3 associated with Waardenburg syndrome type I, *Hum Mutat* 3:205, 1994.
4. Fitzpatrick TB: History and significance of white macules, earliest visible sign of tuberous sclerosis, *Ann NY Acad Sci* 615:26, 1991.
5. Alper JC, Holmes LB: The incidence and significance of birthmarks in a cohort of 4,641 newborns, *Pediatr Dermatol* 1:58, 1983.
6. Osborne JP, Fryer A, Webb D: Epidemiology of tuberous sclerosis, *Ann NY Acad Sci* 615:125, 1991.
7. Roach ES, Smith M, Huttenlocher P, et al: Diagnostic criteria: tuberous sclerosis complex, *J Child Neurol* 2:221, 1992.
8. Sampson JR, Scahill SJ, Stephenson JBP, et al: Genetic aspects of tuberous sclerosis in the west of Scotland, *J Med Genet* 26:28, 1989.
9. Jannsen B, Sampson J, van der Est M, et al: Refined localization of TSC1 by combined analysis of 9q34 and 16p13 data in 14 tuberous sclerosis families.
10. Dhar S, Kanwar AJ, Kaur S: Nevus depigmentosus in India: experience with 50 patients, *Pediatr Dermatol* 10:299, 1993.
11. Jimbow K, Fitzpatrick TB, Szabo G, Hori Y: Congenital circumscribed hypomelanosis: a characterization based on electron microscopic study of tuberous sclerosis, nevus depigmentosus, and piebaldism, *J Invest Dermatol* 64:50, 1975.
12. Sybert VP: Hypomelanosis of Ito: A description, not a diagnosis, *J Invest Dermatol* 103:141S, 1994.
13. Mountcastle EA, Diestelmeier MR, Lupton GP: Nevus anemicus, *J Am Acad Dermatol* 14:628, 1986.
14. Halder RM, Grimes PE, Cowan CA, et al: Childhood vitiligo, *J Am Acad Dermatol* 16:948, 1987.

15. Jaisankar TJ, Baruah MC, Garg BR: Vitiligo in children, *Int J Dermatol* 31:621, 1992.

16. Le Poole IC, van den Wijngaard RMJGJ, Westerhof W, et al: Presence or absence of melanocytes in vitiligo lesions: an immunohistochemical investigation, *J Invest Dermatol* 100:816, 1993.

17. Cui J, Arita Y, Bystryn JC: Cytolytic antibodies to melanocytes in vitiligo, *J Invest Dermatol* 100:812, 1993.

18. Norris DA, Kissinger RM, Naughton GK, Bystryn JC: Evidence for immunologic mechanisms in human vitiligo: patients' sera induce damage to human melanocytes in vitro by complement-mediated damage and antibody-dependent cellular cytotoxicity (ADCC), *J Invest Dermatol* 90:783, 1988.

19. Nordlund JJ, Halder RM, Grimes P: Management of vitiligo, *Dermatol Clinics* 11:27, 1993.

20. Oetting WS, King RA: Molecular basis of oculocutaneous albinism, *J Invest Dermatol* 103:131S, 1994.

21. Creel DJ, Summers CG, King RA: Visual anomalies associated with albinism, *Ophthalmic Pediatr Genet* 11:193, 1990.

22. Hizawa K, Iida M, Matsumoto T, et al: Cancer in Peutz-Jeghers syndrome, *Cancer* 72:2777, 1993.

23. Srivatsa PJ, Keeney GL, Podratz KC: Disseminated cervical adenoma malignum and bilateral ovarian sex cord tumors with annular tubules associated with Peutz-Jeghers syndrome, *Gynecol Oncol* 53:256, 1994.

24. Rodrigo MR, Cheng CH, Tai YT, O'Donnell D: "Leopard" syndrome, *Anaesthesia* 45:30, 1990.

25. Koopman RJ, Happle R: Autosomal dominant transmission of the NAME syndrome (nevi, atrial myxoma, mucinosis of the skin and endocrine overactivity), *Hum Genet* 86:300, 1991.

26. Huson SM: Recent developments in the diagnosis and management of neurofibromatosis, *Arch Dis Child* 64:745, 1989.

27. Arnsmeier SL, Riccardi VM, Paller AS: Familial multiple café au lait spots, *Arch Dermatol* 130:1425, 1994.

28. Cordova A: The Mongolian spot: a study of ethnic differences and a literature review, *Clin Pediatr* 20:714, 1981.

29. Lynn A, Brozenza SJ, Espinoza CG, Fenske NA: Nevus of Ota acquisita of late onset, *Cutis* 51:194, 1993.

30. Alvarez J, Peteiro C, Toribio J: Linear and whorled nevoid hypermelanosis, *Pediatr Dermatol* 10:156, 1993.

31. Rhodes AR, Albert LS, Barnhill RL, Weinstock MA: Sun-induced freckles in children and young adults. A correlation of clinical and histopathologic features, *Cancer* 67:1990, 1991.

32. Abdel-Malek Z, Swope V, Boissy Y, et al: Cutaneous hyperpigmentary lesions in neurofibromatosis-1 are not due to a functional or structural defect in the melanocyte, *J Invest Dermatol* 100:589, 1993.

33. Gutmann DH: New insights into the neurofibromatoses, *Curr Opin Neurol* 7:166, 1994.

34. Tan OT, Morelli JG, Kurban AK: Pulsed dye laser treatment of superficial benign cutaneous pigmented lesions, *Laser Surg Med* 12:538, 1992.

35. Watanabe S, Takahashi H: Treatment of nevus of Ota with the Q-switched ruby laser, *N Engl J Med* 331:1745, 1994.

36. Goss BD, Forman D, Ansell PE, et al: The prevalence and characteristics of congenital pigmented lesions in newborn babies in Oxford, *Paediatr Perinat Epidemiol* 61:448, 1990.

37. Angelucci D, Natali PG, Amerio PI, et al: Rapid perinatal growth mimicking malignant transformation in a giant congenital melanocytic nevus, *Hum Pathol* 22:297, 1991.

38. Carrol CB, Ceballos P, Perry AE, et al: Severely atypical medium-sized congenital nevus with widespread satellitosis and placental deposits in a neonate: the problem of congenital melanoma and its simulants, *J Am Acad Dermatol* 30:825, 1994.

39. Rigel DS, Friedman RJ: The management of patients with dysplastic and congenital nevi, *Dermatol Clin* 3:251, 1985.

40. Quaba AA, Wallace AF: The incidence of malignant melanoma (0-15 years of age) arising in "large" congenital nevocellular nevi. *Plastic Reconstr Surg* 78:174-181, 1986.

41. Gari LM, Rivers JK, Kopf A: Melanomas arising in large congenital nevi: a prospective study, *Pediatr Dermatol* 5:151, 1988.

42. Gallagher RP, Rivers JK, Yang CP, et al: Melanocytic nevus density in Asian, IndoPakistani and white children: the Vancouver mole study, *J Am Acad Dermatol* 25:507, 1991.

43. Marghoob AA, Kopf AW, Rigel DS, et al: Risk of cuta-

neous malignant melanoma in patients with "classic" atypical-mole syndrome, *Arch Dermatol* 130:993, 1994.

44. Gallagher RP, McLean DI, Yang CP, et al: Suntan, sunburn, and pigmentation factors and the frequency of acquired melanocytic nevi in children, *Arch Dermatol* 126:770, 1990.

45. Fritschi L, McHenry P, Green A, et al: Naevi in schoolchildren in Scotland and Australia, *Br J Dermatol* 130:599, 1994.

46. Gallagher RP, McLean DI, Yang CP, et al: Anatomic distribution of acquired melanocytic nevi in white children, *Arch Dermatol* 126:466, 1990.

47. Meyer LJ, Zone JJ: Genetics of cutaneous melanoma, *J Invest Dermatol* 103:112S, 1994.

48. Swerdlow AJ, English J, MacKie RM, et al: Benign melanocytic naevi as a risk factor for malignant melanoma, *Br Med J* 292:1555, 1986.

49. Holly EA, Kelly JW, Shpall SN, Chiu SH: Number of melanocytic nevi as a major risk factor for malignant melanoma, *J Am Acad Dermatol* 17:459, 1987.

50. Augustsson A: Melanocytic naevi, melanoma, sun exposure, *Acta Derm Venereol (Stockh)* 166(suppl):1, 1991.

51. Green A: Sun exposure and the risk of melanoma, *Austr J Dermatol* 25:99, 1984.

52. Stuart CA, Pate CJ, Peters EJ: Prevalence of acanthosis nigricans in an unselected population, *Am J Med* 87:269, 1989.

53. Schwartz RA: Acanthosis nigricans, *J Am Acad Dermatol* 31:1, 1994.

18

Immobile and Hypermobile Skin

Certain skin changes are distinguished by palpation rather than by visual assessment of morphology. Skin mobility and elasticity are two qualities that are distinguished by this method.

Skin that is immobile is fixed to the underlying fascia and sometimes to muscle or bone. A growth or nodule that is fixed to the underlying fascia might indicate a malignant tumor in childhood. Far more common, however, are fibrous thickenings that attach the dermis to the fascia, as in the localized forms of scleroderma. Testing for this feature is performed by grasping the skin with the thumb and forefinger and determining its movement. Hypermobile skin is often associated with hypermobile joints and brings to mind the various forms of the Ehlers-Danlos syndrome.

SKIN THICKENINGS

Skin may become thickened and immobile in certain areas. Nodules are not formed, but the thickened, slightly raised, or slightly depressed area can be appreciated on palpation.

LOCALIZED SCLERODERMA (MORPHEA)

Clinical features

Circumscribed areas of scleroderma may occur as solitary or multiple oval lesions, or as a linear lesion.[1,2] Sixty percent of the children will have solitary linear lesions on the extremities (Fig. 18-1), forehead, or chest.[1,2] Atrophy of an extremity, digital contracture, or facial hemiatrophy (Parry-Romberg syndrome) may occur.[1,2] Linear lesions of the forehead often extend into the frontal scalp, producing a scarring hair loss (*en coup de sabre*)[1,2] (Fig. 18-2). The immobile area will be exaggerated by having the child wrinkle the forehead. The surface of the immobile, bound-down skin of morphea is often shiny and hypopigmented, and it may be surrounded by a violaceous hue (lilac) or a brown border[1,2] (Fig. 18-3). About one third of children with morphea have arthralgias. Guttate morphea may present with a depressed, dusky appearing, slightly thickened area that is not completely bound down[1-3] (Fig. 18-4). Often this is confused with atrophoderma, but some of the lesions will evolve to more typical bound-down circumscribed morphea. Some children have lesions

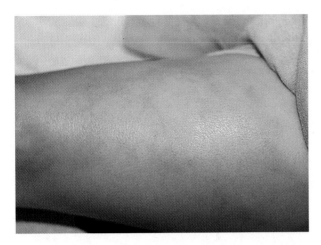

Fig. 18-1
Linear morphea (scleroderma). White, bound-down plaque extending down the back of the thigh of an adolescent female.

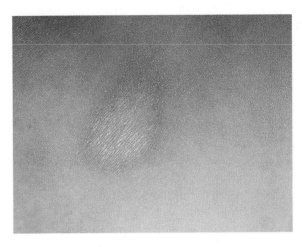

Fig. 18-3
Lilac borders with white center of an "active" lesion of guttate morphea.

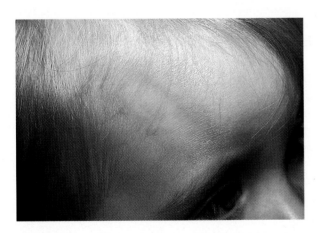

Fig. 18-2
Linear scleroderma of the forehead in a child.

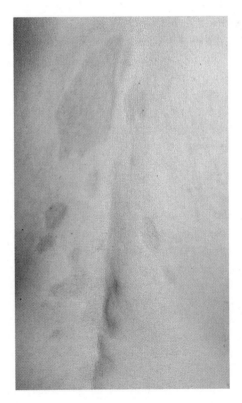

Fig. 18-4
Slightly depressed, tan, slightly bound-down lesions of early morphea.

of guttate morphea and linear morphea simultaneously or have guttate morphea lesions accompanied by lesions of acrodermatitis chronica atrophicans.[1-3] Concurrent lesions of morphea and lichen sclerosus et atrophicus (LS&A) have also been noted in childhood. Dysesthesias of lesions or spinal radiculopathies have also been recognized in children with morphea, particularly when a distribution of cutaneous lesions on the back assumes a "Christmas tree" or a dermatomal distribution.[1-3] It is exceedingly rare for childhood morphea to progress to progressive systemic sclerosis (PSS).[1-3] PSS is rare in childhood and usually presents with severe acral and orofacial sclerosis.[3] If Raynaud's phenomenon is present, the erythrocyte sedimentation rate is elevated, or the antinuclear antibody (ANA) test is positive, the possibility of progression to systemic sclerosis is increased.[3]

The so-called subcutaneous morphea represents eosinophilic fasciitis. There is often diffuse thickening of the skin in an irregular surface pattern, leading to a "lumpy-bumpy" skin appearance.[4,5] Children with eosinophilic fasciitis often progress to scleroderma-like fibrosis of the skin with sparing of distal areas.[5]

Differential diagnosis

LS&A shows many features that overlap those of morphea, but its characteristic epidermal thinning and lichenoid papules help differentiate it from morphea. Atrophoderma may mimic morphea.

The dusky lesions of early morphea often appear slightly depressed, and only with the evolution of lesions such that some become "bound down" will the diagnosis be certain. An excisional skin biopsy down to and including fascia may be diagnostic.[1-3]

Pathogenesis

The mechanism of the disease is unknown, but evidence from Europe implicating a *Borrelia* infection by positive serology, presence of a spirochete by immunoperoxidase staining of affected skin biopsies, and recovery of a spirochete by culture of morphea lesions is intriguing,[6] although it has not been confirmed in North America.[2,3] The associated neurologic symptoms and coexistence with known *Borrelia* infections, such as acrodermatitis chronica atrophicans, strengthen the possible role of some spirochetal infection producing the condition. An inflammatory stage precedes the sclerotic stage and is characterized by a predominantly lymphocytic infiltrate around dermal blood vessels and collagen bundles.[1-3] In the sclerotic stage, thickened dermal collagen replaces the subcutaneous fat. Injury to the underlying muscle fibers, with separation and inflammation of muscle,

occurs in linear forms. In eosinophilic fasciitis, thickening and inflammation of the fascia is diagnostic.[4,5] The inflammation often demonstrates an excess of eosinophils. Fibrous replacement of the subcutaneous fat may be minimal.

Treatment

There is no specific treatment. Symptomatic relief may be achieved with the use of topical lubricants three times daily or topical glucocorticosteroids twice daily. Whether penicillin or other antispirochetal therapy is indicated in North American patients is yet to be determined. Systemic therapies such as oral prednisone, D-penicillamine, cyclophosphamide, and chlorambucil have more side effects than benefit.[1-3]

Patient education

The duration of lesion activity is 3 to 5 years, followed by softening of the skin. Residual pigmentary changes may last several years longer.[1-3] Atrophy of the limbs or facial hemiatrophy will persist.

Follow-up visits

Examination at 3-month intervals is useful to determine whether systemic symptoms or signs have appeared. A repeat ANA test for laboratory evidence of systemic collagen vascular disease is useful.

LICHEN SCLEROSUS ET ATROPHICUS

Clinical features

White papules and immobile plaques occur primarily in the anogenital area in grade-school or adolescent girls.[7,8] LS&A is 10 times more common in girls[7] (Fig. 18-5). Purpura, vesicles, and telangiectasia may be seen within the plaques in the genital area. As the lesions age, the skin surface becomes thinned and finely wrinkled (Fig. 18-6). Bleeding may occur.[7,10] Ulcerations and excoriations may be superimposed on these primary lesions. The anogenital lesions in girls tend to surround both the vulva and the anus in a figure-eight pattern.[7,8] Itching and burning of the skin are frequent complaints. Painful defecation, con-

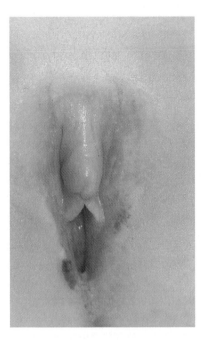

Fig. 18-5
Lichen sclerosus et atrophicus of a child's vulva.

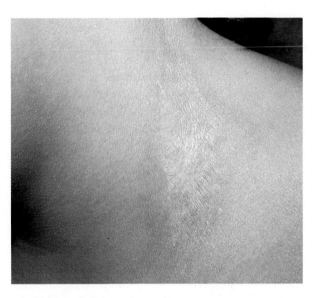

Fig. 18-6
Extragenital lichen sclerosus et atrophicus of the neck.
Telangiectasia and fine wrinkling within the white area.

stipation, bloody stools, and encopresis may be reported.[7]

Extragenital lesions appear as asymptomatic white papules on the upper back or upper chest (Fig. 18-6) and occasionally on the face or extremities.[7,8] About half of the patients with anogenital lesions will also have distal lesions. The isomorphic phenomenon occurs in LS&A, and lesions may develop in surgical scars or other sites of skin trauma. Coexistence of LS&A with morphea is observed in children.[7-9] Familial cases have been documented, and it may be useful to examine siblings or parents.[9]

Differential diagnosis

Skin immobility suggests localized scleroderma, but atrophic skin, the white color, and papular lesions help distinguish it from scleroderma. Anogenital lesions may be confused with sexual abuse, and abuse investigations may be incorrectly initiated.[7,8] In LS&A the hymen is never involved, whereas it may reveal injury in sexual abuse.[7] Also, candidiasis, intertrigo, or irritant dermatitis may be confused with LS&A. Atrophic areas of lichen planus may mimic LS&A, but the purple papular border of lichen planus is a useful differentiating feature.

Pathogenesis

In LS&A the dermis is sclerotic and thickened and the epidermis is thinned and atrophic.[7-9] A bandlike accumulation of lymphocytes is present in the middermis, and features of epidermal injury are also seen. Atrophy of the epidermis and hydropic degeneration of the basal epidermal cells are present.[9] Hyperkeratosis occurs, so that the stratum corneum layer is much thicker than the remainder of the epidermis.[9] Edema and homogenization of collagen in the upper dermis are also seen. As the lesions progress, the collagen of the lower dermis thickens, mimicking circumscribed scleroderma. The mechanism of this inflammatory disease is unknown, although, like morphea, some investigators have linked LS&A to *Borrelia* infections.

Treatment

Spontaneous clearing within 2 years of the onset has been described in half the cases.[7] There is no specific treatment. Itching often responds to low-potency topical glucocorticosteroid ointments applied three times daily. Topical lubricants may relieve the symptoms. Prophylactic topical antibiotic ointments, and cleanliness of the anogenital area, are useful in preventing superimposed infection. Whether penicillin or other antispirochetal drugs will help is yet to be determined. Androgen creams offer no benefit and may virilize the child. For bleeding telangiectatic vessels, the vascular-specific pulsed dye laser at 585 nm has been useful.[10]

Patient education

It is helpful to explain to patients that the course is irregularly progressive, although lesions may remain stable for long periods. One should emphasize that by puberty two thirds of children will have spontaneous clearing.[7] Patients should be informed that areas of whitish thickening (leukoplakia) may appear on the mucosa or adjacent mucosal surfaces, and that these may rarely progress to carcinoma. Carcinomas have been reported in childhood, but they are exceedingly rare.[7-9]

Follow-up visits

Yearly examinations are useful to monitor the progress of the disease and examine lesions for possible malignant changes, which require biopsy.

EHLERS-DANLOS SYNDROME

Clinical features

Ehlers-Danlos syndrome is a phenotype in which there is excessive stretching of skin and joints.[11,12] Ten different subtypes of Ehlers-Danlos syndrome have been described, with most forms having autosomal dominant inheritance (Table 18-1).[11,12] Types I through IV constitute the majority of children affected.[11,12] The increase in skin stretchability is often spectacular; however, the skin returns to its normal position (Fig. 18-7). Skin fragility is a major problem, and slow healing is very common.[12] Skin injury often results in large hematomas that heal with a fibrotic nodule covered by thin, wrinkled epidermis.[11] These are usually prominent over the lower part of the legs (Fig. 18-8). These nodules may calcify. Wound dehiscence is observed in at least a third of lesions.[12] Easily visible veins and epistaxis are also noted. Hyperextensible joints may result in subluxation of the joints, particularly of the shoulders, elbows, hips, and knees, and flat feet, kyphosis, and scoliosis may occur (Fig. 18-9). Back pain may become a problem with age, and weakness, muscle cramps, and arthritis may eventuate.[12] Jaw pain or jaw clicking is common.[12]

Hematemesis and bleeding in the lower intestine may occur. Menorrhagia may be seen. Aortic aneurysms, arteriovenous fistula, retinal detachment,

Table 18-1

Subtypes of Ehlers-Danlos Syndrome and Their Clinical Features

Subtype/inheritance		Skin/joints	Other
I	Dominant	Hyperextensible, lax skin and joints	Hernias, scars, varicosities
II	Dominant	Soft, bruisable; lax hands and feet	
III	Dominant	Normal skin, lax joints	
IV	Recessive	Thin, prominent veins,	Bowel and/or aortic rupture
	Dominant	Pale skin, echymoses	
V	X-linked	Hypermobile skin, scarring, bruising	Floppy mitral valves
VI	Recessive	Hyperextensible skin, lax joints	Blue sclerae
VII	Recessive	Soft, hyperextensible skin, hip dislocation, lax joints	Short stature
VIII	Dominant	Fragile skin, lax joints	Periodontitis
IX	X-linked	Lax skin and joints	Pectus excavatum
X	Recessive	Soft, lax skin and joints	Bruising

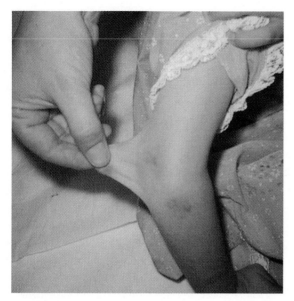

Fig. 18-7
Hyperextensible skin in a child with Ehlers-Danlos syndrome.

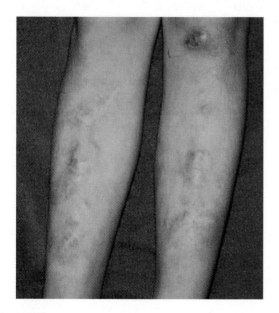

Fig. 18-8
Large scars and pseudotumors of anterior aspect of the lower legs of a child with Ehlers-Danlos syndrome.

and lens abnormalities and myopia have been described.[11,12] Premature births and miscarriages are common.[12]

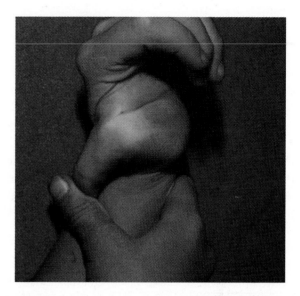

Fig. 18-9
Hyperextensible, lax joints of a child with Ehlers-Danlos syndrome.

Differential diagnosis
The hyperextensible skin is characteristic and usually is not confused with other disorders.

Pathogenesis
The common problem in all 10 subtypes is faulty formation of collagen.[13] Since collagen limits the stretchability of skin, joints, and blood vessels, defective collagen results in hyperextensible skin and joints and fragile blood vessels. Type I patients have disorganized dermal collagen bundles with bizzare shapes, and types II and III demonstrate somewhat more organized collagen bundles but with increased amounts of matrix substances within them.[14] For the most common types I, II, and III, no molecular or biochemical defect has yet been pinpointed.[13,14] In two subtypes, deficiencies of enzymes necessary for cross-linking collagen molecules have been identified. In type IV, four separate defects in synthesis of type III collagen have been identified, two at the messenger RNA (mRNA) level, two at the structural protein level.[13] Molecular biology techniques are likely to clarify the mechanisms of types currently unknown.

Treatment

Protective measures to prevent skin trauma, particularly during the toddler stage, are most useful. Pediatric orthopedic and ophthalmologic care is recommended. Otherwise, no satisfactory treatment is available.

Patient education

Informed genetic counseling should be given if a parent is affected. The expectation of premature birth should be emphasized. The skeletal and eye difficulties that may occur as the child grows should also be stressed.

Follow-up visits

Yearly ophthalmologic and orthopedic examinations are recommended.

References

1. Krafchik BR: Localized cutaneous scleroderma, *Semin Dermatol* 11:65, 1992.
2. Uziel Y, Krafchik BR, Silverman ED, et al: Localized scleroderma in childhood: a report of 30 cases, *Semin Arthritis Rheum* 23:328, 1994.
3. Ansell BM, Falcini F, Woo P: Scleroderma in childhood, *Clin Dermatol* 12:299, 1994.
4. Miller JJ III: The fasciitis-morphea complex in children, *Am J Dis Child* 146:733, 1992.
5. Farrington ML, Haas JE, Nazar-Stewart V, et al: Eosinophilic fasciitis in children frequently progresses to scleroderma-like cutaneous fibrosis, *J Rheumatol* 20:128, 1993.
6. Aberer E, Kollegger H, Kristofeitsch W, et al: Neuroborreliosis in morphea and lichen sclerosus et atrophicus, *J Am Acad Dermatol* 19:820, 1988.
7. Loening-Burke V: Lichen sclerosus et atrophicus in children, *Am J Dis Child* 145:1058, 1991.
8. Ridley CM: Genital lichen sclerosus (lichen sclerosus et atrophicus) in childhood and adolescence, *J R Soc Med* 86:69, 1993.
9. Sahn EE, Bluestein EL, Oliva S: Familial lichen sclerosus et atrophicus in childhood, *Pediatr Dermatol* 11:160, 1994.
10. Rabinowitz LG: Lichen sclerosus et atrophicus treatment with the 585-nm flashlamp-pumped pulsed dye laser, *Arch Dermatol* 129:381, 1993.
11. Yeowell HN, Pinnell SR: The Ehlers-Danlos syndromes, *Semin Dermatol* 12:229, 1993.
12. Ainsworth SR, Aulicino PL: A survey of patients with Ehlers-Danlos syndrome, *Clin Orthop* 286:250, 1993.
13. Tilstra DJ, Byers PH: Molecular basis of hereditary disorders of connective tissue, *Annu Rev Med* 45:149, 1994.
14. Hausser I, Anton-Lamprecht I: Differential ultrastructural aberrations of collagen fibrils in Ehlers-Danlos syndrome types I-IV as a means of diagnostics and classification, *Hum Genet* 93:394, 1994.

19

Genodermatoses

There are hundreds of hereditary skin diseases, and the discussion of all of them is beyond the scope of this book. The most common genodermatoses are considered in other chapters: the neurocutaneous disorders in Chapter 17, genetic nail disorders in Chapter 16, genetic hair disorders in Chapter 15, photodermatoses in Chapter 10, and vascular lesions in Chapter 14. There are uncommon types of hereditary skin diseases that may be encountered in practice. These conditions are considered here because they are important in the differential diagnosis of more common conditions, and they are lifelong problems for the affected individuals. Included in this chapter are the disorders of keratinization, including the ichthyoses and Darier's disease, the mechanobullous diseases, and ectodermal dysplasias. Acrodermatitis enteropathica is also included in this chapter, although it is separate from the three major categories.

ICHTHYOSIS

Ichthyosis is a term used to describe excessive scaling of the skin, which may be "fish scale–like." Although normal infants born after 40 to 42 weeks of gestation will display some thin scales and mild peeling of skin, as will the dysmature infant, the scaling in the forms of ichthyosis is usually generalized and the scales are thick. Four major hereditary types of ichthyosis have been described and characterized[1] (Fig. 19-1). Lamellar ichthyosis and bullous ichthyosis usually present at birth with severe scaling.[1,2] Ichthyosis vulgaris and X-linked ichthyosis may be present in the neonate or may be expressed later in childhood.[1-3]

Clinical features
Ichthyosis vulgaris
Ichthyosis vulgaris is inherited as an autosomal dominant disease that may be as frequent as 1 in 250 individuals.[1,2] Fine scales usually become prominent by 6 months to 2 years of age[2,3] (Fig. 19-1). The scales are most prominent over the lower legs (Fig. 19-2) and buttocks. Dry, follicular, horny plugs (keratosis pilaris) are present on the extensor extremities and may be widespread. Palms and soles show an increased number of skin creases. The entire skin surface is dry. Water retention by the stratum corneum is minimal.[4] Occasionally, children may have associated

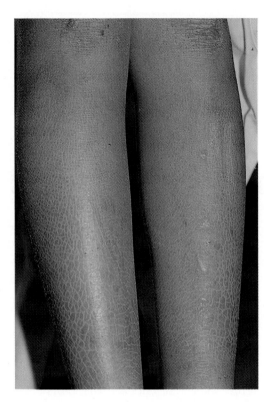

Fig. 19-1
Ichthyosis vulgaris. Scales over the lower legs in a toddler.

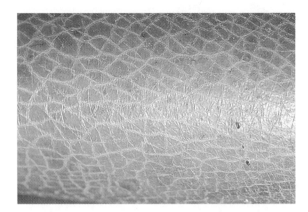

Fig. 19-2
Ichthyosis vulgaris. Prominent scales over the lower legs in a 12-year-old.

atopic dermatitis.[2] The skin in ichthyosis vulgaris usually remains normal throughout the newborn period.

X-linked ichthyosis

X-linked ichthyosis may appear at birth but usually presents in infancy with scales over the posterior neck, upper trunk, and extensor surfaces of the extremities[1,2] (Fig. 19-3). As the child ages, the scales often become thicker and dirty-yellow or brown. The antecubital and popliteal fossae may be spared (Fig. 19- 4). Scaling is usually mild during the first 30 days of life and the skin is a normal color. Palms and soles are spared, in contrast to the other forms of ichthyosis.[1,2] An associated steroid sulfatase deficiency has been described with X-linked ichthyosis.[5]

Lamellar ichthyosis and congenital nonbullous ichthyosiform erythroderma

Although both conditions appear to be an autosomal recessive trait, two separate disease entities may

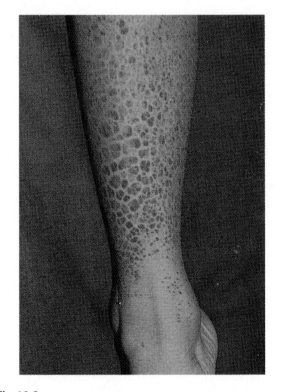

Fig. 19-3
X-linked ichthyosis. Large, dark, platelike scales on the lower leg.

exist.[1,2] The nonbullous congenital ichthyosiform erythroderma individuals have generalized fine scales on erythematous skin.[1,2] The lamellar ichthyosis patients have larger, darker, platelike scales with or without erythematous skin. With either condition the

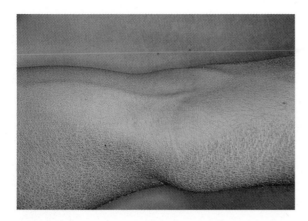

Fig. 19-4
X-linked ichthyosis. Darkened scales with sparing of the ante-cubital fossa.

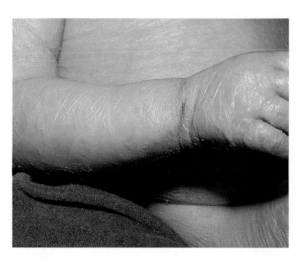

Fig. 19-5
Lamellar ichthyosis. Thickened, shiny skin without erythema in a child.

affected baby can be born with a collodion membrane. Severe water and electrolyte imbalance may develop.[6] The erythroderma may fade during childhood in some of the infants (Fig. 19-5). Ectropion and eclabium may be present and appear shortly after birth in patients with lamellar ichthyosis.[1,2,7] The palms and soles in these patients may be greatly thickened. Skin biopsy after the collodion membrane is shed will demonstrate hyperkeratosis but is otherwise not diagnostic.[1,2,7]

Bullous ichthyosis (congenital bullous ichthyosiform erythroderma, epidermolytic hyperkeratosis)

Epidermolytic hyperkeratosis (EHK), an autosomal dominant disorder, is characterized by extensive scaling at birth, erythroderma, and recurrent episodes of bullae formation[1,2,6,7] (Figs. 19-6, 19-7, and 19-8). The blisters represent lysis of the epidermal granular layer, and secondary infection with *Staphylococcus aureus* becomes a major difficulty in the neonatal period and during infancy. As the child ages, the involvement becomes more limited in extent. By school age, thick, warty, dirty-yellow scales with malodorous excessive bacterial colonization of the skin will have developed on the palms, soles, elbows, and knees (Fig. 19-9). Skin biopsy will reveal enlargement of the granular cell layer with bizarre vacuolization of the epidermal granular cells.[2,7,8] A related autosomal

dominant condition called *bullous ichthyosis of Siemens* demonstrates similar but milder findings with more superficial bullae.[7] Widespread epidermal nevi that show the pathologic changes of EHK, such as ichthyosis histrix and systematized epidermal nevi, may show histologic changes similar to EHK.[7,8]

Differential diagnosis

At birth, lamellar ichthyosis and bullous ichthyosis may be difficult to distinguish from one another. The hereditary pattern and skin biopsy may help.[7] If an individual with ichthyosis has corneal opacities, and sparing of the palms and soles, it is likely to be X-linked ichthyosis. If an ectropion and eclabium are present, it is likely to be lamellar ichthyosis; and recurrent bullous episodes will distinguish EHK. Measurement of steroid sulfatase activity in red blood cells may be useful in the diagnosis of X-linked ichthyosis.[5]

Ichthyosis vulgaris in its mild form may be difficult to distinguish from dry skin, but the extensive distribution of scales, particularly scaling over the buttocks and lower legs, increased palmar creases, and skin biopsy will differentiate ichthyosis vulgaris from dry skin.[8] Scaling disorders similar to lamellar ichthyosis are present in many ichthyosis syndromes associated with neurologic disease.[1]

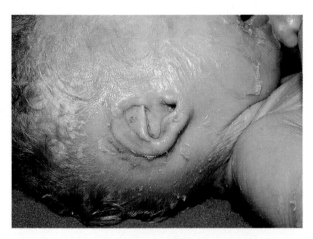

Fig. 19-6
Lamellar ichthyosis. Thickened scales in scalp and shiny, thickened skin of the ear and face in a toddler.

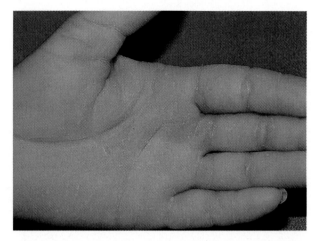

Fig. 19-8
Epidermolytic hyperkeratosis. Hyperkeratosis of the palms and deep fissures at creases.

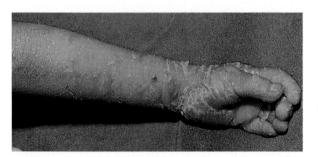

Fig. 19-7
Epidermolytic hyperkeratosis. Thickened scales plus numerous erosions on the arm of a child.

Pathogenesis

Skin biopsy in the ichthyosis syndromes will often be of diagnostic value. In ichthyosis vulgaris there is a thin or absent granular cell layer in addition to the hyperkeratosis.[2,6] X-linked ichthyosis demonstrates hyperkeratosis with an otherwise normal-appearing epidermis.[2,6] Vacuolization and separation of the granular cell layer with blister cavity formation are associated with the hyperkeratosis in bullous ichthyosis.[2,6,7] Similar findings in the more superficial epidermis are found in bullous ichthyosis of Siemens.[7,8] Lamellar ichthyosis may demonstrate hyperkeratosis, acanthosis, and a mild chronic inflammatory infiltrate.[2,6]

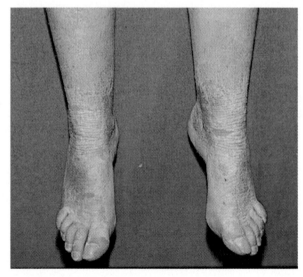

Fig. 19-9
Epidermolytic hyperkeratosis. Thickened, malodorous skin on the legs and ankles.

Increased epidermal turnover has been demonstrated in lamellar ichthyosis and bullous ichthyosis, such that excessive numbers of stratum corneum cells are produced.[2] In contrast, X-linked ichthyosis and ichthyosis vulgaris demonstrate normal epidermal turnover, and the accumulated scale is thought to be due to faulty shedding of the stratum corneum.

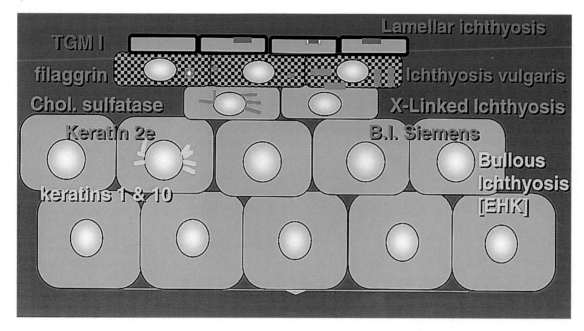

Fig. 19-10
Gene mutations in the ichthyoses.

Molecular diagnosis is most useful, if available (Fig. 19-10). In ichthyosis vulgaris, gene abnormalities of profillagrin and fillagrin have been identified.[9] In X-linked ichthyosis, mutations in the gene coding for steroid sulfatase deficiency are described.[9] In bullous ichthyosis, mutations in the genes encoding the paired keratins 1 and 10 have been uncovered.[10,11] These keratin proteins are expressed in differentiated keratinocytes, and with mutations develop an unstable keratin scaffolding within the suprabasilar keratinocytes. The cytoskeleton collapses, resulting in separation of affected cells from one another and blister formation.[8] In bullous ichthyosis of Siemens, mutations in the gene encoding keratin 9, a cytoskeletal protein expressed superficial to the granular layer, have been identified.[9] In lamellar ichthyosis, mutations in the gene encoding transglutaminase 1 have been found.[13] Transglutaminase 1 is important in the cross-linking of proteins forming the cornified envelope of the differentiated keratinocyte, and the failure to form the envelope may result in loss of regulation of keratinocyte proliferation. Epidermal nevi with pathology of EHK may represent mosaicism for EHK, with the affected skin showing the gene mutation for keratins 1 or 10 and the unaffected intervening skin displaying normal keratins.[14]

Treatment

There is no satisfactory treatment for the ichthyoses. In ichthyosis vulgaris and X-linked ichthyosis, hydration of the skin twice daily, and the generous use of lubricants, will control the dryness and scaling. The use of α-hydroxy acids such as lactic acid, 5% ointment, citric acid 5% ointment, or 12% ammonium lactate lotion applied once or more daily may be helpful in the more severe ichthyoses, although many such patients do as well with bland lubricants alone. In bullous ichthyoses, systemic antistaphylococcal antibiotics are required to treat the infectious episodes.

In ichthyosis great caution must be used in applying therapeutic agents to the skin of an affected infant or child. Because of the larger surface area per body weight, systemic toxicity and side effects can be seen, and acidosis can occur secondary to topical therapy.

Recognize that both the active medication and the vehicle for the medication could cause significant toxicity in the infant with ichthyosis.

The synthetic retinoids given orally have shown promise in the management of ichthyosis but their use is restricted by long-term effects on growing bones.[15,16]

Patient education

The genetic nature of the ichthyoses should be emphasized, as well as the methods of controlling these disorders. Good supportive relationships should be established with these patients.

Follow-up visits

A visit 1 week after discharge from the newborn nursery is useful in evaluating therapy. Thereafter, routine visits for pediatric care and additional visits may be necessary, depending on the severity of the ichthyosis.

MECHANOBULLOUS DISEASES

Epidermolysis bullosa

At least 18 distinct hereditary types of epidermolysis bullosa (EB) have been described,[17] and recent molecular genetic studies have resulted in the identification of mutations in the responsible keratinocyte genes.[10,18] EB can be divided into nonscarring and scarring types.[17] The nonscarring types include those with intraepidermal separation and junctional separation, whereas the scarring (dystrophic) forms include the subepidermal types. The disease is uncommon but potentially life-threatening to newborns and infants. Correct diagnosis in the newborn period can be difficult and depends on a combination of clinical, histologic, and molecular biology techniques.[17] In all 18 forms of EB, evolution of clinical lesions during the first 30 days of life may confuse the clinician. Family history of childhood blistering diseases is often absent, and the clinician must depend on the findings in the affected baby.[17,18] Extreme care must be taken to obtain a biopsy of an induced blister and not an old or established blister. Induction of a blister with a pencil eraser or a suction device is the most reliable method.[17,18] A shave biopsy taken from the normal skin into the induced blister is preferred. Optimally, the biopsy specimen should be examined by light and electron microscopy plus immunofluorescent mapping.[17]

Nonscarring types

Clinical features of epidermolysis bullosa simplex EB simplex (EBS) is dominantly inherited and may be generalized or localized.[17,18] The most common form is localized to the hands and feet (Fig. 19-11) and often is not present at birth (recurrent eruption of the hands and feet [Weber-Cockayne disease]). Blisters of the hands and feet first occur in late childhood or adolescence, when the child experiences minor frictional trauma (Fig. 19-12). It often has its onset in warm weather.

EBS may also be generalized with lesions present at birth or more likely the appearance of blisters at 6 to 12 months of age.[17] They are more numerous on the distal extremities but may also be seen on elbows and knees. It is autosomal dominant and worsens in warm weather. In the Koebner type of generalized EBS the lesions are discrete (Fig. 19-13) and in the Dowling-Meara type they are grouped[10,17] (Fig. 19-14).

EBS superficialis appears at birth without intact blisters but with rather superficial areas of peeling of

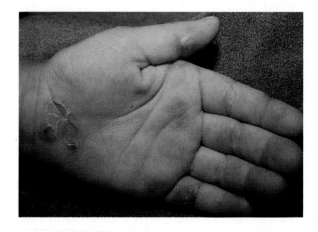

Fig. 19-11
Epidermolysis bullosa simplex. Weber-Cockayne type. Minor trauma on playground equipment induced blisters of the palms.

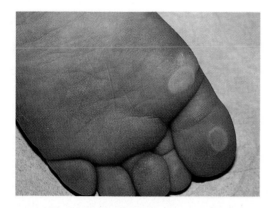

Fig. 19-12

Epidermolysis bullosa simplex. Weber-Cockayne type. Painful blisters on the foot of a child after a run.

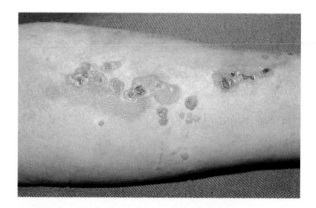

Fig. 19-14

Epidermolysis bullosa simplex. Dowling-Meara type. Grouped blisters on the leg of a child.

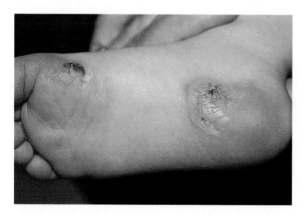

Fig. 19-13

Epidermolysis bullosa simplex. Koebner type. Discrete blisters on the toddler's foot.

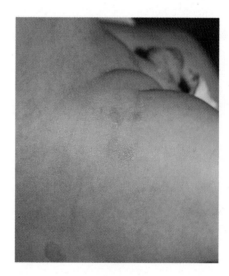

Fig. 19-15

Epidermolysis bullosa simplex superficialis. Superficial erosions on the hip of an infant where diaper tapes adhered to the skin.

the skin[17] (Fig. 19-15). It persists in a mild form to adult life and requires heat plus trauma to produce lesions.

Clinical features of junctional epidermolysis bullosa A generalized often fatal form (Herlitz) and a milder form are recognized.[17,18] Both will present at birth with very few lesions (Fig. 19-16). Mucous membrane lesions appear within the first month of life in the lethal form and are absent or minimal in the milder form. Oral mucosa becomes severely affected in the lethal form (Fig. 19-17), interfering with eating and often resulting in failure to thrive.[17,18] There may develop nonhealing granulation tissue over bony prominences such as the spine, ear, or midface[17] (Fig. 19-18). Secondary bacterial infection can be severe. The majority of lesions heal without scarring, but lateral extension of large bullae can result in hemorrhage and healing with scarring.

Clinical features of scarring (dystrophic) forms of epidermolysis bullosa In EB of the recessive dystrophic type, hemorrhagic bullae appear on the skin at birth or shortly after[17,18] (Fig. 19-19). Removal of the blister roof leaves a raw, bleeding base

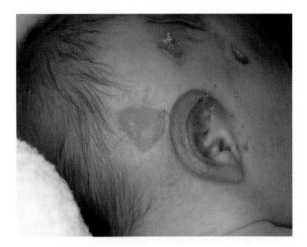

Fig. 19-16
Junctional epidermolysis bullosa. Newborn with a few scattered blisters.

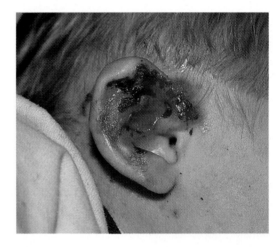

Fig. 19-18
Junctional epidermolysis bullosa. Nonhealing granulation tissue at blister site on a child's ear.

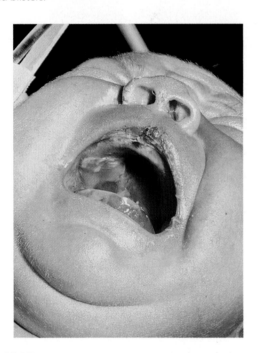

Fig. 19-17
Junctional epidermolysis bullosa. Severe oral erosions in an infant.

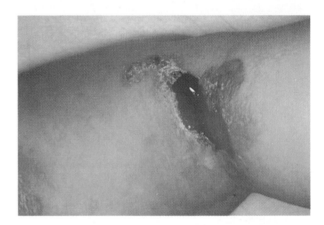

Fig. 19-19
Dystrophic epidermolysis bullosa, recessive. Hemorrhagic blister on a newborn.

that heals with scar formation. Healing scars often entrap islands of epithelium, producing milia that appear as tiny white cysts within scars[17] (Fig. 19-20). Scarring is sufficiently severe to result in replacement of nails and pseudowebbing of all digits, leading eventually to a clublike appearance of the hands and feet[17] (Fig. 19-21). Scarring alopecia of the scalp will develop. Severe scarring of the eyelid may occur.[18] Blisters and erosions of the oral mucosa result in limitation of eating, immobilization of the tongue, and esophageal stricture with resultant dysphagia in 76% of patients.[17,18,20] Laryngeal bullae will produce respiratory stridor.[17] The teeth may be malformed and carious (Fig. 19-22). Anemia due to chronic blood

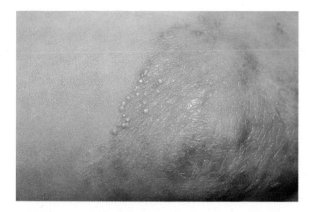

Fig. 19-20
Recessive dystrophic epidermolysis bullosa. Multiple white milia at the border of a scar.

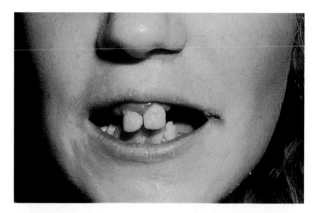

Fig. 19-22
Recessive dystrophic epidermolysis bullosa. Loss of teeth and restriction of mouth opening in a child.

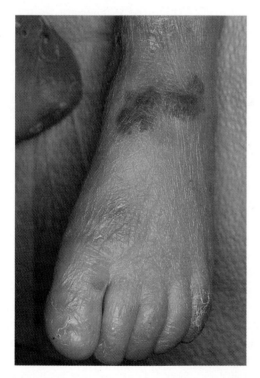

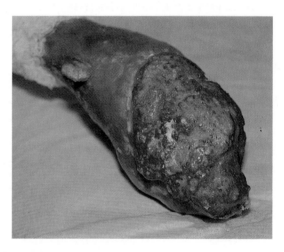

Fig. 19-23
Recessive dystrophic epidermolysis bullosa. Huge verrucous growth on the hand of an adolescent represents squamous cell carcinoma.

Fig. 19-21
Recessive dystrophic epidermolysis bullosa. Loss of toenails, pseudowebbing of digits, and new blisters.

loss and malnutrition occur and failure to thrive will commonly develop.[17,20] Secondary bacterial or candidal infection of the skin is frequent. In adolescent years, squamous cell carcinoma may arise in atrophic scars of the skin (Fig. 19-23) or in leukplakia areas of the mucous membranes.[17]

In EB of the dominant dystrophic type, hemorrhagic bullae are seen at birth, and erosions due to intrauterine blister formation may be observed at delivery.[17,18] Intrauterine erosions are frequently found over the dorsa of the feet and the anterior lower legs. As the child ages, atrophic scars and milia appear (Fig. 19-24). Mucous membrane involvement is less common than in the recessive dystrophic type and

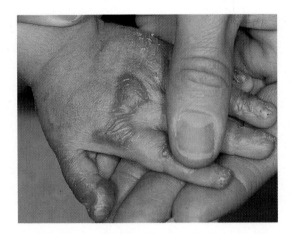

Fig. 19-24
Dominant dystrophic epidermolysis bullosa. Blister, scar formation, milia, and loss of a fingernail in an infant.

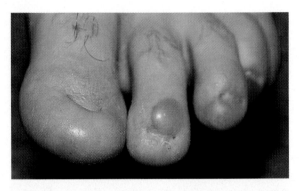

Fig. 19-25
Dominant dystrophic epidermolysis bullosa. Loss of toenails and active blisters but no pseudowebbing in an adolescent.

when present, quite mild.[17,20] Ichthyosis, keratosis pilaris, thickened nails, and hyperhidrosis may develop. Nails may be shed and replaced by scars (Fig. 19-25), but pseudowebbing does not occur.[17] Scarring alopecia is absent, and anemia and failure to thrive are rarely seen.[17,20] A variant, also dominantly inherited, characterized by white atrophic lesions without clinical blister formation, is designated the albopapuloid form.[17] Numerous milia and hypopigmented scars are seen predominantly on the trunk rather than on the extremities.

Differential diagnosis The ease of blistering skin by suction or friction will differentiate EB from friction blisters or spontaneous blistering disease.[17] At birth, obstetric injuries are frequently confused because of the hemorrhagic blisters and eroded, raw areas.[17] Urinary uroporphyrins will distinguish porphyria cutanea tarda from EB. The forms of EB may be differentiated from one another by the inheritance pattern, with a skin biopsy specimen examined by electron microscopy or by molecular genetic analysis.[17,18]

Pathogenesis Almost all forms of EB are inherited.[17,18] The mechanism of the disease is known to be due to gene mutations encoding three major structural proteins: keratins 5 and 14 in EBS, laminin 5 in junctional EB, and type VII collagen in dystrophic

forms of EB[10,18] (Fig. 19-26). They are distinguished by ultrastructural examination of the skin biopsy specimen. Recurrent bullous eruption of the hands and feet demonstrates a separation of epidermal cells just above the basal layer. EBS superficialis demonstrates a separation within the granular layer of epidermis.[17] It is the most superficial blister formation of all the forms of EB. EBS separates the basal cells within the basal layer. In junctional EB, the separation occurs just below the plasma membrane of the basal cells and above the basal lamina of the dermis.[17,18]

The two scarring forms show a separation below the basal lamina in the dermis. In EB dystrophica, recessive type, the anchoring fibrils, which support the basal lamina, are missing.[17]

Mutations of genes encoding for either of the paired keratins 5 and 14 have been demonstrated for EBS.[10,18] The mutated proteins form a faulty keratin scaffolding, and the basal cell collapses and separates from adjacent cells. Mutations of genes encoding for laminin 5 are found in junctional EB.[18,22-24] This results in lack of binding of the basal keratinocyte to type IV collagen though anchoring filaments. Mutations of genes encoding for type VII collagen are found in dystrophic forms of EB, leading to loss of anchoring fibrils.[18,24]

Treatment Treatment is symptomatic and supportive.[25] One of the U.S. centers for EB may be consulted for a comprehensive care program. For the

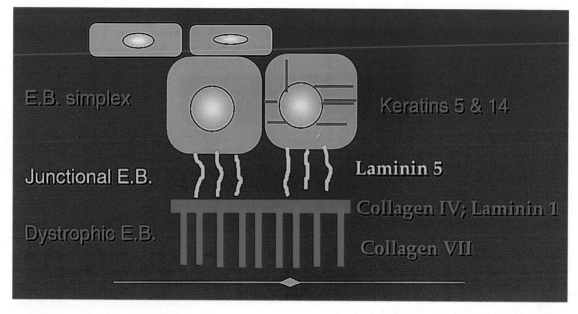

Fig. 19-26
Gene mutations in epidermolysis bullosa.

scarring and junctional forms, skilled nursing and general health care are required. For the newborn infant, small, frequent feedings with a soft nipple are indicated. Gentle handling; soft, loose-fitting clothing; gentle sponge baths; cotton diapers; and a sheepskin pad for the crib should be instituted. Large blisters can be opened with sterile scissors and the roof allowed to collapse by gently compressing out the fluid. Blisters and erosions should have a topical antibiotic (mupirocin) applied gently to the surface (a wooden tongue depressor is useful). Rotating topical antibiotics over months will be useful to reduce the likelihood of bacterial resistance.[25]

For infants and children a passive physical therapy program should be instituted. Water beds, egg crate padding, or sheepskin are useful for sleep.[25] Keeping the room cool will reduce blistering and the accompanying pruritus. Wound dressings, such as Vigilon, Second Skin, and DuoDerm, may be useful for large nonhealing erosions. Keratinocyte-cultured autografts have been successful in severe nonhealing areas. If anemia is present, vitamin supplements and iron may be required. Protein and caloric requirements may be twice that recommended for size because of ongoing skin or mucosal losses, Fluids should be lukewarm, and acidic juices avoided. Ensure or other nutritional supplements may be considered. Whole-grain breads and cereals may reduce constipation, which can be a major problem. A multidisciplinary approach is required in the scarring forms to deal with problems such as esophageal strictures, dental disease, pseudodactyly, laryngeal disorders, urethral meatal stenosis, conjunctival scarring, and psychosocial problems.

In recurrent bullous eruption of the hands and feet, resistance to friction may improve by painting the hands and feet one to two times a week with tincture of benzoin or spray preparations such as Tuff-Skin.

Patient education Much support is required for parents and patients with these disorders, which are chronic, frustrating, and in the dystrophic form, severely debilitating. Patients should be provided with a checklist of steps to reduce friction and instructed by persons skilled in nursing techniques. The lay support group DEBRA of America, Inc. (451 Clarkson Ave., Suite 6101, Brooklyn, NY 11203) has excellent information available for parents and a North American network of local support groups to help families with children who have EB.

Follow-up visits A regular schedule of visits is required to monitor anemia and secondary infections. After birth, visits should be weekly or biweekly. Routine immunizations and well baby care are needed.

Ectodermal dysplasias

There are dozens of ectodermal dysplasias, but the ones most frequently seen include incontinentia pigmenti, anhidrotic and hidrotic forms of ectodermal dysplasia, Goltz syndrome, the palmoplantar keratodermas, and Darier's disease. Ectodermal dysplasias have defects of skin, hair, teeth, nails, and sweating. Skin defects include ichthyosis changes, pigmentary abnormalities, and hypoplasias or aplasias. Sparse or absent scalp or other hair may be found. Ichthyosis with sparse hair is a frequent combination and is seen in Conradi's disease, Netherton's syndrome, and the keratitis-ichthyosis deafness syndrome, for example. Teeth may be cone-shaped, sparse, or absent. Nails may be thickened, thinned, or hypoplastic. Sweating is usually diminished, but hypohidrosis may be patchy and difficult to detect.

Incontinentia pigmenti

Clinical features Four distinct stages of skin changes occur in incontinentia pigmenti. First, linear rows of blisters on the extremities are seen[27] (Fig. 19-27). These blistering episodes recur over the first 3 months of life and are replaced by warty linear areas that may last until 1 year of age[27] (Fig. 19-28). Rows of brown pigmentation are then left (Fig. 19-29). In addition, swirls of brown pigmentation are found on the trunk and in areas where the blisters and warty lesions did not occur[27,28] (Fig. 19-30). The pigmentation fades as the child ages and is usually not seen after adolescence. Hypopigmented scarred areas may develop afterward.

Incontinentia pigmenti is thought to be an X-linked trait, lethal to the male, which explains the female predominance in this disorder.[27-29] Mental retardation, seizures, microcephaly, and other central nervous system (CNS) disorders occur in up to 30% of the reported patients,[27] although it is the authors' experience that the association is much less. Ocular and skeletal anomalies may also be noted.

Differential diagnosis In the blistering stage, herpes simplex or bullous impetigo may be confused with incontinentia pigmenti, but the linear arrangement of its blisters and appropriate cultures will distinguish it from these two disorders. The warty phase may mimic linear epidermal birthmarks or warts. The

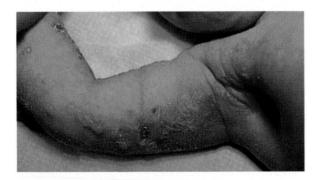

Fig. 19-27
Incontinentia pigmenti. Linear vesicles and crust in an affected newborn girl.

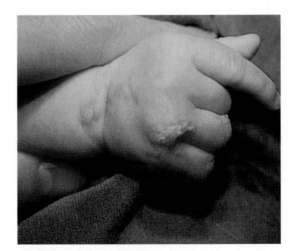

Fig. 19-28
Incontinentia pigmenti. Warty linear growths at the site of previous blisters.

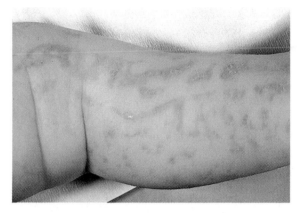

Fig. 19-29
Incontinentia pigmenti. Whorled pigmentation of extremity in sites of previous blisters.

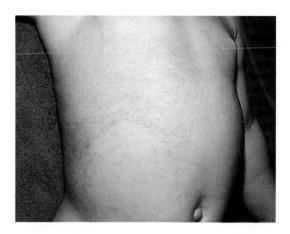

Fig. 19-30
Incontinentia pigmenti. Whorled brown pigmented streaks on the abdominal skin where no prior blisters were noted.

hyperpigmentation is uniquely arranged in whorls and is unlikely to be confused with other causes of hyperpigmentation.

Pathogenesis Skin biopsy demonstrates an inflammatory dermatitis with subcorneal vesicles filled with numerous eosinophils.[28] The warty stage merely demonstrates hyperkeratosis and chronic inflammation in the dermis. In the pigmentary stage, melanin is found free in the dermis or engulfed by dermal macrophages, which accounts for the term *incontinentia pigmenti*.[27,28] Two distinct genes have been implicated, one mapped to Xp11.21 and the other to Xq28.[29] The etiology of this acute dermatitis and its peculiar linear arrangement is not known.

Treatment There is no satisfactory treatment.

Patient education It should be emphasized that the disorder is inherited, and the expected future cutaneous stages should be described.

Follow-up visits Routine infant care visits should be scheduled. Additional visits may be necessary, depending on the complications that arise.

Hypohidrotic and hidrotic ectodermal dysplasia

Clinical features Two common forms of ectodermal dysplasia have been recognized: the anhidrotic form and the hidrotic form.[30] In each there is sparse scalp hair. In addition, a number of other uncommon and rare forms of ectodermal dysplasias

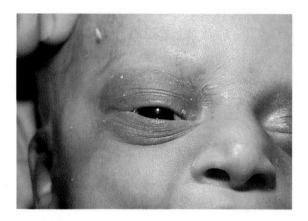

Fig. 19-31
Hypohidrotic ectodermal dysplasia. Absence of the eyebrows and eyelashes and darkened eyelids in a newborn.

have thin or absent hair.[30] Absence of the eyebrows and eyelashes in the newborn may be an important clue to the diagnosis[30,31] (Fig. 19-31). Other clinical findings may be less obvious.

In anhidrotic ectodermal dysplasia, sweating is reduced or completely absent.[30,31] Such infants may present with fever of unknown origin or recurrent high fevers. The faces of such children are very distinctive, with everted lips, prominent frontal ridges, a saddle nose, and absence of eyebrows and eyelashes.[30,31] Temporary and permanent teeth are reduced in number or may be entirely absent. If teeth erupt, they are often cone-shaped (see Fig. 15-17), and this may be observed by dental radiographs even in the preeruptive stage. Atrophic rhinitis and frequent upper respiratory tract symptoms may lead to the mistaken diagnosis of respiratory allergy.[30] Scalp hair is seldom totally absent but is very sparse and is often the first concern of the parents. Fingernails and toenails are normal in at least half of the cases but may be thin or brittle. A careful genetic history should be obtained.

The hidrotic form is characterized by nail dystrophy as the most prominent clinical finding. The nails are thickened, slow growing, and brittle. Thick nails may be apparent early in infancy. In one third of the families, the only feature present is nail disease. As in the anhidrotic form, the scalp hair is thin and sparse and eyebrows are thin, but sweating is normal. Teeth are often normal. The palms and soles may be diffusely thickened, and thickening over the knuckles, knees, and elbows may be prominently observed.

Differential diagnosis   The major conditions to be considered in the differential diagnosis are listed in Box 15-5 on p. 251. The findings of disorders of nails, skin, and teeth in the same patient, in addition to the hair loss, will suggest ectodermal dysplasia. Within a single family with ectodermal dysplasia, the features may be quite variable. To diagnose abnormalities of sweating, a combination of tests may be required.[32] Sweat pore counting using silicone rubber plastic imprints and silver nitrate staining is reliable but does not take into account functional sweating, which can be quantitated by *0*-phthaldialdehyde stains of induced sweating.[32]

Pathogenesis   Anhidrotic ectodermal dysplasia is inherited in an X-linked recessive pattern linked to the Xq12 region or, rarely, an autosomal recessive pattern.[31] The hidrotic form is inherited as autosomal dominant and has been observed in a large French-Canadian family, surnamed Clouston. In the anhidrotic form, sweat glands are absent or rudimentary, as are scalp hair follicles, sebaceous glands, and the mucous glands of the respiratory passages. Lack of sweating results in poor thermal control and high fevers. Lack of hair follicles is expressed as sparse hair, and lack of respiratory mucus produces frequent infections and watery rhinorrhea. A disorder of keratinization is thought to be important in the hidrotic form to explain the nail disease and hyperkeratosis of the palms and soles.

Treatment   Fever control through the use of cool compresses is vital in the newborn or infant with recurrent fevers. There is no specific therapy otherwise available.[30] The use of wigs and dental corrective devices may be necessary.

Patient education   Genetic counseling is very useful, as is the explanation of the cause of the febrile responses and respiratory symptoms in the infant.

Follow-up visits   At least one follow-up visit within 4 weeks of the initial visit is most useful to reexplain the genetic factors and the symptoms of disease.

Focal dermal hypoplasia (Goltz syndrome)

Clinical features   The hallmarks of Goltz syndrome are linear red, swirly streaks in the skin that represent the areas of focal dermal hypoplasia[32,33] (Fig. 19-32). Atrophy, scarring areas, hypopigmentation (Fig. 19-33), and telangiectasias are seen. There may be yellow nodules in a linear pattern.[33] Small papillomatous growths on periorificial or intertriginous areas are found.[32] In the oral mucosa or perineal area, they may be mistaken for warts. Nails may be hypoplastic, short, or brittle. Hair is sparse. Teeth are sparse and enamel defects frequent.[33]

Syndactyly, polydactyly, and a variety of other bony malformations are seen (Fig. 19-34). Lip pits, hemihypoplasia of the tongue, cleft lip, strabismus, colobomas, cataracts, neurosensory hearing loss, and mental retardation are common.[32,33]

Differential diagnosis   Many other ectodermal dysplasias will demonstrate some features in common with Goltz syndrome but will not show the characteristics of focal dermal hypoplasia.[33] Sometimes aplasia cutis congenita or intrauterine erosions of EB are confused, but a skin biopsy will distinguish. In focal dermal hypoplasia, a normal epidermis overlies subcutaneous fat, with a rudi-

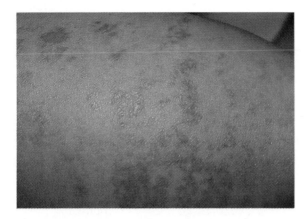

Fig. 19-32
Focal dermal hypoplasia. Linear and whorled red streaks on a female infant.

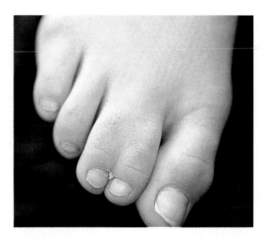

Fig. 19-34
Focal dermal hypoplasia. Syndactyly of the toes in a child.

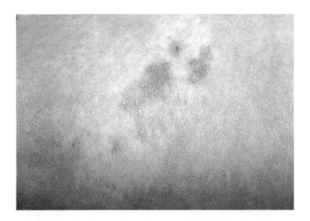

Fig. 19-33
Focal dermal hypoplasia. Atrophic and scarred skin with hypopigmented patch in a child.

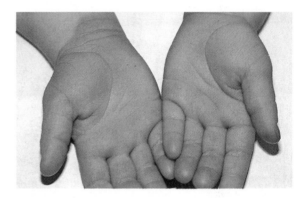

Fig. 19-35
Diffuse palmoplantar keratoderma. All of this child's palmar skin is thickened.

mentary dermis present. In aplasia cutis the epidermis is absent or effaced and subcutaneous fat diminished, and in dystrophic EB the sweat glands and hair follicles are present in a normal dermis with a loss of epidermis.

Pathogenesis An X-linked dominant inheritance pattern is described with many sporadic cases. In a variant with microophthamia, a deletion of Xp22 is described.[33]

Treatment There is no available treatment. A multidisciplinary genetics clinic may be of great assistance in assessment.

Patient education The genetics of the disease should be discussed, including the likelihood of a great variety of bony, eye, and CNS disturbances.

Follow-up visits The frequency of review should be determined by the associated defects.

Hereditary palmoplantar keratodermas
Some children are born with thickening of the palms and soles. There are many genetic types, and they are seen in three main phenotypic patterns: diffuse, involving the entire surface (Fig. 19-35); round and linear (Fig. 19-36); or multiple discrete 1- to 2-mm

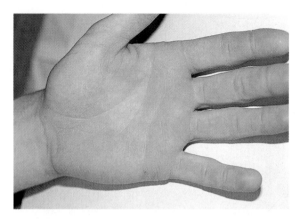

Fig. 19-36
Oval and linear palmoplantar keratoderma. Child's palms have linear and oval plaques of thickening.

Fig. 19-38
Keratosis follicularis. Numerous keratotic papules on an adolescent's upper back.

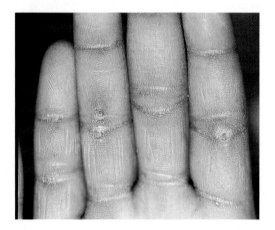

Fig. 19-37
Punctate palmoplantar keratoderma. Adolescent has discrete thickened areas on palms.

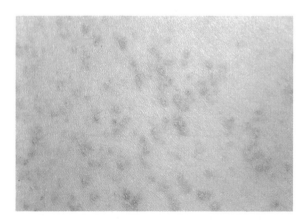

Fig. 19-39
Keratosis follicularis. Discrete brown, "greasy-feeling" keratotic papules.

papules[35] (Fig. 19-37). In the diffuse forms with pathologic changes of EHK, gene mutations in keratins have been detected.[10]

Keratosis follicularis (Darier-White disease)

Clinical features   Keratosis follicularis is characterized by skin-colored to red-brown keratotic 2- to 5-mm papules on the face, neck, scalp, chest, back (Fig. 19-38), and proximal extremities.[35] The skin changes usually begin between the ages of 5 and 10 years, but the age of onset is variable (Fig. 19-39). Over the tops of the hands are skin-colored flat-topped papules, and 0.1-mm punctate papules may be seen on the palms. There are longitudinal streaks of the nails, which terminate in a wedge-shaped split in the free end of the nail. Heat sensitivity is severe, with exacerbations in hot weather or following sun exposure. Severe bacterial or herpes simplex skin infections may occur. Hypopigmented macules on the

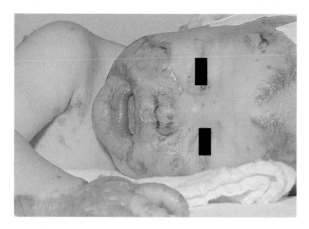

Fig. 19-40
Acrodermatitis enteropathica. Perioral erosions, scalp crusting, and hand erosions in an infant.

trunk and extremities are seen. The course often worsens during adolescence.[36]

Differential diagnosis Keratosis pilaris can mimic keratosis follicularis. The lesions of keratosis pilaris are often much smaller, white, and likely to be dome-shaped. A biopsy may be required to distinguish. Keratosis follicularis has focal areas of acantholytic dyskeratosis, whereas keratosis pilaris reveals a follicular keratotic plug in the body hair channel.

Pathogenesis The disease is considered a disorder of keratinization and has been linked to chromosome 12q.[37] The clumping of keratins and cell-cell separation observed on pathology indicate a likely defect in a protein necessary for the cytoskeletal integrity.

Treatment Keeping the skin surface cool, sometimes with wet dressings, is helpful. Oral retinoids, such as isotretinoin, 0.5 to 1.0 mg/kg/day during hot months, may be useful. Oral antibiotics for bacterial superinfections should be used.

Acrodermatitis enteropathica

Clinical features Acrodermatitis enteropathica is an autosomal recessive disorder of zinc transport.[38,39] It is not apparent at birth but begins at 1 to 2 months of age, with acral skin erosions, intermittent diarrhea, and failure to thrive.[39] The erosions appear as red, moist areas over the distal extremities, including the hands and feet, and in the perioral and perineal areas (Fig. 19-40). Often the cutaneous features precede the diarrhea by several weeks to several months. As the disorder continues, weight loss occurs, as well as photophobia, apathy, irritability, anorexia, anemia, alopecia, thrush, and paronychia due to *Candida albicans*. If the child survives the complications of malnutrition, the skin lesions become erythematous plaques with silvery scales that mimic psoriasis.[39]

The diagnosis is made by measuring serum or plasma zinc levels.[39,40] There are many sources of zinc contamination in rubber stoppers and glass tubes and other blood-collecting devices that produce falsely high zinc levels. Thus the diagnosis may be obscured. Therefore blood samples should be collected in acid-washed sterile plastic tubes, using acid-washed plastic syringes.

Zinc deficiency can also be seen in premature and term infants who are fed a diet deficient in zinc. Occasionally human breast milk can be low in zinc, allowing zinc deficiency in the totally breast-fed infant.[39] Acquired zinc deficiency can be seen in organic acidurias, during hyperalimentation, and in a variety of severe gastrointestinal disturbances.[38]

Differential diagnosis The lesions are often mistaken for mucocutaneous candidiasis associated with immunodeficiency, such as found in human immunodeficiency virus (HIV) infection. Plasma or serum zinc levels will distinguish between the two. Often, protein-calorie malnutrition states are considered, but lesions usually develop in such patients after 6 months of age, and the nutritional history may distinguish between the two. Histiocytosis X will present with intertriginous erosions in infancy. Acquired zinc deficiency states, such as seen with prolonged parenteral hyperalimentation, will mimic acrodermatitis enteropathica. Necrolytic migratory erythema seen with a glucagonoma will also mimic.[38]

Pathogenesis Depletion of body zinc stores due to faulty transport of zinc is responsible for the symptoms and signs of acrodermatitis enteropathica.[39,40] It is not known whether this is due to the lack of a zinc carrier protein or to some defect of zinc absorption in the intestine. Zinc is stored in the same tissues as iron and serves as an important cofactor for a variety of enzymes such as alkaline phosphatase and carbonic anhydrase. The zinc deficiency is the result of depletion of total body stores. It is thought that zinc deficiency results in impairment of metalloenzyme activity, which produces the clinical features.[39,40]

Treatment   Oral zinc sulfate, 5 mg/kg/day given twice daily, produces rapid clinical improvement.[39] Apathy disappears within 24 hours, and the skin lesions and diarrhea resolve within 7 to 14 days. Photophobia, alopecia, and growth failure are reversed over the ensuing months.

Patient education   The hereditary inability to absorb zinc should be explained. It is not known whether lifetime maintenance with supplemental zinc is required.

Follow-up visits   A visit 2 weeks after diagnosis is useful to repeat zinc level determinations and evaluate the response. The measurement of plasma or serum zinc levels at monthly intervals is useful to monitor supplemental zinc requirements.

References

1. Bale SJ, Doyle SZ: The genetics of ichthyosis: a primer for epidemiologists, *J Invest Dermatol* 102:49s, 1994.

2. Schwayder T, Ott F: All about ichthyosis, *Pediatr Clin North Am* 38:835, 1991.

3. Rabinowitz LG, Esterly NB: Atopic dermatitis and ichthyosis vulgaris, *Pediatr Rev* 15:220, 1994.

4. Mukerjee S, Gupta AB: A statistical study on the in vivo sorption and desorption of water in ichthyosis vulgaris, *J Dermatol* 21:78, 1994.

5. Paller AS: Laboratory tests for ichthyosis, *Dermatol Clin* 12:99, 1994.

6. Buyse L, Hraves C, Marks R, et al: Collodion baby dehydration: the danger of high transepidermal water loss, *Br J Dermatol* 129:86, 1993.

7. Niemi KM, Kanerva L, Kuokkanen K, et al: Clinical light and electron microscopic features of recessive congenital ichthyosis type I, *Br J Dermatol* 130:626, 1994.

8. Anton-Lamprecht I: Ultrastructural identification of basic abnormalities as clues to genetic disorders of the epidermis, *J Invest Dermatol* 103:6s, 1994.

9. Burton JL: Keratin genes and epidermolytic hyperkeratosis. *Lancet* 344:1103, 1994.

10. Fuchs E, Coulombe P, Cheng J, et al: Genetic basis of epidermolysis bullosa simplex and epidermolytic hyperkeratosis, *J Invest Dermatol* 103:25s, 1994.

11. DiGiovanna JJ, Bale SJ: Epidermolytic hyperkeratosis: applied molecular genetics, *J Invest Dermatol* 102:390, 1994.

12. Kremer H, Zeeuwen P, McLean WH, et al: Ichthyosis bullosa of Siemens is caused by mutations in the keratin 2a gene, *J Invest Dermatol* 103:286, 1994.

13. Huber M, Rettler I, Bernasconi K, et al: Mutations of keratinocyte transglutaminase in lamellar ichthyosis, *Science* 267:525, 1995.

14. Paller AS, Syder AJ, Chan YM, et al: Genetic and clinical mosaicism in a type of epidermal nevus, *N Engl J Med* 331:1408, 1994.

15. Steijlen PM, Van Dooren-Greebe RJ, Van de Kerkhof PC: Acitretin in the treatment of lamellar ichthyosis, *Br J Dermatol* 130:211, 1994.

16. Paige DG, Judge MR, Shaw DG, et al: Bone changes and their significance with ichthyosis on long-term etretinate therapy, *Br J Dermatol* 127:387, 1992.

17. Fine J-D, Bauer EA, Briggaman RA, et al: Revised clinical and laboratory criteria for subtypes of inherited epidermolysis bullosa, *J Am Acad Dermatol* 24:119, 1991.

18. Uitto J, Christiano AM: Inherited epidermolysis bullosa, *Dermatol Clin* 11:549, 1993.

19. Lin AN, Murphy F, Brodie SE, et al: Review of ophthalmologic findings in 204 patients with epidermolysis bullosa, *Am J Ophthalmol* 118:384, 1994.

20. Travis SPL, McGrath JA, Turnbull AJ, et al: Oral and gastrointestinal manifestations of epidermolysis bullosa, *Lancet* 340:1505, 1992.

21. Fine J-D: Laboratory tests for epidermolysis bullosa, *Dermatol Clin* 12:123, 1994.

22. Aberdam D, Galliano MF, Vailly J, et al: Herlitz's junctional epidermolysis bullosa is linked to mutations in the gene (LAMC2) for the gamma 2 subunit of nicein/kalinin (LAMININ 5), *Nat Genet* 6:299, 1994.

23. Gil SG, Brown TA, Ryan MC, et al: Junctional epidermolysis bullosis: defects in expression of epiligrin/nicein/kalinin and integrin B 4 that inhibit hemidesmosome formation, *J Invest Dermatol* 103:31s, 1994.

24. Uitto J, Pulkkinen L, Christiano AM: Molecular basis of the dystrophic and junctional forms of epidermolysis bullosa: mutations of the type VII collagen and kalinin (laminin 5) gene, *J Invest Dermatol* 103:39s, 1994.

25. Pessar A, Verdicchio JF, Caldwell D: Epidermolysis bullosa: the pediatric dermatological management and therapeutic update, *Adv Dermatol* 3:99-120, 1988.

26. Allman S, Haynes L, MacKinnon P, et al: Nutrition in dystrophic epidermolysis bullosa, *Pediatr Dermatol* 9:231, 1992.

27. Landy SJ, Donnai D: Incontinentia pigmenti (Bloch-Sulzberger syndrome), *J Med Genet* 30:53, 1993.

28. Ashley JR, Burgdorf WHC: Incontinentia pigmenti: pigmentary changes independent of incontinence, *J Cutan Pathol* 14:248, 1987.

29. Gorski JL, Burright EN: The molecular genetics of incontinentia pigmenti, *Semin Dermatol* 12:255, 1993.

30. Masse JF, Perusse R: Ectodermal dysplasia, *Arch Dis Child* 71:1, 1994.

31. Zonana J, Jones M, Clarke A, et al: Detection of de novo mutations and analysis of their origin in families with X linked hypohidrotic ectodermal dysplasia, *J Med Genet* 31:287, 1994.

32. Berg D, Weingold DH, Abson KG, et al: Sweating in ectodermal dysplasia syndromes, *Arch Dermatol* 126:1075, 1990.

33. Kilmer SL, Grix AW Jr, Isseroff RR: Focal dermal hypoplasia: four cases with widely varying presentations, *J Am Acad Dermatol* 28:839, 1993.

34. Moore DJ, Mallory SB: Goltz syndrome, *Pediatr Dermatol* 6:251, 1989.

35. Lucker GPH, Van De Kerkhof PCM, Steijlen PM: The hereditary palmoplantar keratoses: an updated review and classification, *Br J Dermatol* 131:1, 1994.

36. Burge S: Darier's disease—the clinical features and pathogenesis, *Clin Exp Dermatol* 19:193, 1994.

37. Ikeda S, Wakem P, Haake A, et al: Localization of the gene for Darier disease to a 5-cm interval on chromosome 12q, *J Invest Dermatol* 103:478, 1994.

38. Black CK, Piette WW: The multisystem spectrum of necrolytic migratory erythema, *Curr Opin Dermatol* 1:87, 1995.

39. Van Wouve J: Clinical and laboratory diagnosis of acrodermatitis enteropathica, *Eur J Pediatr* 149:2, 1989.

40. Sandstrom B, Cederblad A, Lindblad BS, et al: Acrodermatitis enteropathica, zinc metabolism, copper status and immune function, *Arch Pediatr Adolesc Med* 148:980, 1994.

20

Drug Eruptions

The diagnosis of a drug eruption is usually only suspected and not confirmed with absolute certainty.[1] Evaluation of the possibility of a drug eruption depends on the patient's previous experience with specific drugs and the experience of the general population with drugs to which the patient has been exposed. The morphology of the patient's lesions, and the relative frequency of similar-type reactions in the general population, are of assistance. Specific medications have a higher frequency of drug eruptions and specific types of a drug eruption than other medications.[2] These are listed in Boxes 20-1 through 20-7. The timing of the eruption in relationship to the commencement of drug therapy may assist in establishing the association of the drug with the eruption. The clinician should look for alternate explanations for the eruption, which include infection or the primary illness. Depending on the type of eruption and the drug involved, rechallenge to that drug in the future may be indicated to confirm the diagnosis, but rechallenge is usually not done because of concern about a more severe reaction. Removal of the suspected drug from the patient may or may not assist in more rapid resolution of the drug eruption. Fortunately the incidence of adverse drug reactions in infants and children appears to be less than in adults.[3,4]

DRUG ERUPTIONS

Clinical features
Morbilliform drug eruptions
Cutaneous drug reactions often have specific patterns. The morbilliform (so-called maculopapular eruption) or exanthematous eruption is probably the most common of all drug-induced eruptions in children. The term *morbilliform* means measleslike because of the development of a maculopapular erythematous rash that becomes confluent (Figs. 20-1 and 20-2). This rash often starts on the trunk and extends onto the extremities. It is frequently symmetric and often has areas of totally normal skin that are surrounded by the eruption (Fig. 20-3). The initial macules may become papular, and then large plaques may form from the confluence of the individual lesions. The patient may have associated fever as well as malaise and arthralgias. Box 20-1 lists drugs associated with morbilliform drug eruptions.

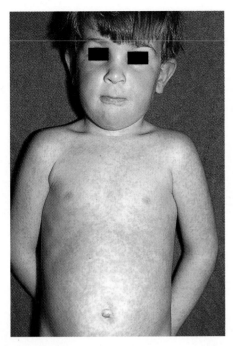

Fig. 20-1
Morbilliform drug eruption. Trimethoprim-sulfamethoxazole--induced eruption with discrete macules and papules on the trunk and confluent erythema on the face.

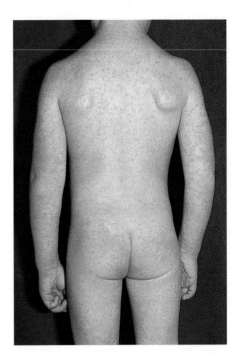

Fig. 20-2
Morbilliform drug eruption. Trimethoprim-sulfamethoxazole--induced eruption with confluence of lesions on the upper arms and buttocks.

Urticarial drug eruptions

Drug eruptions associated with hives are called *urticarial drug eruptions*. These present as edematous, flat, erythematous papules that usually last less than 24 hours (Fig. 20-4). New lesions appear almost continuously. The lesions may begin as small discrete papules that become confluent large figurate plaques (Fig. 20-5). Occasionally, the edema can be so intense in the center of the erythematous papules and plaques that the center appears less erythematous than the periphery, giving a target appearance. Lesions may resolve, leaving a macular blue-brown appearance that looks like a bruise. The absence of epidermal injury and more typical urticarial papules and plaques on the rest of the body confirm that this is an urticarial drug eruption and not erythema multiforme. Box 20-2 lists the drugs associated with urticarial drug eruptions.

If the lesions show a deep dermal component with induration and swelling of the subcutaneous tissue,

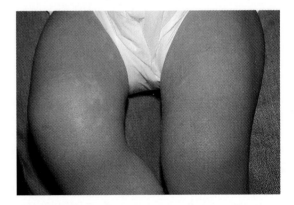

Fig. 20-3
Morbilliform drug eruption. Confluent intense erythema with islands of normal skin in a patient treated with both phenobarbital and trimethoprim-sulfamethoxazole.

the reaction is called *angioedema*. If angioedema involves the mucous membranes, it can become life-threatening secondary to airway obstruction.

Box 20-1   Drugs associated with morbilliform drug eruption

Analgesics, antipyretics, antirheumatics
- Gold
- Nonsteroidal antiinflammatory drugs (NSAIDs)
    - Ibuprofen
    - Meclofenamate sodium
    - Piroxicam
    - Sulindac
    - Zomepirac sodium

Antibiotics
- Amoxicillin
- Ampicillin
- Cephalosporins
- Chloramphenicol
- Erythromycin
- Gentamicin sulfate
- Isoniazid
- Penicillins
- Sulfonamides
- Trimethoprim
- Trimethoprim and sulfamethoxazole

Drugs acting on the central nervous system
- Barbiturates
- Carbamazepine
- Phenytoin

Other
- Allopurinol

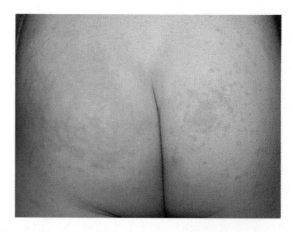

Fig. 20-4
Mixed urticarial and morbilliform drug eruption. Trimethoprim-sulfamethoxazole–induced urticarial plaques on the left buttock with maculopapular lesions on the right buttock.

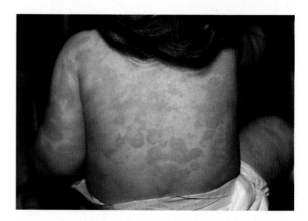

Fig. 20-5
Urticarial drug eruption. Large urticarial plaques in a child treated with cefaclor.

Serum-sickness–like reaction

Serum-sickness–like reactions clinically initially appear to resemble urticaria often accompanied by angioedema (Fig. 20-6). The child may develop fever, pruritus, arthritis, and/or arthralgias. The large urticarial plaques may resolve with dusky to purple centers, giving the skin a bruised appearance. The affected child may appear severely ill and be very uncomfortable. Cephalosporins are most commonly reported to cause this type of drug eruption.[5,6]

Fixed drug eruptions

Fixed drug eruptions may present as solitary or multiple, sharply demarcated, erythematous lesions that go on to give an intense macular hyperpigmentation[7] (Fig. 20-7). The initial lesions may appear edematous, like urticaria, or become bullous (Fig. 20-8). Over several days the edema and erythema will frequently decrease within the lesion, leaving a macular hyperpigmentation with sharply demarcated outlines in a figurate pattern. Rechallenges with the same medication may cause lesions in precisely the same spot as

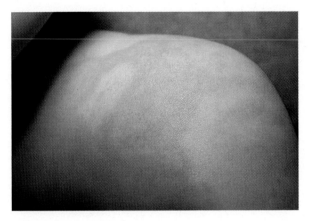

Fig. 20-6
Serum-sickness–like reaction to cefaclor. The urticarial lesions resolve with a dusky, bruised appearance. Note the swelling and edema involving the knee.

Box 20-2   Drugs commonly associated with urticarial drug eruptions

Analgesics, antipyretics, antirheumatics
  Acetylsalicylic acid
Antibiotics
  Amoxicillin
  Ampicillin
  Cephalosporins
  Penicillins
  Sulfonamides
  Trimethoprim and sulfamethoxazole
Other
  Horse serum

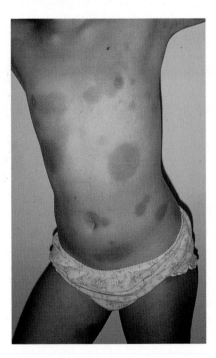

Fig. 20-7
Fixed drug eruption. Trimethoprim-sulfamethoxazole–induced oval erythematous macules with diffuse hyperpigmentation within several lesions.

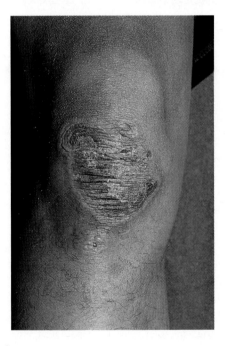

Fig. 20-8
Fixed drug eruption. Bullous reaction to tetracycline. The lesions have a necrotic hyperpigmented epidermis with sharp demarcation of normal and involved skin.

Box 20-3   Drugs associated with fixed drug eruptions

Barbiturates
Carbamazepine
Phenazone derivatives (phenylbutazone)
Phenolphthalein
Sulfonamides
Tetracycline
Trimethoprim
Trimethoprim and sulfamethoxazole

Box 20-4   Drugs associated with vasculitis

Allopurinol
Barbiturates
Gold
Horse serum
Penicillins
Sulfonamides
Thiazide derivatives

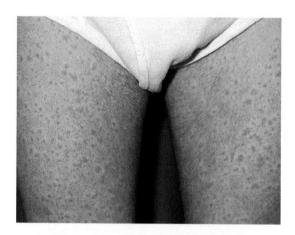

Fig. 20-9
Vasculitis. Amoxicillin-induced lesions on legs.

well as lesions on new locations. Box 20-3 lists the drugs commonly causing fixed drug eruptions.

Vasculitis

Palpable purpuric lesions associated with cutaneous necrotizing vasculitis can be associated with drugs. The vasculitis is usually on the lower extremities in dependent areas but can occur anywhere on the body (Fig. 20-9). The lesions may begin as soft, small erythematous papules or urticarial papules that blanch when pressure is applied over the skin. Over several hours to days the lesions become firm and dark red-blue or purple. Box 20-4 lists drugs associated with vasculitis.

Exfoliative dermatitis

Diffuse erythema followed by bullae and loss of large sheets of epidermis can be associated with drugs. This is called *Lyell's syndrome* or toxic epidermal necrolysis. Specific clinical classifications have been developed that may give prognostic and epidemiologic information in the future.[8-10] Drugs commonly associated with this condition are listed in Box 20-5. This eruption usually presents as morbilliform or urticarial eruptions that show desquamation or become bullous within several hours or several days[11] (Fig. 20-10). This condition is considered in depth in Chapter 11.

Differential diagnosis
Morbilliform drug eruptions

Morbilliform eruptions usually begin within a week of therapy, but with the penicillins it may be 2 weeks or more after therapy has begun before the eruption is seen. The onset of the eruption may occur after the drug is stopped. Morbilliform eruptions may fade over time, even with continuation of the responsible medication.[12] The eruption typically lasts 7 to 14 days and may be associated with pruritus during that time. Morbilliform eruptions are difficult to separate from viral exanthems.

Urticarial drug eruptions

Urticarial lesions are usually pruritic, and at times it is difficult to separate an urticarial eruption from a morbilliform eruption early in the course of the condition (Fig. 20-4). Urticarial lesions may occur

Box 20-5 Drugs associated with exfoliative dermatitis

Allopurinol
Barbiturates
Hydantoin derivatives
Penicillins
Phenazone derivatives (phenylbutazone)
Sulfonamides
Sulindac

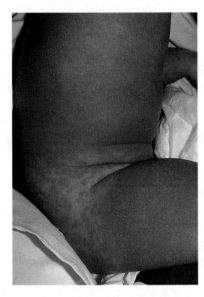

Fig. 20-10
Exfoliative dermatitis. Dusky blue-red edematous lesions with focal epidermal necrosis and areas of noninvolvement. The epidermal necrosis is not sufficient to give a bullous reaction.

immediately after exposure to the drug or within several days. The individual urticarial lesions usually resolve over 24 hours, with new lesions arising. In the morbilliform drug eruption, individual lesions expand over several days, giving more of a confluent macular-type eruption, whereas urticarial plaques are raised and indurated. Urticarial lesions commonly occur in children and are not associated with drugs (see Chapter 13).

Serum-sickness–like reaction

The serum-sickness–like reaction to drugs is not usually associated with circulating immune complexes, proteinuria, and lymphadenopathy as seen in a true serum-sickness reaction. The eruption usually begins 7 or more days after the drug is first given. The eruption may also begin after the cephalosporin was stopped. In contrast, Kawasaki disease usually has involvement of the lips, conjunctiva, and mucous membranes.

Fixed drug eruptions

The fixed drug eruption will usually occur within several days of the drug exposure. Biopsy of the fixed drug lesion will often help to confirm the diagnosis. Rechallenge with the suspected medication may cause recurrences of similar lesions in the identical spot. The area of hyperpigmentation may take several months to resolve.

Vasculitis

Drug-induced vasculitis can occur quickly after drug exposure or following prolonged drug use. Since drugs are one of many causes for cutaneous vasculitis, other conditions inducing these lesions must be considered. Sepsis with bacterial emboli, and many viruses, can cause palpable purpura with very similar cutaneous appearances. Biopsy of an individual lesion can confirm the small-vessel vasculitis but cannot confirm the cause of the vasculitis.

Exfoliative dermatitis

Toxic epidermal necrolysis can be confirmed by a biopsy that demonstrates full-thickness epidermal necrosis and separation of the epidermis from the dermis. As with vasculitis, the biopsy can confirm the condition but not the cause.

Other conditions that must be included in the differential diagnosis of drug eruptions include graft-versus-host disease. Viral or bacterial exanthems need to be recognized to characterize the cutaneous eruption as a response of the illness and not as an adverse response to the therapy.[13]

Pathogenesis

Drug reactions can occur secondary to immunologic reactions or nonimmunologic reactions.[14-18] Immunologic reactions require host immunologic pathways and are called *drug allergies*. The ability of a drug to elicit an immune reaction depends on many characteristics. Most drugs are small organic molecules with molecular weights less than 1000 daltons. Because of their size they are unable to elicit immune responses unless they bind to a larger molecule, which is usually a protein macromolecule. In this situation the drug functions as a hapten. Most drugs have little ability to form covalent bonds with macromolecules and are unable to form this type of immunologic antigen.

The host reacts to drugs in different manners. The body may respond differently to a drug given intravenously or a drug applied topically. Patients may have variation in their ability to absorb or metabolize a given drug. The patient infected with infectious mononucleosis may be more likely to develop a morbilliform eruption to ampicillin.

The body's immunologic response to drugs may be immunoglobulin E (IgE) dependent, which can be associated with pruritus, urticaria, bronchial spasm, and laryngeal edema. Drug eruptions may be associated with serum sickness caused by circulating immune complexes. Cytotoxic drug reactions can occur where the drug combines with the tissue, and that combination then becomes the target for antibodies or cellular-mediated cytotoxicity.

Nonimmunologic drug reactions can result through various modalities. Aspirin, opiates, and radiocontrast medications may directly release mast cell mediators, resulting in urticaria. Overdosage of a medicine may cause adverse cutaneous side effects by direct injury to cutaneous cells. Genetic inability to detoxify certain chemical compounds results in toxic metabolites that can also damage cutaneous cells.

Secondary side effects of chemotherapy can include alopecia or particular types of rashes secondary to thrombocytopenia. Antibiotics can destroy the normal bacterial flora, allowing overgrowth of other organisms. Drugs may interact to compete for binding sites or cause metabolic changes. In addition certain drugs, such as lithium, which exacerbates acne and psoriasis, can exacerbate preexisting dermatologic diseases.

Drug-induced urticaria can also be caused by either IgE mechanisms or circulating immune complexes. The IgE-dependent urticaria reactions usually occur within 36 hours of drug exposure, but they can occur within minutes. The eruption associated with circulating immune complexes is a type of serum-sickness reaction. It usually begins 4 to 12 days after exposure to the drug, at which time an equilibrium has been achieved between antibody and drug antigen, allowing for the formation of immune complexes. The serum-sickness–type reaction is often accompanied by fever, hematuria, and arthralgia. Liver and neurologic injury may occur.

The pathophysiology of drug-associated cutaneous vasculitis is not clear, but immune complexes may be responsible. The lesions usually begin to resolve several days or weeks after the offending drug is removed.

Treatment

Removal of the offending drug is the usual first therapy. Drug eruption is easily diagnosed when one can identify a specific pattern of drug eruption with a known timely exposure to only a single medication, and that medication has been frequently associated with that specific type of eruption. The infant or child exposed to multiple medications over a short period offers a more difficult diagnostic and therapeutic dilemma. Depending on the severity of the drug reaction, none of the drugs, the most likely drug, or all of the drugs may need to be removed. Boxes 20-1 through 20-5 are useful in identifying which drugs are most likely to cause the various types of eruptions.

Morbilliform eruptions may fade with time, without drug removal, especially when associated with amoxicillin or ampicillin. Urticarial eruptions may respond to antihistamine therapy. Because of fear that continued offending drug therapy can be associated with anaphylaxis or toxic epidermal necrolysis, attempts at drug removal are usually made.

Anaphylaxis associated with urticarial eruptions and angioedema is a medical emergency. Immediate therapy should be started with 1:1000 aqueous epinephrine, 0.2 to 0.5 ml given subcutaneously, and intravenous fluids. Antihistamines and systemic steroids may also be required to maintain an adequate airway while the symptoms subside.

Treatment of exfoliative drug eruptions requires various levels of care.[19] Severe involvement will require burn center care.[20] Most centers do not use systemic steroids, but cyclosporin has been used in life-threatening situations.[21,22] Early referral to the appropriate center may be lifesaving.

Patient education

The parents should be informed of the possible association of the cutaneous eruption and the specific drugs involved. The risk for the child from subsequent exposure to the specific or similar medications needs to be explained. For severe reaction the child may be instructed to wear a bracelet or necklace to alert examining health care workers to the suspected allergy. The parents should be informed of alternative forms of therapy that would avoid the offending agent.

Follow-up visits

Follow-up visits are necessary to confirm the resolution of the eruption and recognize the response of the original illness that required drug therapy. The frequency and timing of the visits will depend on the severity of the original illness and the drug eruption.

The patient's medical records should document the possible drug-associated eruption to attempt avoidance of future exposures to the drug or related compounds. For penicillin-associated reaction, skin testing may be indicated to attempt to predict the future possibility of hypersensitivity reactions to the penicillins.[23]

PHOTOSENSITIVE DRUG ERUPTIONS

Drug photosensitivity reactions can be either phototoxic or photoallergic. In either situation a combina-

tion of topical or systemic medication and exposure to light is necessary.

Photoallergic reactions are less common than phototoxic reactions. The photoallergic reaction involves an immunologic response to a chemical (drug) that is altered by ultraviolet light. The body recognizes the altered form as a foreign antigen and develops an immunologic delayed hypersensitivity response. This process requires sufficient drug and light to produce adequate antigen for immunization.

Phototoxic reactions involve direct cutaneous injury by a drug after the drug is changed by light energy. Increased light energy or increased amount of drug increases the risk of a phototoxic reaction.

Clinical features

Photosensitive eruptions are characterized by more intense dermatitis in the areas of greatest sun exposure. Often the face, upper trunk, and extensor surfaces of the arms are involved. The lesions are usually erythematous and edematous with associated papules, vesicles, or oozing, weeping lesions. Increased skin fragility and scarring may be seen.[24] Lesions may resolve with marked hyperpigmentation that may remain for months (Fig. 20-11).

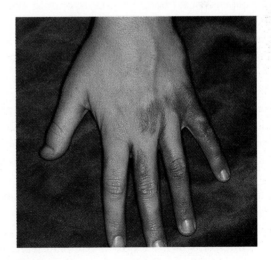

Fig. 20-11
Phototoxic reaction to psoralen-containing plant that caused marked hyperpigmentation of the hand.

Box 20-6   Drugs associated with phototoxic reactions

Coal tar derivatives
Furocoumarins in plants
Furosemide
Griseofulvin
Ibuprofen
Methotrexate
Nalidixic acid
Naproxen
Nifedipine
Para-aminobenzoic (PABA) esters
Phenothiazines
Psoralen
Sulfonamides
Tetracycline
Thiazides
Tretinoin

Box 20-7   Drugs associated with photoallergic reaction

Fragrances
PABA esters
Perfume
Phenothiazines
Sulfonamides

Phototoxic reactions are often are painful, similar to a severe sunburn. Photoallergic reactions may be painful or have severe pruritus in the areas of the most intense sun exposure. Phototoxic reactions are dose dependent for both the amount of drug and the amount of light exposure. In addition to sunlight, fluorescent lamps or sunlight that comes through window glass may produce photosensitive drug reactions.

Pathogenesis
Common drugs associated with phototoxic and photoallergic reactions are listed in Boxes 20-6 and 20-7. The histologic picture for photoallergic contact dermatitis and phototoxic reaction is similar, with associated epidermal spongiosis, dermal edema, and inflammatory response. True phototoxicity is pathologically more like sunburn than a dermatitis.

The photosensitivity may be confirmed by a photopatch test in which the drug is readministered and multiple intensities of ultraviolet light exposure are given. Photosensitive reactions are usually in the ultraviolet A range. Photosensitive reactions often

resolve with marked hyperpigmentation that may take several months for resolution.

Treatment
The specific diagnosis is suggested by involvement of the light-exposed areas of the skin. A history of a combination of drug and light exposure will strongly support the diagnosis.

Treatment involves removal of the offending drug. The acute dermatitis can be treated as listed in Chapter 10 for sunburn. If a true photoallergic reaction exists with severe pruritus, systemic steroids may be necessary for more rapid relief.

Patient education
The cause of the photosensitivity should be fully described to the family and child. If the drug that caused a phototoxic reaction is required, it may be continued if the ultraviolet light intensity can be decreased to a level that is not adequate to cause significant dermatitis. Children who develop a phototoxic reaction to psoralen-containing plants, such as celery or limes, should avoid the combination of plant exposure and sun exposure. If possible, the photosensitizing drug should be totally withdrawn. If hyperpigmentation occurs, it may require months to resolve.

Follow-up visits
A follow-up visit in 1 week may be necessary to confirm the resolution of significant dermatitis. Additional follow-up visits for photopatch testing to confirm the diagnosis depend on the severity of the reaction and the medical necessity to confirm the diagnosis.

References

1. Breathnach SM, Hintner H: *Adverse drug reactions in the skin*, Oxford, 1992, Blackwell Scientific.

2. Bruinsma W: *The guide to drug eruptions*, ed 4, Norwood, NJ, 1987, American Overseas Book Co.

3. Kramer MS, Hutchinson TA, Flegel KM, et al: Adverse drug reactions in general pediatric outpatients, *J Pediatr* 106:305, 1985.

4. Soumerai SB, Ross-Degnan D: Drug prescribing in pediatrics: challenges for quality improvement, *Pediatrics* 86:782, 1990.

5. Hebert AA, Sigman ES, Levy ML: Serum sickness-like reactions from cefaclor in children, *J Am Acad Dermatol* 25:805, 1991.

6. Lowery N, Kearns GL, Young RA, Wheeler JG: Serum sickness-like reactions associated with cefprozil therapy, *J Pediatr* 125:325, 1994.

7. Zanolli MD, McAlvany J, Krowchuk DP: Phenolphthalein-induced fixed drug eruption: a cutaneous complication of laxative use in a child, *Pediatr* 91:1199, 1993.

8. Bastuji-Garin S, Rzany B, Stern RS, et al: Clinical classification of cases of toxic epidermal necrolysis, Stevens-Johnson syndrome, and erythema multiforme, *Arch Dermatol* 129:92, 1993.

9. Roujeau JC: The spectrum of Stevens-Johnson syndrome and toxic epidermal necrolysis: a clinical classification, *J Invest Dermatol* 102:28S, 1994.

10. Kaufman DW: Epidemiologic approaches to the study of toxic epidermal necrolysis, *J Invest Dermatol* 102:31S, 1994.

11. Roujeau JC, Stern RS: Severe adverse cutaneous reactions to drugs, *N Engl J Med* 331:1272, 1994.

12. Croydon EAP, Wheeler AW, Grimshaw JJ, et al: Prospective study of ampicillin rash: report of a collaborative study group, *Br Med J* 1:7, 1973.

13. Haverkos HW, Amsel Z, Drotman DP: Adverse virus-drug interactions, *RID* 13:698, 1991.

14. Shear NH, Spielberg SP: Pharmacogenetics and adverse drug reactions in the skin, *Pediatr Dermatol* 1:165, 1983.

15. Wintroub BU, Stern R: Cutaneous drug reactions: pathogenesis and clinical classification, *J Am Acad Dermatol* 13:167, 1985.

16. Shear NH, Spielber SP: Anticonvulsant hypersensitivity syndrome, *J Clin Invest* 82:1826, 1988.

17. Handfield-Jones SE, Jenkins RE, Whittaker SJ, et al: The anticonvulsant hypersensitivity syndrome, *Br J Dermatol* 129:175, 1993.

18. Chosidow O, Bourgault I, Roujeau JC: Drug rashes, what are the targets of cell-mediated cytotoxicity?, *Arch Dermatol* 130:627, 1994.

19. Prendiville JS, Hebert AA, Greenwald MJ, Esterly NB: Management of Stevens-Johnson syndrome and toxic epidermal necrolysis in children, *J Pediatr* 115:881, 1989.

20. Heimbach DM, Engrav LH, Marvin JA, Harnar TJ: Toxic epidermal necrolysis: a step forward in treatment, *JAMA* 257:2171, 1987.

21. Renfro L, Grant-Kels JM, Daman LA: Drug-induced toxic epidermal necrolysis treated with cyclosporin, *Int J Dermatol* 28:441, 1989.

22. Hewitt J, Ormerod AD: Toxic epidermal necrolysis treated with cyclosporin, *Clin Exp Dermatol* 17:264, 1992.

23. Gadde J, Spence M, Wheeler B, Adkinson NF: Clinical experience with penicillin skin testing in a large inner-city STD clinic, *JAMA* 270:2456, 1993.

24. Levy ML, Barron KS, Eichenfield A, Honig PJ: Naproxen-induced pseudoporphyria: a distinctive photodermatitis, *J Pediatr* 117:660, 1990.

Semipermeable wound dressings may offer additional cutaneous pain relief and protection, but additional studies must be done to analyze the potential for associated risk with bacterial growth under the dressings.[2,4]

TRANSIENT SKIN DISEASE

Milia
Clinical features
Milia are multiple, white, 1-mm to 2-mm papules seen over the forehead, cheeks, and nose of infants (Fig. 21-3). They may be present in the oral cavity as well, where they are called *Epstein's pearls*. About 40% of newborns have milia on the skin and 60% on the palate.[7] The cystic spheres rupture onto the skin surface and exfoliate their contents within a few weeks of birth.

Differential diagnosis
Molluscum contagiosum, an acquired viral infection, may mimic milia but does not usually appear in the immediate neonatal period. Sebaceous gland hyperplasia also occurs over the nose and cheeks of infants but is yellow, rather than whitish.

Pathogenesis
On histologic examination, milia appear as superficial epithelial cysts in the upper dermis, just beneath the epidermis. The cyst cavity is filled with keratin.

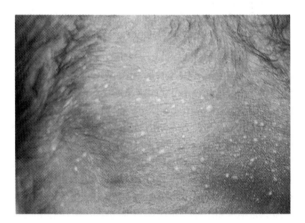

Fig. 21-3
Milia. Multiple white papules seen over the forehead of an infant.

Sebaceous gland hyperplasia
Clinical features
Tiny (1 mm) yellow macules or yellow papules are seen at the opening of each pilosebaceous follicle over the nose and cheeks of newborns (Fig. 21-4). These occur in about 50% of infants.[7] They recede completely by 4 to 6 months of age.

Differential diagnosis
Milia may mimic sebaceous hyperplasia, but are white and cystic in appearance.

Pathogenesis
Maternal androgenic stimulation is responsible for the increase in sebaceous gland volume, sebaceous cell size, and the total number of sebaceous cells.

Mottling
Clinical features
A lacelike pattern of dusky erythema appears over the extremities and trunk of neonates when exposed to a temperature decrease. This phenomenon may be sen-

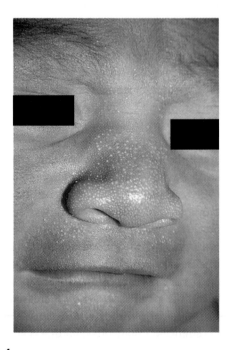

Fig. 21-4
Sebaceous gland hyperplasia on the nose and upper lip of a neonate.